Imaging the Hospitalized Patient

Editors

TRAVIS S. HENRY
VINCENT M. MELLNICK

RADIOLOGIC CLINICS
OF NORTH AMERICA

www.radiologic.theclinics.com

Consulting Editor
FRANK H. MILLER

January 2020 • Volume 58 • Number 1

ELSEVIER

1600 John F. Kennedy Boulevard • Suite 1800 • Philadelphia, Pennsylvania, 19103-2899

http://www.theclinics.com

RADIOLOGIC CLINICS OF NORTH AMERICA Volume 58, Number 1
January 2020 ISSN 0033-8389, ISBN 13: 978-0-323-75428-6

Editor: John Vassallo (j.vassallo@elsevier.com)
Developmental Editor: Donald Mumford

Radiologic Clinics of North America (ISSN 0033-8389) is published bimonthly by Elsevier Inc., 360 Park Avenue South, New York, NY 10010-1710. Months of issue are January, March, May, July, September, and November. Periodicals postage paid at New York, NY and additional mailing offices. Subscription prices are USD 513 per year for US individuals, USD 980 per year for US institutions, USD 100 per year for US students and residents, USD 594 per year for Canadian individuals, USD 1253 per year for Canadian institutions, USD 703 per year for international individuals, USD 1253 per year for international institutions, USD 100 per year for Canadian students/residents, and USD 315 per year for international students/residents. To receive student and resident rate, orders must be accompanied by name of affiliated institution, date of term and the signature of program/residency coordinatior on institution letterhead. Orders will be billed at individual rate until proof of status is received. Foreign air speed delivery is included in all *Clinics* subscription prices. All prices are subject to change without notice. **POSTMASTER:** Send address changes to *Radiologic Clinics of North America*, Elsevier Health Sciences Division, Subscription Customer Service, 3251 Riverport Lane, Maryland Heights, MO63043. **Customer Service: Telephone: 1-800-654-2452** (U.S. and Canada); **1-314-447-8871** (outside U.S. and Canada). **Fax: 1-314-447-8029. E-mail: journalscustomerservice-usa@elsevier.com (for print support); journalsonlinesupport-usa@elsevier.com (for online support)**.

Reprints. For copies of 100 or more of articles in this publication, please contact the Commercial Reprints Department, Elsevier Inc., 360 Park Avenue South, New York, New York 10010-1710. Tel.: +1-212-633-3874; Fax: +1-212-633-3820; E-mail: reprints@elsevier.com.

Radiologic Clinics of North America also published in Greek Paschalidis Medical Publications, Athens, Greece.

Radiologic Clinics of North America is covered in *MEDLINE/PubMed (Index Medicus), EMBASE/Excerpta Medica, Current Contents/Life Sciences, Current Contents/Clinical Medicine, RSNA Index to Imaging Literature, BIOSIS, Science Citation Index,* and *ISI/BIOMED*.

Printed in the United States of America.

Contributors

CONSULTING EDITOR

FRANK H. MILLER, MD, FACR
Lee F. Rogers MD Professor of Medical Education, Chief, Body Imaging Section and Fellowship Program, Medical Director, MRI, Department of Radiology, Northwestern Memorial Hospital, Northwestern University Feinberg School of Medicine, Chicago, Illinois, USA

EDITORS

TRAVIS S. HENRY, MD
Associate Professor of Clinical Radiology, Cardiac and Pulmonary Imaging Section, Director, Cardiothoracic Imaging Fellowship, University of California San Francisco, San Francisco, California, USA

VINCENT M. MELLNICK, MD
Associate Professor, Radiology, Chief, Abdominal Imaging Section, Co-Director, Emergency Radiology, Abdominal Imaging Section, Mallinckrodt Institute of Radiology, Washington University in St. Louis, St Louis, Missouri, USA

AUTHORS

ABDULLAH ALABOUSI, MD, FRCPC
Department of Radiology, St. Joseph's Healthcare Hamilton, McMaster University, Hamilton, Ontario, Canada

MOSTAFA ALABOUSI, MD
Department of Radiology, McMaster University, Hamilton, Ontario, Canada

SANJEEV BHALLA, MD
Professor of Radiology, Mallinckrodt Institute of Radiology, St Louis, Missouri, USA

ALBERTO COSSU, MD
Scuola di Specializzazione di Radiodiagnostica, Università degli Studi di Ferrara, Azienda Ospedaliera Universitaria S. Anna di Ferrara, Arcispedale Sant'Anna, Ferrara Centralino, Italy

JUDITH A. GADDE, DO, MBA
Department of Radiology and Imaging Services, Emory University School of Medicine, Atlanta, Georgia, USA

SAMIR HAROON, MD
Department of Radiology, Boston University Medical Center, Boston, Massachusetts, USA

TRAVIS S. HENRY, MD
Associate Professor of Clinical Radiology, Cardiac and Pulmonary Imaging Section, Director, Cardiothoracic Imaging Fellowship, University of California San Francisco, San Francisco, California, USA

MICHAEL D. HOPE, MD
Chief of Radiology, San Francisco VA Health Care System, Associate Professor of Radiology, Department of Radiology and Biomedical Imaging, University of California, San Francisco, Department of Radiology, San Francisco Veterans Affairs Medical Center, San Francisco, California, USA

MICHAEL HOROWITZ, MD, PhD
Fellow, Cardiothoracic Radiology, University of California, San Diego, La Jolla, California, USA

MALAK ITANI, MD
Assistant Professor of Radiology, Mallinckrodt Institute of Radiology, Washington University in St Louis School of Medicine, St Louis, Missouri, USA

KATHLEEN JACOBS, MD
Assistant Professor, Cardiothoracic Radiology, University of California, San Diego, La Jolla, California, USA

KIMBERLY G. KALLIANOS, MD
Assistant Professor of Clinical Radiology, Department of Radiology and Biomedical Imaging, University of California, San Francisco, San Francisco, California, USA

JEFFREY P. KANNE, MD
Professor and Chief of Thoracic Imaging, Department of Radiology, University of Wisconsin School of Medicine and Public Health, Madison, Wisconsin, USA

SETH KLIGERMAN, MD
Associate Professor, Division Chief of Cardiothoracic Radiology, University of California, San Diego, La Jolla, California, USA

JOANNA EVA KUSMIREK, MD
Assistant Professor, Department of Radiology, University of Wisconsin School of Medicine and Public Health, Madison, Wisconsin, USA

CHRISTINA A. LeBEDIS, MD, MS
Department of Radiology, Boston University Medical Center, Boston, Massachusetts, USA

MARIA DANIELA MARTIN ROTHER, MD
Assistant Professor, Department of Radiology, University of Wisconsin School of Medicine and Public Health, Madison, Wisconsin, USA

VINCENT M. MELLNICK, MD
Associate Professor, Radiology, Chief, Abdominal Imaging Section, Co-Director, Emergency Radiology, Abdominal Imaging Section, Mallinckrodt Institute of Radiology, Washington University in St. Louis, St Louis, Missouri, USA

ALEXANDER MERRITT, MD
Department of Radiology, Boston University Medical Center, Boston, Massachusetts, USA

CRISTOPHER A. MEYER, MD
Professor, Department of Radiology, University of Wisconsin School of Medicine and Public Health, Madison, Wisconsin, USA

ABIGAIL MILLS, MD
Radiology Resident, Mallinckrodt Institute of Radiology, Washington University in St Louis School of Medicine, St Louis, Missouri, USA

JOANNA MOSER, MBChB, FRCR
Radiology Department, St George's University Hospitals, NHS Foundation Trust and School of Medicine, London, United Kingdom

MARK E. MULLINS, MD, PhD, FACR
Department of Radiology and Imaging Services, Emory University School of Medicine, Atlanta, Georgia, USA

KEVIN NEAL, MD
Instructor of Radiology, Cardiothoracic Radiology Fellow, Mallinckrodt Institute of Radiology, St Louis, Missouri, USA

ANSU NORONHA, MD
Section of Gastroenterology, Department of Medicine, Boston University Medical Center, Boston, Massachusetts, USA

RYAN B. O'MALLEY, MD
Department of Radiology, Abdominal Imaging, University of Washington, Seattle, Washington, USA

MICHAEL N. PATLAS, MD, FRCPC, FCAR, FSAR
Department of Radiology, McMaster University, Hamilton General Hospital, Hamilton, Ontario, Canada

HAMZA RAHIMI, MD
Department of Radiology, Boston University Medical Center, Boston, Massachusetts, USA

DEMETRIOS A. RAPTIS, MD
Assistant Professor of Radiology, Mallinckrodt Institute of Radiology, St Louis, Missouri, USA

JONATHAN W. REVELS, DO
Department of Radiology, Body and Thoracic
Imaging, University of New Mexico,
Albuquerque, New Mexico, USA

DONGHOON SHIN, MD, MS
Department of Radiology, Boston University
Medical Center, Boston, Massachusetts,
USA

**KONSTANTINOS STEFANIDIS, MD, MSc,
PhD**
Radiology Department, King's College
Hospital, NHS Foundation Trust, London,
United Kingdom

JENNIFER W. UYEDA, MD
Assistant Professor, Department of Radiology,
Brigham and Women's Hospital, Boston,
Massachusetts, USA

ALINA UZELAC, DO
Associate Clinical Professor, Neuroradiology,
Department of Radiology, Zuckerberg San
Francisco General Hospital, University of

California, San Francisco, California,
USA

ABHINAV VEMULA, MD
Section of Gastroenterology, Department of
Medicine, Boston University Medical Center,
Boston, Massachusetts, USA

IOANNIS VLAHOS, MBBS, BSc, MRCP, FRCR
Radiology Department, St George's University
Hospitals, NHS Foundation Trust and School of
Medicine, London, United Kingdom

ELIZABETH WEIHE, MD
Associate Professor, Cardiothoracic
Radiology, University of California, San Diego,
La Jolla, California, USA

BRENT D. WEINBERG, MD, PhD
Department of Radiology and Imaging
Services, Emory University School of Medicine,
Atlanta, Georgia, USA

HEISHUN YU, MD
Instructor, Department of Radiology, Brigham
and Women's Hospital, Boston,
Massachusetts, USA

Contents

Bowel wall thickening in the hospitalized patient can be due to myriad etiologies. Familiarity with the optimal study protocols and a structured approach for evaluation are important. Understanding the pathology and knowing the imaging features of most common entities (ischemia, shock bowel, hemorrhage, infection, graft-versus-host disease, and fluid overload) enable radiologists to provide unique value to clinical management.

Gastrointestinal tract perforation involving the stomach, duodenum, small intestine, or large bowel occurs as a result of full-thickness gastrointestinal wall injury with release of intraluminal contents into the peritoneal or retroperitoneal cavity. Most cases are associated with high mortality and morbidity, requiring urgent surgical evaluation. Initial patient presentations can be nonspecific with a broad differential, which can delay timely management. This article provides brief overviews of different causes of perforation. Various imaging modalities and protocols are discussed, along with direct and indirect imaging findings of perforation. Specific findings associated with different causes are also described to aid in the diagnosis.

Abdominal pain is a common cause for emergency department visits in the United States, and biliary tract disease is the fifth most common cause of hospital admission. Common causes of acute hepatobiliary include gallstones and its associated complications and multiple other hepatobiliary etiologies, including infectious, inflammatory, vascular, and neoplastic causes. Postoperative complications of the biliary tract can result in an acute abdomen. Imaging of the hepatobiliary tree is integral in the diagnostic evaluation of acute hepatobiliary dysfunction, and imaging of the biliary tree requires a multimodality approach utilizing ultrasound, computed tomography, nuclear medicine, and MR imaging.

Acute kidney injury (AKI) is characterized by a decline in the glomerular filtration rate. AKI affects up to 20% of hospitalized patients, and is even more common among intensive care unit admissions. Complications of AKI are related to uremia (encephalopathy, neuropathy, pericarditis), volume overload (pulmonary edema), and electrolyte disturbances (hyperkalemia). In addition to having increased associated morbidity and mortality, patients who develop AKI may never fully recover their baseline kidney function. Imaging can play a valuable role in the work-up of AKI. This article discusses the utility of imaging in characterizing AKI in adult patients in a hospital setting.

Alberto Cossu, Maria Daniela Martin Rother, Joanna Eva Kusmirek, Cristopher A. Meyer, and Jeffrey P. Kanne

Imaging plays a central role in the evaluation of patients following cardiothoracic surgery, both for monitoring in the early postoperative period and for assessing for suspected complications. Patients with postsurgical complications can develop a range of signs and symptoms, from hypotension and tachycardia, as the result of severe bleeding, to fever and leukocytosis because of infection. The radiologist is an important member of the care team in the postoperative period, helping identify and manage complications of cardiothoracic surgery. This article reviews the common complications of cardiothoracic surgery focusing on the role of imaging and clues to diagnosis.

Seth Kligerman, Michael Horowitz, Kathleen Jacobs, and Elizabeth Weihe

Patients hospitalized in the intensive care unit (ICU) often have multiple support lines and devices that need routine imaging evaluation by radiologists. In patients with cardiogenic shock or depressed cardiac function, mechanical circulation support devices are used in combination with medical therapies to improve patient outcomes and sometimes can stabilize patients for surgical intervention. This article discusses some of the more commonly encountered mechanical circulation devices seen in ICU patients, including intra-aortic balloon pumps, Impella devices, extracorporeal membrane oxygenation cannulas, and ventricular assist devices. Normal appearance and commonly encountered device-related complications that can be diagnosed on imaging are reviewed.

Judith A. Gadde, Brent D. Weinberg, and Mark E. Mullins

A brief introduction is provided of the different imaging modalities encountered in the intensive care unit (ICU). The spectrum of intracranial pathology as well as potential postsurgical complications is reviewed, with a focus on pearls and pitfalls. A brief overview also is provided of imaging of the spine in an ICU patient.

Alina Uzelac

Neuroimaging is an invaluable diagnostic tool for sorting through the vast array of etiologies that underlie altered mental status (AMS). Head computed tomography (CT) without contrast is the primary modality for evaluation of AMS and should be complemented by MR imaging in cases of negative CT but high clinical concern. Studies to maximize brain imaging efficiency and improve the yield of positive scans through the utilization of clinical and laboratory pre-scan diagnostics are ongoing. However, imaging remains the gold standard due to its rapidity with which certain diagnoses can be made or excluded.

PROGRAM OBJECTIVE
The objective of the *Radiologic Clinics of North America* is to keep practicing radiologists and radiology residents up to date with current clinical practice in radiology by providing timely articles reviewing the state of the art in patient care.

TARGET AUDIENCE
Practicing radiologists, radiology residents, and other healthcare professionals who provide patient care utilizing radiologic findings.

LEARNING OBJECTIVES
Upon completion of this activity, participants will be able to:
1. Review commonly encountered cardiovascular support devices seen in ICU patients, proper placement as well as commonly encountered device related complications that can be diagnosed on imaging.
2. Discuss neuroimaging of patients in the ICU, potential complications, pearls, and pitfalls.
3. Recognize complications of cardiothoracic surgery, the role of imaging and clues to diagnosis.

ACCREDITATION
The Elsevier Office of Continuing Medical Education (EOCME) is accredited by the Accreditation Council for Continuing Medical Education (ACCME) to provide continuing medical education for physicians.

The EOCME designates this journal-based CME activity for a maximum of 12 *AMA PRA Category 1 Credit*(s)™. Physicians should claim only the credit commensurate with the extent of their participation in the activity.

All other healthcare professionals requesting continuing education credit for this enduring material will be issued a certificate of participation.

DISCLOSURE OF CONFLICTS OF INTEREST
The EOCME assesses conflict of interest with its instructors, faculty, planners, and other individuals who are in a position to control the content of CME activities. All relevant conflicts of interest that are identified are thoroughly vetted by EOCME for fair balance, scientific objectivity, and patient care recommendations. EOCME is committed to providing its learners with CME activities that promote improvements or quality in healthcare and not a specific proprietary business or a commercial interest.

The planning committee, staff, authors and editors listed below have identified no financial relationships or relationships to products or devices they or their spouse/life partner have with commercial interest related to the content of this CME activity:

Abdullah Alabousi, MD, FRCPC; Mostafa Alabousi, MD; Sanjeev Bhalla, MD; Alberto Cossu, MD; Judith A. Gadde, DO, MBA; Samir Haroon, MD; Travis S. Henry, MD; Michael D. Hope, MD; Michael Horowitz, MD, PhD; Malak Itani, MD; Kathleen Jacobs, MD; Kimberly G. Kallianos, MD; Jeffrey P. Kanne, MD; Alison Kemp; Seth Kligerman, MD; Joanna Eva Kusmirek, MD; Pradeep Kuttysankaran; Christina A. LeBedis, MD, MS; Maria Daniela Martin Rother, MD; Vincent M. Mellnick, MD; Alexander Merritt, MD; Cristopher A. Meyer, MD; Frank H. Miller, MD, FACR; Abigail Mills, MD; Joanna Moser, MBChB, FRCR; Mark E. Mullins, MD, PhD, FACR; Donald Mumford; Kevin Neal, MD; Ansu Noronha, MD; Ryan B. O'Malley, MD; Michael N. Patlas, MD, FRCPC, FCAR, FSAR; Hamza Rahimi, MD; Demetrios A. Raptis, MD; Jonathan W. Revels, DO; Donghoon Shin, MD, MS; Konstantinos Stefanidis, MD, MSc, PhD; Jennifer W. Uyeda, MD; Alina Uzelac, DO; John Vassallo; Abhinav Vemula, MD; Ioannis Vlahos, MBBS, BSc, MRCP, FRCR; Elizabeth Weihe, MD; Brent D. Weinberg, MD, PhD; HeiShun Yu, MD.

UNAPPROVED/OFF-LABEL USE DISCLOSURE
The EOCME requires CME faculty to disclose to the participants:
1. When products or procedures being discussed are off-label, unlabelled, experimental, and/or investigational (not US Food and Drug Administration [FDA] approved); and
2. Any limitations on the information presented, such as data that are preliminary or that represent ongoing research, interim analyses, and/or unsupported opinions. Faculty may discuss information about pharmaceutical agents that is outside of FDA-approved labelling. This information is intended solely for CME and is not intended to promote off-label use of these medications. If you have any questions, contact the medical affairs department of the manufacturer for the most recent prescribing information.

TO ENROLL
To enroll in the *Radiologic Clinics of North America* Continuing Medical Education program, call customer service at 1-800-654-2452 or sign up online at http://www.theclinics.com/home/cme. The CME program is available to subscribers for an additional annual fee of USD 330.

METHOD OF PARTICIPATION
In order to claim credit, participants must complete the following:
1. Complete enrolment as indicated above.
2. Read the activity.

3. Complete the CME Test and Evaluation. Participants must achieve a score of 70% on the test. All CME Tests and Evaluations must be completed online.

CME INQUIRIES/SPECIAL NEEDS

For all CME inquiries or special needs, please contact elsevierCME@elsevier.com.

RADIOLOGIC CLINICS OF NORTH AMERICA

RELATED SERIES

Magnetic Resonance Imaging Clinics
Neuroimaging Clinics
PET Clinics

Preface
Multisystem Imaging of the Critically Ill Patient

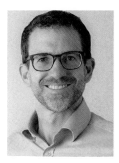 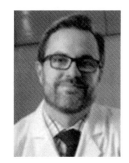

Travis S. Henry, MD   Vincent M. Mellnick, MD
Editors

Hospitalized patients present a unique challenge to radiologists. In the era of ever-increasing subspecialization, it is important to take a step back and recognize that the critically ill patient often has disease that affects multiple organ systems, or multiple concurrent disorders that prompt imaging. In addition to systemic conditions with multiple findings, surgical changes, support devices, medications, and their side effects may all cause imaging findings in the hospitalized patient. The effects of these conditions may be readily apparent, but providing a precise diagnosis requires awareness from the interpreting radiologist. Recognition of these abnormalities can literally mean the difference between life and death in patients whose condition is tenuous. Critically ill patients also often require special examination considerations, ranging from contrast administration concerns to accounting for artifacts that may result from altered mental status or implanted devices.

The aim of this issue of *Radiologic Clinics of North America* is to provide a high-yield and up-to-date multispecialty review of the critically ill patient across different imaging disciplines and modalities with the goal of providing all radiologists with an up-to-date approach to diagnosis and management of some of the sickest patients we will encounter. Some articles are designed to provide an approach for commonly encountered abnormalities (eg, imaging of bowel wall thickening; gastrointestinal tract perforation; neuroimaging pearls and pitfalls; approach to abnormal chest computed tomographic contrast enhancement; imaging of the misplaced central venous catheter); other articles address common indications for imaging (eg, acute hepatobiliary dysfunction; acute renal failure; altered mental status; diffuse lung disease), and some articles review postoperative findings both expected and unexpected (eg, abdominal postoperative complications; early postoperative complications of cardiothoracic surgery; imaging of cardiac support devices).

It is our hope that all radiologists, from the generalist to the subspecialist, will learn from these articles and, it is hoped, improve the way that critically ill patients are diagnosed and managed.

Travis S. Henry, MD
Cardiac and Pulmonary Imaging Section
University of California San Francisco
505 Parnassus Avenue
M-396
San Francisco, CA 94143, USA

Vincent M. Mellnick, MD
Abdominal Imaging Section
Mallinckrodt Institute of Radiology
Washington University in St. Louis
510 South Kingshighway Boulevard
St Louis, MO 63110, USA

E-mail addresses:
travis.henry@ucsf.edu (T.S. Henry)
mellnickv@mir.wustl.edu (V.M. Mellnick)

Radiol Clin N Am 58 (2020) xiii
https://doi.org/10.1016/j.rcl.2019.10.001
0033-8389/20/© 2019 Published by Elsevier Inc.

Imaging of Bowel Wall Thickening in the Hospitalized Patient

Abigail Mills, MD, Vincent M. Mellnick, MD, Malak Itani, MD*

KEYWORDS

- Bowel wall thickening • Bowel thickening • Computed tomography • Radiology • Imaging
- Hospitalized patient

KEY POINTS

- Bowel wall thickening in the hospitalized patient is a nonspecific finding that can be encountered in a wide range of pathologic conditions. Proper evaluation starts with an optimal targeted study protocol.
- A pattern-based approach for image analysis consists of assessing length and sites of involvement, any changes to the fold pattern, the severity and attenuation of wall thickening, bowel contents, bowel dilation, and ancillary findings in the mesentery, vessels, and other organs.
- It is important for the radiologist to integrate imaging features with clinical findings and laboratory analysis to reach the most sensible diagnosis.
- Radiologists should be familiar with the most common entities causing bowel wall thickening in the hospitalized patients and with red flags that should be promptly brought to clinical attention.

INTRODUCTION

Hospitalized patients, especially in tertiary and quaternary care facilities, often have complex medical histories with multiple comorbidities. Due to nonspecific and variable clinical manifestations and, in many cases, detrimental consequences when diagnosis is delayed, bowel pathology should be considered during work-up of abdominal symptoms, including nausea, vomiting, gastrointestinal bleeding, and abdominal pain. Hospitalized patients may have abnormal bowel due to vascular, infectious, inflammatory, neoplastic, or other etiologies. It is important to remember the broad range of conditions effecting the bowel, particularly in critically ill patients, in whom an accurate physical examination and history may be difficult to obtain. Whether the cause for admission or not, acute conditions of the bowel can be life-threating and may be difficult to diagnose, in part due to their overlapping imaging appearances. One important manifestation of gastrointestinal disease, bowel wall thickening, is a nonspecific finding that can be seen with a variety of pathologies but also can be a valuable tool to allow radiologists to provide an appropriate differential diagnosis. With the increasing use of cross-sectional imaging in these settings, radiologists are also relied on to be familiar with the utility and limitations of different imaging modalities to evaluate the gastrointestinal tract. This article describes the characterization of bowel wall thickening in the hospitalized patient in different clinical contexts and provides pictorial examples

Disclosure Statement: The authors have nothing to disclose.
Mallinckrodt Institute of Radiology, Washington University in St. Louis School of Medicine, 510 South Kingshighway Boulevard, PO Box 8131, St Louis, MO 63110, USA
* Corresponding author.
E-mail address: mitani@wustl.edu
twitter: @ItaniMalak (M.I.)

Radiol Clin N Am 58 (2020) 1–17
https://doi.org/10.1016/j.rcl.2019.08.006
0033-8389/20/© 2019 Elsevier Inc. All rights reserved.

of common relevant pathologies with the goal of aiding radiologists in diagnosing these conditions, thereby adding value in clinical management.

NORMAL ANATOMY AND IMAGING TECHNIQUE

The small and large bowel is made up of multiple layers, including, from internal to external, the mucosa, submucosa, muscularis propria, and serosa (intraperitoneal) or adventitia (retroperitoneal).[1] Retroperitoneal segments of bowel include the second and third portions of the duodenum, the ascending and descending colon, and the rectum. The histology of the wall layers is varied throughout the alimentary tract depending on function. Although the mucosa is best evaluated with direct visualization through endoscopy or less frequently with fluoroscopic examinations, computed tomography (CT), MR imaging, and ultrasound assess all layers of bowel and can show differential enhancement of the individual layers.

All imaging modalities have important uses in the abdomen, although some offer more useful information in the setting of bowel pathology than others. Considerations for choosing a modality include not only bowel visualization but also availability, radiation dose, cost, and patient stability.

Ultrasound is not often used to evaluate the bowel in hospitalized patients due to its focused nature, but it has been well established in certain populations, including pediatric patients with intussusception and pregnant patients with appendicitis. Contrast-enhanced ultrasound is gaining popularity in the work-up of inflammatory bowel disease in children, especially in Europe and Canada. Additionally, ultrasound may be used to target percutaneous procedures, including placement of tubes and potentially biopsy of exoenteric bowel wall masses. Due to its inability to visualize the entire gastrointestinal tract and its well-known operator dependency, however, ultrasound has limited use in this clinical context.

The ability to perform portable radiographic studies is an advantage for critically ill patients who are too unstable for transport. Although there are some occasions when bowel conditions have typical aunt-Minnie appearances on abdominal radiographs, such as the lead-pipe colon in ulcerative colitis (**Fig. 1**), abdominal radiographs most often have limited utility in the setting of bowel wall thickening because of their poor resolution of superimposed structures. Fluoroscopic examinations with intraluminal contrast agents have historically been used for the evaluation of bowel

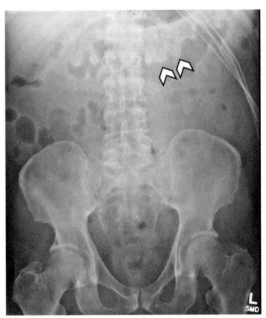

Fig. 1. Typical colonic thumbprinting pattern reflecting colonic wall thickening most pronounced in the transverse colon. Extensive edema of the haustrations results in luminal protrusions with round contour (*arrowheads*) resembling thumbs.

pathology and remained the only way to image the bowel lumen for several decades. Similar to radiography, fluoroscopy provides limited information about submucosal and extraluminal disease and also has the added limitations of the need for patient cooperation, prolonged imaging times, and often the requirement that the radiologist obtains the images to ensure an adequate study. High-quality barium fluoroscopic examinations also may not be possible in hospitalized patients due to the need for preparation and gaseous distention as well as concern for possible leak into the peritoneal cavity in surgical patients. Thus, although the high spatial resolution and dynamic aspect of fluoroscopy make it useful for evaluation of abnormal mucosa, small fistulous tracts, and early leaks (**Fig. 2**), these benefits do not make up for the technical challenges, and the use of fluoroscopy in evaluating bowel pathology has been declining.[2]

Because of the limitations of fluoroscopy in the hospitalized patient, cross-sectional imaging with CT and MR imaging is often called on to provide more comprehensive information about abdominal pathology, including the bowel wall. These modalities allow for evaluation of all bowel wall layers, associated structures such as mesenteric vessels, and the remainder of the abdomen, which could suggest alternative diagnoses. MR imaging

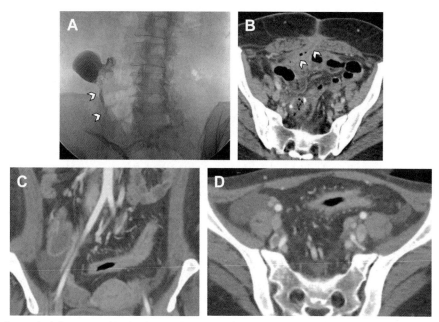

Fig. 2. Persistent draining wound in the lower abdomen of a patient with Crohn disease. (*A*) Sinus tract injection under fluoroscopy demonstrated a patent enterocutaneous fistula (*arrowheads*). (*B*) CT scan done 1 month prior demonstrated the sinus tract but no clear communication. (*C, D*) Typical bowel wall thickening with white attenuation pattern in Crohn disease consistent with active inflammatory phase in the proximal sigmoid colon. Prominent vasa recta produce the comb sign.

is desirable due to its superior contrast resolution and lack of ionizing radiation, which makes it a safe choice in pediatric and pregnant populations and in patients who need repetitive imaging for chronic conditions, such as inflammatory bowel disease,[3] but these advantages need to be balanced with the need for the hospitalized patient to be still and cooperate with breathing instructions. Patients with claustrophobia, end-stage renal disease precluding contrast, and implantable devices present challenges for performing an MR imaging as well. Because of these concerns, contrast-enhanced CT of the abdomen and pelvis has emerged as the most commonly ordered modality for the work-up of bowel pathology in the hospitalized patient given its availability and speed of acquisition compared with MR imaging. Because of the above-mentioned, limitations with other imaging modalities, this article largely focuses on CT imaging for this patient population.

IMAGING PROTOCOLS

Protocol selection is an important consideration when performing CT to evaluate the patient with abnormal bowel. Although a noncontrast study can provide some information about bowel wall thickening, it remains a limited examination (**Fig. 3**). The importance of administering intravenous contrast cannot be overstated, because it allows for evaluation of bowel wall hyperenhancement and hypoenhancement, mesenteric vasculature, and solid organs. Generally patients with glomerular filtration rate greater than 30 mL/min per 1.73 m^2 and no contrast allergy can safely receive contrast, and detailed guidelines are routinely updated by the American College of Radiology (ACR).[4] For a patient with an acute abdominal presentation requiring an emergency department visit or admission to an inpatient unit, a common practice is to perform single acquisition CT with intravenous contrast in the portal venous phase. For the patient with known or highly suspected bowel pathology, however, CT protocols can be optimized to specifically evaluate for inflammatory bowel disease, bowel ischemia, and acute gastrointestinal bleed (**Table 1**). Detailed clinical history allows a radiologist to choose the appropriate protocol. These protocols call for variable timing of one or more postcontrast phase(s). Some require initial noncontrast imaging, which can be helpful for evaluating enhancement as well as documenting the presence of hyperdense material that otherwise could be confused for contrast extravasation. Dual-energy CT can potentially obviate a separate precontrast acquisition by allowing virtual noncontrast imaging.

The value added by the routine use of oral contrast in abdominal and pelvic CT, especially

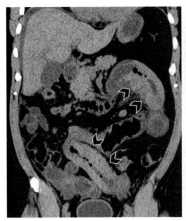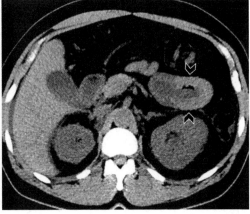

Fig. 3. Despite its limited utility, noncontrast CT can still provide valuable information. Coronal reformatted (*left*) and axial (*right*) images demonstrate hyperdense wall thickening (*arrowheads*) corresponding to multifocal intramural small bowel wall hematoma in this patient receiving a supratherapeutic dose of warfarin with international normalized ratio value of 6.75.

in the inpatient and emergency setting, is not as well-established as that of intravenous contrast and has been a controversial topic until recent ACR guidelines recommended against its routine use in the emergency setting.[5] In the 1980s, it was widely accepted that positive (radiopaque) enteric contrast was necessary for adequate visualization of the abdominal organs and that negative (radiolucent) contrast was helpful in evaluating intraluminal disease.[6] Over the past few decades, however, arguments against oral contrast have emerged, especially in the acute setting, including increased wait time for the patients before the scan, potential risk of aspiration of oral contrast material, and reportedly being the least pleasant portion of the CT examination for patients.[7] The use of oral contrast likely was more valuable when CT slices were thicker and the image quality was relatively poor,[7] but with modern computerized display and the ability to scroll through sequential images, radiologists can identify the continuity of structures to discern bowel loops from lymph nodes or soft tissue lesions. Even with the use of oral contrast, uniform opacification of the gastrointestinal tract is hard to achieve. Furthermore, with the growing overweight and obese population, many adult patients have enough visceral fat to provide spatial resolution between bowel loops and abdominal structures. A 2015 study by Alabousi and colleagues[8] showed that omitting oral contrast for patients with body mass index greater than 25 kg/m² presenting with acute abdominal pain resulted in no delayed or missed diagnoses.

In the authors' institution, CT studies are performed without oral contrast except in select

Table 1
Bowel-specific computed tomography protocols

Protocol	Components and Timing	Slice Thickness
Mesenteric ischemia/ gastrointestinal bleed	Oral contrast: none Intravenous contrast rate: 4 mL/s Phases: noncontrast Arterial 35 s fixed delay or 5 s after aorta trigger Portal venous 60–90 s fixed delay	Noncontrast: axial 3 mm Arterial: axial 2 mm, coronal 3 mm Portal venous: axial 3 mm
Small bowel obstruction	Oral contrast: none Intravenous contrast rate: 3 mL/s Phase: portal venous 60 s fixed delay	Axial 2 mm, coronal 3 mm
CT enterography	Oral contrast: dilute 0.1% barium sulfate suspension Intravenous contrast rate: 3 mL/s Phase: portal venous 60 s	Axial 3 mm, coronal 3 mm

scenarios. Prompt imaging is important in the acutely ill patient, and the potential value of oral contrast often does not justify a 30-minute to 90-minute imaging delay. Positive oral contrast may obscure the bowel mucosa and evaluation of enhancement. Circumstances in which the authors use intraluminal contrast include positive oral contrast for suspected extraluminal leak in postsurgical patients (fluoroscopy is an alternative study in this group) and suspected traumatic bowel injury if initial trauma CT was equivocal, negative oral contrast (such as water or dilute 0.1% wt/wt barium sulfate suspension) for CT enterography, and carbon dioxide insufflation for CT colonography. Regarding negative oral contrast agents, dilute barium sulfate has been shown to provide better distention of the stomach, small bowel, and colon and better visualization of bowel wall features compared with water alone and/or water containing methylcellulose.[9,10] Additionally, the low radiographic density of neutral or negative oral contrast minimizes attenuation artifact on CT scans.[11] Pediatric or thin patients may also require oral contrast to improve visibility of the gastrointestinal tract and separate it from fluid collections and/or masses.

Several other important factors should be considered when developing imaging protocols. Thinner slices provide better spatial resolution, but thicker slices result in better signal to noise ratio; therefore, slice thickness must be optimized to the specific anatomy in question. A 3-mm to 5-mm slice thickness typically is used. Reconstructions in coronal and sagittal planes are routinely generated and useful for following the bowel. Additional reconstructions, such as 3-dimensional volumetric images, maximum intensity projection images, curved reconstructions, and oblique and double oblique views, may be performed, particularly for assessment of the mesenteric vasculature.

Variables relating to intravenous contrast, namely contrast volume, rate of injection, and timing of image acquisition, also must be adjusted depending on the patient and clinical question. A larger volume of contrast media results in greater tissue enhancement and may be needed in larger patients. This also should be balanced, however, with potential risk for postcontrast acute kidney injury. Increasingly, dual-energy CT applications are used to artificially lower the kilovoltage after scanning to improve the conspicuity of lower quantities of iodinated contrast media. A faster injection rate (3–5 mL/s) allows for improved vascular opacification, but it results in a short temporal window for image acquisition in specific phases and usually requires a larger caliber (14–20 gauge) and more proximal (antecubital or

central) intravenous access. This is needed for evaluating patients with suspected gastrointestinal (GI) bleeding or bowel ischemia, in whom vascular assessment is critical. A slower injection rate is technically easier and is sufficient for parenchymal and venous imaging because those phases last for a relatively longer time. Once contrast has been injected, images can be obtained at a fixed delay or at a time that is individualized to each patient. Individualized options are generally used for vascular imaging and for patients with compromised cardiac output and include test-bolus and bolus-tracking methods. The bolus-tracking method is generally used for abdominal imaging when contrast timing is of utmost importance. Images are obtained at a reference level (usually the aorta) and repeated after injecting the full dose of contrast. When enhancement reaches a predetermined threshold, image acquisition is triggered. Alternatively, the test-bolus method involves generating a time-enhancement curve from low radiation images obtained with a small contrast volume that is then used to calculate the appropriate imaging delay. It models a patient's cardiovascular response and often is seen in the setting of cardiac CT angiography.[12]

IMAGING FINDINGS—APPROACH TO DIAGNOSIS

Bowel wall thickening in the hospitalized patient is a nonspecific finding that can be encountered in a wide range of pathologic conditions. This necessitates a systemic approach for evaluation of bowel wall thickening, which consists of assessing the length and sites of involvement; the pattern of enhancement; any changes to the pattern of haustration or valvulae conniventes; the severity and attenuation of wall thickening, bowel contents, bowel dilation; and any ancillary features outside the bowel, such as mesenteric findings.[13,14]

Normal small and large bowel thickness is variable and depends on bowel distention. In the colon, a normal wall measures up to 6 mm to 8 mm if the lumen is decompressed and 0 mm to 2 mm with increasing distention.[15] The small bowel wall should measure no more than 3 mm if the lumen is decompressed and 0 mm to 2 mm if the bowel is distended.[16] Because bowel wall thickness varies with the degree of distention and because decompressed bowel loops can be difficult to delineate from one another, accurately diagnosing bowel wall thickening on imaging can pose a challenge. Many factors, including but not limited to the clinical context, distribution and severity of bowel wall thickening, pattern of enhancement, and bowel wall attenuation as well as mesenteric and other associated nonenteric findings, are important to note when evaluating bowel wall thickening. These factors provide the basis for the selection of imaging studies and protocols available for the work-up of bowel pathology.

Sites and Length of Involvement

The traditional approach to evaluating small bowel pathology using barium studies relied on the length of involvement as a major variable in the diagnostic approach to bowel wall thickening. Different disease processes tend to involve the bowel in variable patterns, with the most common patterns being segmental versus diffuse involvement.[17] The length and site of involvement can help in narrowing the differential considerations (Table 2). The more prevalent pathologies in hospitalized patients, including infectious, inflammatory, and ischemic processes, tend to involve longer segments of bowel. Exceptions include skip lesions in Crohn disease and noncontiguous ischemic bowel, such as in watershed areas. In contrast, systemic processes, such as graft-versus-host disease (GVHD), celiac disease, and lupus, and edema, generally involve long segments of the bowel.

Enhancement and Fold Pattern

The bowel wall attenuation is one of the most useful clues for differential diagnosis and can be a reflection of the pathophysiology of the underlying process, either due to its intrinsic attenuation or that of increased or decreased enhancement (Fig. 4; Table 3).[18] Reliable attenuation difference

is defined as at least 10 Hounsfield units and preferably 20 Hounsfield units above that of the reference structure, which is usually skeletal muscle. White attenuation, which describes full-thickness transmural enhancement of the bowel wall, can be seen with severe active inflammation or with leaky capillaries. Less commonly, diffuse hyperattenuation of the bowel wall can be secondary to acute submucosal hemorrhage and is best seen on noncontrast images. Gray enhancement reflects a lower level of enhancement than skeletal muscle, making it difficult to differentiate the layers of bowel wall. Submucosal edema of the bowel usually results in the water target sign, which describes enhancing inner (mucosa) and outer (muscularis propria and/or serosa) wall layers.[19] Bowel wall fat and gas generally are easy to appreciate and differentiate (Fig. 5).

Changes to the normal folds (valvulae conniventes or plica circulares) of the small bowel or colonic haustrations are not commonly encountered but can be very specific findings. This feature has historical basis from small bowel fluoroscopy studies. Normally, the small bowel folds are composed of both mucosa and submucosa, and they are more closely spaced and thicker in the jejunum and gradually become more spaced and thinner in the ileum.[17] Reversal of the jejunal and ileal fold pattern is characteristic of celiac disease. Fold thickening can be focal or diffuse, and it can be smooth or nodular irregular. In hospitalized patients, smooth diffuse thickening can be seen with edema or third spacing, whereas focal smooth thickening can be seen with hemorrhage. Nodular or irregular fold thickening in the hospitalized patients favor an infectious etiology. Other less common causes of nodular thickening include malignancy or autoimmune diseases, such as amyloidosis and mastocytosis.[17]

Degree of Wall Thickening

The extent of bowel wall thickening is a useful feature for differentiating underlying etiologies, although it is not always directly related to the severity of the pathology. In bowel ischemia, arterial occlusion can result in paper-thin bowel wall, whereas venous occlusion can result in congested bowel with marked wall thickening. Pronounced wall thickening is often seen in cases of pseudomembranous colitis, which typically spares the small bowel, and Crohn disease, which can cause acute inflammation superimposed on areas of chronic thickening and fibrosis. Nodular wall thickening can be more concerning for an underlying neoplastic process, whereas smooth wall thickening often is benign.

Table 2 Length of involvement	
Length of Bowel Involvement	Differential Diagnosis
<5 cm	Adenocarcinoma
5–10 cm	Diverticulitis, Crohn disease, ischemia
10–30 cm	Ischemia, submucosal hemorrhage, radiation enterocolitis, infection, Crohn disease, lymphoma
Diffuse colonic involvement	Ulcerative colitis
Diffuse small and large bowel involvement	Infection, edema, lupus

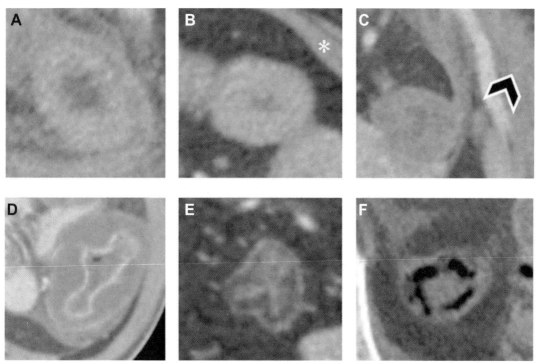

Fig. 4. Different patterns of bowel wall enhancement. (*A*) White enhancement involving the jejunum in a patient with Crohn disease and (*B*) a second patient with immunotherapy related enteritis. Note the hyperenhancement of the entire jejunal wall compared with the adjacent abdominal wall muscles (*asterisk*). (*C*) Gray enhancement seen in a patient with rectosigmoid adenocarcinoma in a coronal reformatted image; this can be compared with the adjacent partially visualized iliopsoas muscle (*arrowhead*). (*D*) Water target sign seen in an immunocompromised acute myeloid leukemia patient with pseudomembraneous colitis. (*E*) Bowel wall fat deposition in an obese patient with no known bowel pathology or acute symptoms. (*F*) Pneumatosis intestinalis in a patient with ischemic enteritis.

Additional Findings

In addition to direct evaluation of the bowel wall, indirect findings can offer invaluable clues to the diagnosis. Note should be made of the bowel contents. In patients with diarrhea, bowel loops usually are fluid filled with possible ileus. Intraluminal fat can be seen in patients with steatorrhea secondary to pancreatic insufficiency (pancreatitis or cystic fibrosis) or malabsorption (celiac disease). Feculent material in the small bowel, or the pseudofeces sign, signifies stasis of ingested material in the small bowel and can be seen with bowel obstruction but is nonspecific. Intraluminal hyperdense blood products, ingested foreign bodies, and gallstones also are pertinent findings. Specific changes to the bowel contour also can be helpful indicators of disease etiology. For example, pseudosacculations along the antimesenteric wall are appreciated with Crohn disease. Finally, the proximity of bowel loops to each other should be evaluated. In chronic inflammatory bowel disease, mesenteric fat hypertrophy causes separation of adjacent bowel loops, whereas fibrotic processes

and desmoplastic reactions that occur with carcinoid tumors or sclerosing mesenteritis can cause tethering of adjacent bowel loops. Close approximation of adjacent loops can also imply a fistulous connection.

Assessment of the mesenteric vessels should be an integral component of evaluating bowel wall thickening in the hospitalized patient. In cases of ischemia, patency of the mesenteric arteries and veins should be confirmed, and the radiologist should carefully search for gas in the mesenteric and portal veins, because it is associated with poor outcomes. Mesenteric vascular patency is relevant in cases of infection and inflammation, in addition to postoperative patients and hypercoagulable states, including neoplasms because all these situations present a risk of mesenteric venous thrombosis.[20] Images of the heart, when included, might uncover a source for arterial emboli (**Fig. 6**). Enlarged mesenteric lymph nodes can guide the differential toward infectious, inflammatory, and neoplastic etiologies, whereas mesenteric edema and vascular engorgement

Table 3
Enhancement pattern

Enhancement Pattern	Differential Diagnosis
White attenuation	• **Acute inflammatory bowel disease** (hyperemia/vasodilation leads to enhancement) • **Shock bowel** (hypoperfusion causes increased permeability of intramural vessels and interstitial leakage of contrast) • **Reperfusion after ischemia** • **Intramural hematoma** after trauma or in an anticoagulated patient
Gray attenuation	• Chronic (fibrotic) Crohn disease • Ischemia • Neoplasm (including adenocarcinoma, metastases, and gastrointestinal stromal tumor)
Water target sign	• **Infection** • Portal hypertension (isolated right colitis/portal colopathy) • **Typhlitis** (necrotizing inflammation of the cecum) • **Ischemia** • **Acute inflammatory bowel disease**
Fat target sign	• Obesity (most common) • Chronic inflammatory bowel disease • Reaction to chemotherapy • Celiac disease
Pneumatosis intestinalis	• **Ischemia with impending bowel perforation** • Trauma • **Infection** • Benign causes: pulmonary disease, medications (steroids, chemotherapy), connective tissue disease (scleroderma), inflammatory bowel disease, recent colonoscopy[18]

Pathologies that are more commonly encountered in hospitalized patients are in bold.

can be seen in cases of closed loop obstruction, hemorrhage, venous ischemia, and mesenteric edema.

COMMON ENTITIES

The wide spectrum of pathology affecting the small bowel and causes of bowel wall thickening is beyond the scope of this review. A few entities, however, represent a majority of causes of bowel wall thickening in hospitalized patients and are important for every radiologist to be aware of.

Acute Mesenteric Ischemia

Acute mesenteric ischemic is a life-threatening condition that is characterized by insufficient bowel perfusion and accounts for approximately 1% of acute abdomen hospitalizations.[21] It has a nonspecific presentation; however, one useful clinical feature is severe abdominal pain that is out of proportion to the physical examination findings. Key laboratory abnormalities that may be encountered include elevated lactate and anion-gap metabolic acidosis.[22] The overall mortality rate of 60% to 80%[23] highlights the importance

of prompt recognition and accurate classification by the radiologists.

The etiologies of this condition can be classified as occlusive mesenteric ischemia, nonocclusive mesenteric ischemia, small vessel disease, or small bowel obstruction. Occlusive mesenteric ischemia refers to cases in which the superior mesenteric artery or vein is occluded. Nonocclusive mesenteric ischemia describes shock bowel from hypoperfusion and is described later. Small vessel disease–related ischemia can be caused by chemotherapy, radiation, or vasculitis. Finally, small bowel obstruction increases pressure within the bowel wall and can lead to resistance to blood flow. The risk of ischemia is increased in cases of closed-loop obstruction.

The CT appearance of bowel ischemia varies depending on etiology. In cases of arterial occlusive ischemia, a filling defect can often be identified in the superior mesenteric artery and/or its branches, and the damage often is slower than venous occlusive ischemia. Radiologic appearance of arterial occlusive ischemia depends on time after onset. In the early phase, there is dynamic ileus due to failure of the muscles to relax,

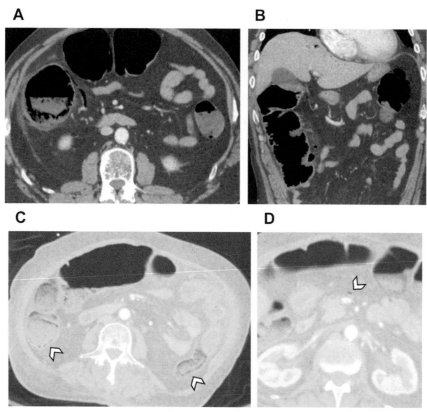

Fig. 5. Irregular wall thickening in a patient with carfilzomib-induced colitis. (*A*) Axial images demonstrate irregular wall thickening of the cecum with surrounding fat stranding. There is gas within the nondependent portions of the cecal wall consistent with pneumatosis intestinalis. In addition, gas is seen tracking within the mesenteric vessels coursing along the right lateral cecal wall. (*B*) Coronal reformatted image demonstrates mesenteric gas medial to the proximal ascending colon, in addition to portal venous gas mostly in the left hepatic lobe. (*C, D*) Displaying CT images with a lung window setting makes detection of abnormally located gas easier, such as in cases of pneumatosis intestinalis (*arrowheads* in *C*), mesenteric and portal venous gas (*arrowheads* in *D*), and pneumoperitoneum.

and CT demonstrates poor or absent enhancement. In the intermediate phase, as venous drainage takes place, the bowel wall becomes paper thin.[24] If there is persistent arterial occlusion, ischemia evolves into infarction. Paradoxically, reperfusion might lead to additional damage rather than healing. At the reperfusion stage, arterial occlusive ischemia has imaging appearance similar to reperfusion injury, discussed later, with hyperenhancing bowel wall thickening and possible associated hemorrhage. Venous occlusive ischemia, in which a filling defect may be seen in the superior mesenteric vein, results in bowel wall thickening and mesenteric venous engorgement due to poor venous drainage. Mucosal enhancement may be normal, increased, or show a target sign. Vasculitides can affect large, medium, or small vessels. Large and medium vessel vasculitides can manifest similarly to occlusive bowel ischemia, whereas small vessel vasculitides may cause mucosal and submucosal

hemorrhage with intervening segments of normal bowel.[25] Radiation-induced or chemotherapy-induced ischemia may be suggested in the appropriate clinical setting and usually is associated with bowel wall thickening with nonspecific enhancement patterns. Radiation usually results in enteritis but can rarely lead to ischemia due to microvascular occlusion. Radiation-induced bowel injury is localized to the radiation port and results in bowel wall thickening with possible strictures and thickened or effaced mucosal folds.[26] Small bowel obstruction is identified by multiple dilated loops of bowel leading to a transition point and a more specific balloons-on-a-string appearance in the setting of closed-loop obstruction. With increased intraluminal pressure, obstruction results in venous outflow obstruction, which is translated to bowel wall thickening and edema on CT. Due to bowel distention, the degree of thickening typically is less pronounced than in mesenteric venous occlusive ischemia (**Fig. 7**). In contrast to

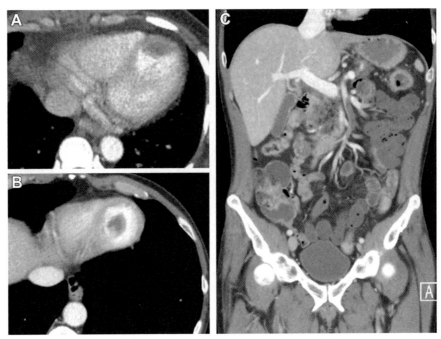

Fig. 6. (*A, B*) Axial images of the chest demonstrating left ventricular filling defects consistent with thrombi, with secondary embolus migration to the superior mesenteric artery (*C*).

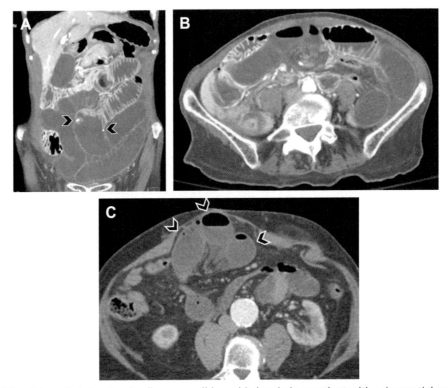

Fig. 7. (*A*) Small bowel obstruction leading to small bowel ischemia in a patient with prior partial small bowel resection. Note the dilated, hypoenhancing loops of bowel in the lower abdomen and pelvis beyond the anastomotic suture line (*arrowheads*). (*B*) Coronal reformatted CT image in the same patient demonstrates swirling of the mesentery and the balloons-on-a-string appearance, suggesting a closed loop obstruction due to an internal hernia, which was confirmed at the time of exploratory laparotomy. (*C*) Closed loop obstruction in a second patient demonstrating a more classic balloons on a string sign (*arrowheads*).

small bowel mesenteric ischemia, ischemic colitis is a distinct entity that can be encountered in the hospitalized patient. It is the most common form of nonocclusive bowel ischemia,[27] although less commonly it can be due to an occlusive etiology. The typical involved segments are watershed areas between the vascular distributions of the superior mesenteric artery and inferior mesenteric artery (splenic flexure) or the inferior mesenteric artery and internal iliac arteries (sigmoid colon). The right colon is a potential watershed area due to underdevelopment of the marginal artery of Drummond in up to 50% of the population.[27] Acute low flow states result in thin nonenhancing bowel wall, whereas later reperfusion injury stage demonstrates wall thickening and edema secondary to inflammation and mucosal ulcerations, with mucosal hyperenhancement or target sign.[28] Other findings include shaggy border of the colonic wall and adjacent mesenteric inflammation. Patients who recover may develop areas of segmental wall thickening and focal strictures that demonstrate transmural enhancement due to fibrosis.[29] Regardless of the etiology of bowel ischemia, pneumatosis intestinalis and mesenteric and portal venous gas are ominous signs and signify microperforations of the bowel wall with potentially irreversible damage (**Fig. 8**).

Hypoperfusion Complex/Shock Bowel and Reperfusion Injury

Shock bowel is the intestinal manifestation of hypoperfusion complex, a constellation of findings that occurs in the setting of hypovolemia and hypotension and reflects radiologic manifestations of volume loss and physiologic stress (fight-or-flight) reaction, including flattening of the inferior vena cava and decreased caliber of the aorta, hypoenhancement of the spleen and liver, hyperenhancement of the adrenal glands, and delayed nephrograms. The small bowel findings are often more prominent than those of other organs due to the vulnerability of intestinal mucosa to ischemia, and the jejunum is more commonly affected than the duodenum and ileum.[30] Bowel hypoperfusion can cause third-spacing losses of fluid into the gastrointestinal tract as the mucosa becomes more permeable and loses its ability to reabsorb fluid.[31] This increased mucosal permeability also allows contrast and fluid to leak into the other bowel wall layers. Therefore, typical findings of shock bowel include fluid-filled, transmurally hyperenhancing, thick-walled loops of bowel giving a white attenuation pattern (**Fig. 9**). Enhancement should be greater than the psoas muscle on contrast-enhanced CT. Alternatively, a target sign may be seen due to bowel wall edema. Free intraperitoneal fluid and mesenteric edema secondary to third-spacing losses also often are present.[32]

Although patients are uniformly hemodynamically unstable, there often are no specific symptoms or direct surgical evidence of shock bowel. Trauma is the most common cause, but cardiac arrest, severe central nervous system injury, septic shock, and diabetic ketoacidosis also can result in hypoperfusion complex.[33] If normal oxygenation of the bowel is maintained via recruitment of capillaries during times of hypotension, CT manifestations of shock bowel can resolve with resolution of hypotension; however, if hypo-oxygenation is severe, reperfusion mechanisms involving oxygen free radicals and inflammatory pathways are activated, leading to tissue injury. This is termed, *reperfusion injury*, and is evidenced by bowel wall thickening and hyperenhancement and

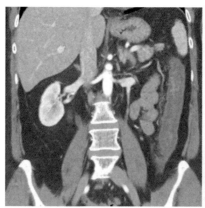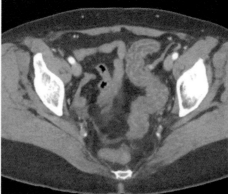

Fig. 8. Coronal reformatted (*left*) and axial (*right*) CT images demonstrating ischemic colitis in a 59-year-old woman with abdominal pain. There is involvement of the descending and sigmoid colon with characteristic sparing of the rectum. There is variable mucosal enhancement in the sigmoid with diffuse submucosal thickening. Colonoscopic biopsy was consistent with ischemic injury.

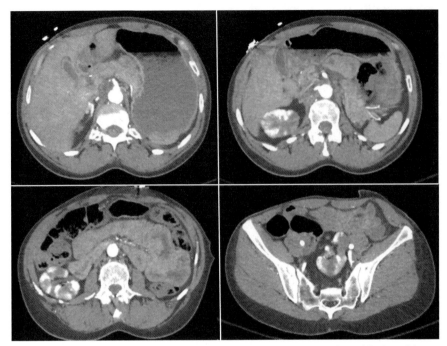

Fig. 9. Hypoperfusion complex after crush injury. The jejunum is thick-walled, fluid-filled, and hyperenhancing, with greater enhancement than adjacent psoas (*top right, bottom left*). Images also demonstrate adrenal hyperenhancement (*top left*), delayed nephrograms, hepatic and splenic hypoperfusion, and a slit-like inferior vena cava. Incidentally noted is a pelvic left kidney (*bottom right*).

possible intraluminal blood filling. If the duration of ischemia is prolonged, this may progress to transmural necrosis.[24]

Hemorrhage

Small bowel intramural hemorrhage is a relatively uncommon cause of abdominal pain but is increasing in incidence in the United States due to an increasing number of patients requiring long-term anticoagulation therapy.[34] Many cases of adult small bowel intramural hemorrhage are associated with anticoagulation; these cases usually affect the jejunum. In contrast, traumatic small bowel intramural hemorrhage is seen most often in the duodenum given its fixed location near the spinal column and is more prevalent in children.[35] Duodenal intramural hemorrhage should raise suspicion for nonaccidental trauma if the clinical history is inconsistent with the diagnosis. Alternatively, vasculitis, pancreatitis, or hematologic disease may be the underlying etiology.[36]

Patients with small bowel intramural hemorrhage present with abdominal pain and vomiting. Because the bleeding is maintained within the bowel wall, gastrointestinal bleeding is not an expected presentation.[37] Blood loss often is not readily apparent on laboratory work-up, but there may be deficiency of clotting factors, such as factor VIII deficiency in the setting of hemophilia, or elevated international normalized ratio, which is usually a sign of supratherapeutic warfarin use. Lactate should not be elevated.

Certain CT imaging findings can help the radiologist discern between intramural hemorrhage and intestinal ischemia. Intramural hemorrhage often causes more pronounced bowel wall thickening but in a shorter segment of bowel than intestinal ischemia (**Fig. 10**). Hemoperitoneum is more likely to be detected in cases of intramural hemorrhage than in intestinal ischemia. Bowel wall enhancement pattern is nonspecific in intramural hemorrhage, with possibilities including increased homogenous enhancement, decreased homogeneous enhancement, and target sign.[38] Noncontrast CT images are helpful to confirm the intrinsic bowel wall hyperdensity in cases of hemorrhage.

Infections

Infectious enteritis can be caused by a wide variety of bacteria, viruses, fungi, and parasites. Patients present with vomiting and/or diarrhea, which may be bloody or nonbloody, crampy abdominal pain, and possible fever and leukocytosis. Symptom onset often is acute, and the patient may report ingestion of questionable food or sick contacts. Immunocompromised patients are at increased

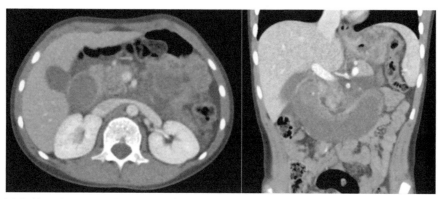

Fig. 10. Axial (*left*) and coronal reformatted (*right*) CT images demonstrating duodenal hematoma in a pediatric patient with Henoch-Schönlein purpura who presented with abdominal pain. The wall of the second, third, and fourth portions of the duodenum is markedly thickened with hypodense fluid. A few hyperdense foci in the wall of the second portion of the duodenum (*right*) are consistent with intramural active extravasation, which required coil embolization by interventional radiology.

risk for atypical infections. Definitive diagnosis requires stool sampling but may be elusive because many causative organisms, such as *Clostridium difficile*, in hospitalized patients cannot be identified on routine stool culture, which is generally considered a low-yield diagnostic test, especially in oncology patients.[39]

Infectious enteritis does not typically warrant radiologic work-up, but some patients may undergo imaging if the diagnosis is unclear. The bowel wall is thick with prominent small bowel folds or thickened colonic haustrations, and there may be bowel wall hyperemia (**Fig. 11**). *Shigella* and *Salmonella* are known to cause a target sign. Often, the bowel is mildly distended and fluid filled. Ileus may develop, but small bowel obstruction is atypical. The distribution of findings can suggest the causative organism: *Giardia*, *Strongyloides*, and *Mycobacterium avium-intracellulare* tend to involve the proximal small bowel; *Yersinia*, *Salmonella*, *Campylobacter*, *Shigella*, and *Anisakis* often affect the distal small bowel; and tuberculosis

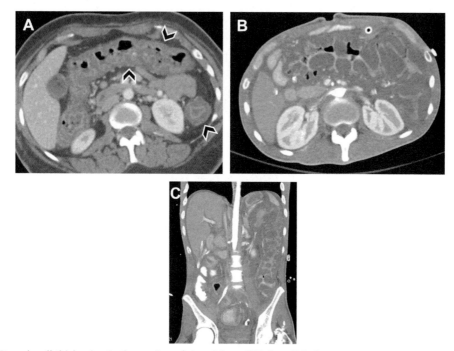

Fig. 11. Bowel wall thickening in the setting of clostridium difficile colitis demonstrating submucosal edema with mucosal hyperenhancement of the colon (*arrowheads* in *A*) in 2 different patients with (*A*) moderate and (*B, C*) severe involvement as shown on (*B*) axial and (*C*) coronal reformatted images.

and amebiasis preferentially involve the terminal ileum.[40] *Salmonella* and *Campylobacter* are the most common causative agents of infectious diarrhea in the United States, whereas *Clostridium difficile* colitis remains one of the most common hospital associated infections.[41,42] Approximately 60% of patients develop pancolitis with diffuse colonic wall thickening and mucosal hyperemia yielding an accordion sign on CT, with 40% developing right-sided colitis.[40] The degree of wall thickening usually is more severe with pseudomembranous colitis than with other etiologies. Neutropenic enteritis affects the right colon in more than half the patients and results in wall thickening with mucosal hyperemia or target sign.[43] Cytomegalovirus is another causative agent of pancolitis in immunocompromised patients.

Graft-Versus-Host Disease

Despite careful analysis prior to transplantation, 40% to 60% of recipients of HLA-identical grafts develop acute GVHD,[44] typically occurring within the first 100 days post–allogenic stem cell transplant (SCT). Chronic GVHD can develop de novo or can represent chronic progression of

acute GVHD.[45] Systemic steroids should be initiated but lead to remission in less than half of patients with acute GVHD.[46] The response to treatment in chronic GVHD is less predictable and can be confounded by infection and other comorbidities.[47]

Diagnosis of GVHD is not always clear on presentation, prompting imaging work-up in many of these patients. As with the aforementioned conditions, the CT findings may be nonspecific and should be evaluated with the clinical history in mind. In acute GVHD, acute inflammation results in mucosal enhancement and often a target sign, with marked bowel wall thickening resulting in luminal narrowing, involving diffusely the small bowel and, in most cases, the colon.[48,49] Bowel loops often are fluid filled due to secretory diarrhea.[49] Mesenteric lymphadenopathy typically is absent, but mesenteric edema is common (**Fig. 12**). The presence of hepatosplenomegaly, periportal edema, and biliary tract thickening and enhancement, in addition to the characteristic bowel findings, can provide further evidence for the diagnosis of GVHD in the appropriate clinical setting. Chronic GVHD, which usually presents within

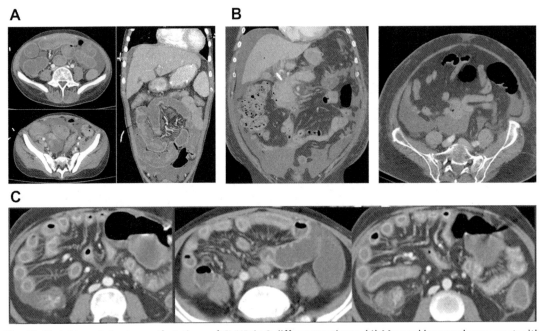

Fig. 12. Variable radiologic manifestations of GVHD in 3 different patients. (*A*) Mucosal hyperenhancement with dilated fluid-filled bowel loops in a patient with sickle cell disease status post-SCT 11 months prior, complicated by GVHD. There is a segmental area of thickening in the terminal ileum. High-density material in the lumen may represent hemorrhage. Mesenteric edema and ascites are present. (*B*) Mild diffuse small bowel wall thickening resulting in borderline narrow lumen in a patient with acute myeloid leukemia and chronic GVHD. A partially visualized biliary stent is present secondary to biliary stricture also caused by GVHD. (*C*) More classic and more pronounced radiologic appearance of GVHD with diffuse mucosal enhancement, mild bowel wall thickening, and narrow-lumen fluid-filled bowel loops.

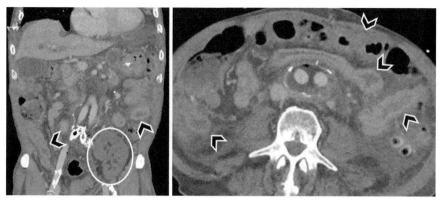

Fig. 13. Coronal reformatted (*left*) and axial (*right*) CT images demonstrate diffuse small and large bowel wall thickening (*arrowheads*) in a patient with hypoproteinemia status post–recent open revision of an abdominal aortic aneurysm and exclusion of renal transplant artery. The left renal transplant is nonenhancing (*circle*). The patient also has ascites and mesenteric edema. Collectively these findings are consistent with anasarca from acute renal failure.

3 years of SCT, has CT findings consistent with long-term bowel inflammation, including segmental strictures and thick mucosal hyperenhancement secondary to hyperemic granulation tissue. The hallmark finding of chronic GVHD is the ribbon bowel sign, which describes a long-segment tubular appearance due to small bowel fold effacement.[49]

Systemic Fluid Overload

Bowel wall edema can be seen with many of the entities described previously, but an important consideration, in the hospitalized patient, is secondary bowel wall thickening due to generalized fluid overload rather than a primary bowel pathology. Many conditions result in third spacing, including congestive heart failure, renal failure, cirrhosis, and hypoproteinemia.[50] Patients in fluid overload complain of shortness of breath, bloating, and diffuse subcutaneous swelling.

Bowel wall edema typically is evidenced by hypodense bowel wall thickening. This finding is seen throughout the entire bowel if edema is secondary to systemic fluid overload. Normal mucosal enhancement and the extent of involvement are important clues, in addition to other imaging findings of fluid overload, including pleural and pericardial effusions, ascites, and anasarca. More specific findings can suggest the primary process, such as cardiomegaly and dilated inferior vena cava and hepatic veins in patients with congestive heart failure, renal atrophy secondary to renal failure, and a shrunken and nodular liver in cases of cirrhosis (**Fig. 13**). Hypoproteinemia usually is encountered in malnourished populations, which in the developed world consist largely of oncologic patients. Nephrotic syndrome is a less common cause of hypoproteinemia and results from protein loss rather than poor intake. Medication-induced fluid overload, which can occur with certain chemotherapeutic

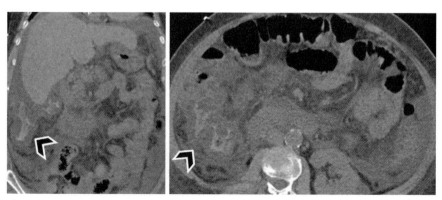

Fig. 14. Marked wall thickening of the hepatic flexure (*arrowheads*) on coronal reformatted (*left*) and axial (*right*) CT images, consistent with portal colopathy in this cirrhotic patient. Appearance was stable for 3 years.

agents,[51] could be considered if other causes of third-spacing are ruled out.

An important imaging distinction is appreciated in cases of portal colopathy, which preferentially affects the right colon instead of the entire bowel and results from portal hypertension, not generalized edema.[52] Portal colopathy could be mistaken for infectious or ischemic colitis if patient history is not considered (Fig. 14). It is important for the radiologist to synthesize imaging findings with clinical history and diagnose secondary bowel wall edema when the criteria are met rather than raise suspicion for a concurrent primary bowel condition.

SUMMARY

Bowel wall thickening in the hospitalized patient can be due to myriad etiologies. Familiarity with the most common causes and their differentiating imaging features, in addition to red flag findings that warrant prompt clinical attention, enables radiologists to provide unique value to clinical management.

REFERENCES

1. Collins JT, Badireddy M. Anatomy, abdomen and pelvis, small intestine. Treasure Island (FL): StatPearls; 2019.
2. Mitka M. GI fluoroscopy declining but still relevant. JAMA 2009;301(2):149.
3. Kilcoyne A, Kaplan JL, Gee MS. Inflammatory bowel disease imaging: current practice and future directions. World J Gastroenterol 2016;22(3):917–32.
4. ACR Manual on Contrast Media. Version 10.3.2018. Available at: https://www.acr.org/-/media/ACR/Files/Clinical-Resources/Contrast_Media.pdf. Accessed May 26, 2019.
5. ACR Appropriateness Criteria Acute Nonlocalized Abdominal Pain. Revised 2018. Available at: https://acsearch.acr.org/docs/69467/Narrative. Accessed May 26, 2019.
6. Hamlin DJ, Burgener FA. Positive and negative contrast agents in CT evaluation of the abdomen and pelvis. J Comput Tomogr 1981;5(2):82–90.
7. Harieaswar S, Rajesh A, Griffin Y, et al. Routine use of positive oral contrast material is not required for oncology patients undergoing follow-up multidetector CT. Radiology 2009;250(1):246–53.
8. Alabousi A, Patlas MN, Sne N, et al. Is oral contrast necessary for multidetector computed tomography imaging of patients with acute abdominal pain? Can Assoc Radiol J 2015;66(4):318–22.
9. Megibow AJ, Babb JS, Hecht EM, et al. Evaluation of bowel distention and bowel wall appearance by using neutral oral contrast agent for multi-detector row CT. Radiology 2006;238(1):87–95.
10. Yaghmai V, Brandwein W, Hammond N, et al. Comparison of water versus VoLumen in multislice CT evaluation of gastrointestinal distension and bowel wall detail in the same patient population. Radiological Society of North America 2006 Scientific Assembly and Annual Meeting. Chicago, IL, 2006, November 26 - December 1, 2006.
11. Berther R, Patak MA, Eckhardt B, et al. Comparison of neutral oral contrast versus positive oral contrast medium in abdominal multidetector CT. Eur Radiol 2008;18(9):1902–9.
12. Bae KT. Intravenous contrast medium administration and scan timing at CT: considerations and approaches. Radiology 2010;256(1):32–61.
13. Wittenberg J, Harisinghani MG, Jhaveri K, et al. Algorithmic approach to CT diagnosis of the abnormal bowel wall. Radiographics 2002;22(5):1093–107 [discussion: 1107–9].
14. Gore R, Smithuis R. Bowel wall thickening CT pattern. 2014. Available at: http://www.radiologyassistant.nl/. Accessed May 26, 2019.
15. Wiesner W, Mortele KJ, Ji H, et al. Normal colonic wall thickness at CT and its relation to colonic distension. J Comput Assist Tomogr 2002;26(1):102–6.
16. Finkelstone L, Wolf EL, Stein MW. Etiology of small bowel thickening on computed tomography. Can J Gastroenterol 2012;26(12):897–901.
17. Levine MS, Rubesin SE, Laufer I. Pattern approach for diseases of mesenteric small bowel on barium studies. Radiology 2008;249(2):445–60.
18. Ho LM, Paulson EK, Thompson WM. Pneumatosis intestinalis in the adult: benign to life-threatening causes. AJR Am J Roentgenol 2007;188(6):1604–13.
19. Ahualli J. The target sign: bowel wall. Radiology 2005;234(2):549–50.
20. Singal AK, Kamath PS, Tefferi A. Mesenteric venous thrombosis. Mayo Clin Proc 2013;88(3):285–94.
21. van den Heijkant TC, Aerts BA, Teijink JA, et al. Challenges in diagnosing mesenteric ischemia. World J Gastroenterol 2013;19(9):1338–41.
22. Dhatt HS, Behr SC, Miracle A, et al. Radiological evaluation of bowel ischemia. Radiol Clin North Am 2015;53(6):1241–54.
23. Oldenburg WA, Lau LL, Rodenberg TJ, et al. Acute mesenteric ischemia: a clinical review. Arch Intern Med 2004;164(10):1054–62.
24. Reginelli A, Genovese E, Cappabianca S, et al. Intestinal ischemia: US-CT findings correlations. Crit Ultrasound J 2013;5(Suppl 1):S7.
25. Sugi MD, Menias CO, Lubner MG, et al. CT findings of acute small-bowel entities. Radiographics 2018;38(5):1352–69.

26. Rha SE, Ha HK, Lee SH, et al. CT and MR imaging findings of bowel ischemia from various primary causes. Radiographics 2000;20(1):29–42.

27. Berritto D, Iacobellis F, Mazzei MA, et al. MDCT in ischaemic colitis: how to define the aetiology and acute, subacute and chronic phase of damage in the emergency setting. Br J Radiol 2016;89(1061): 20150821.

28. Balthazar EJ, Yen BC, Gordon RB. Ischemic colitis: CT evaluation of 54 cases. Radiology 1999;211(2): 381–8.

29. Kim JS, Kim HJ, Hong SM, et al. Post-ischemic bowel stricture: CT features in eight cases. Korean J Radiol 2017;18(6):936–45.

30. Eisenstat RS, Whitford AC, Lane MJ, et al. The "flat cava" sign revisited: what is its significance in patients without trauma? AJR Am J Roentgenol 2002; 178(1):21–5.

31. Chou CK. CT manifestations of bowel ischemia. AJR Am J Roentgenol 2002;178(1):87–91.

32. Lubner M, Demertzis J, Lee JY, et al. CT evaluation of shock viscera: a pictorial review. Emerg Radiol 2008;15(1):1–11.

33. Ames JT, Federle MP. CT hypotension complex (shock bowel) is not always due to traumatic hypovolemic shock. AJR Am J Roentgenol 2009;192(5): W230–5.

34. Abbas MA, Collins JM, Olden KW, et al. Spontaneous intramural small-bowel hematoma: clinical presentation and long-term outcome. Arch Surg 2002;137(3):306–10.

35. LeBedis CA, Anderson SW, Soto JA. CT imaging of blunt traumatic bowel and mesenteric injuries. Radiol Clin North Am 2012;50(1):123–36.

36. Yoldas T, Erol V, Caliskan C, et al. Spontaneous intestinal intramural hematoma: what to do and not to do. Ulus Cerrahi Derg 2013;29(2): 72–5.

37. Birns MT, Katon RM, Keller F. Intramural hematoma of the small intestine presenting with major upper gastrointestinal hemorrhage. Case report and review of the literature. Gastroenterology 1979;77(5): 1094–100.

38. Macari M, Chandarana H, Balthazar E, et al. Intestinal ischemia versus intramural hemorrhage: CT evaluation. AJR Am J Roentgenol 2003;180(1):177–84.

39. O'Connor O, Cooke RP, Cunliffe NA, et al. Clinical value of stool culture in paediatric oncology patients: hospital evaluation and UK survey of practice. J Hosp Infect 2017;95(1):123–5.

40. Childers BC, Cater SW, Horton KM, et al. CT evaluation of acute enteritis and colitis: is it infectious, inflammatory, or ischemic?: resident and fellow education feature. Radiographics 2015;35(7):1940–1.

41. LaRocque R, Harris J. Causes of acute infectious diarrhea and other foodborne illnesses in resource-rich settings. In: Calderwood SB, Bloom A, editors. Waltham (MA): UpToDate; 2019.

42. Kelly C, Lamont J, Bakken J. Clostridioides (formerly Clostridium) difficile infection in adults: treatment and prevention. In: Calderwood SB, Sullivan M, editors. Waltham (MA): UpToDate; 2019.

43. Vogel MN, Goeppert B, Maksimovic O, et al. CT features of neutropenic enterocolitis in adult patients with hematological diseases undergoing chemotherapy. Rofo 2010;182(12):1076–81.

44. Gooptu M, Koreth J. Better acute graft-versus-host disease outcomes for allogeneic transplant recipients in the modern era: a tacrolimus effect? Haematologica 2017;102(5):806–8.

45. Arai S, Arora M, Wang T, et al. Increasing incidence of chronic graft-versus-host disease in allogeneic transplantation: a report from the Center for International Blood and Marrow Transplant Research. Biol Blood Marrow Transplant 2015;21(2):266–74.

46. MacMillan ML, Weisdorf DJ, Wagner JE, et al. Response of 443 patients to steroids as primary therapy for acute graft-versus-host disease: comparison of grading systems. Biol Blood Marrow Transplant 2002;8(7):387–94.

47. Ferrara JL, Levine JE, Reddy P, et al. Graft-versus-host disease. Lancet 2009;373(9674):1550–61.

48. Haber HP, Schlegel PG, Dette S, et al. Intestinal acute graft-versus-host disease: findings on sonography. AJR Am J Roentgenol 2000;174(1):118–20.

49. Lubner MG, Menias CO, Agrons M, et al. Imaging of abdominal and pelvic manifestations of graft-versus-host disease after hematopoietic stem cell transplant. AJR Am J Roentgenol 2017;209(1):33–45.

50. Kattula S, Baradhi KM. Anasarca. Treasure Island (FL): StatPearls; 2019.

51. Torrisi JM, Schwartz LH, Gollub MJ, et al. CT findings of chemotherapy-induced toxicity: what radiologists need to know about the clinical and radiologic manifestations of chemotherapy toxicity. Radiology 2011;258(1):41–56.

52. Macari M, Balthazar EJ. CT of bowel wall thickening: significance and pitfalls of interpretation. AJR Am J Roentgenol 2001;176(5):1105–16.

Imaging of Gastrointestinal Tract Perforation

Donghoon Shin, MD, MS[a],*, Hamza Rahimi, MD[a], Samir Haroon, MD[a],
Alexander Merritt, MD[a], Abhinav Vemula, MD[b], Ansu Noronha, MD[b],
Christina A. LeBedis, MD, MS[a]

KEYWORDS

- Perforation • Ulcer • Pneumoperitoneum • Ischemia • Inflammatory bowel disease
- *Clostridioides difficile* • Appendicitis • Diverticulitis

KEY POINTS

- Gastrointestinal tract perforation in hospitalized patients can occur via variety of causes, including ulcers, trauma, ischemia, iatrogenic, neoplasms, infectious, and inflammatory processes.
- Most gastrointestinal tract perforations are surgical emergencies, but more recently initial conservative medical management has been advocated for clinically stable patients with contained perforation.
- Patient presentation can vary widely depending on the cause, site, and extent of injury, leading to a broad differential diagnosis. Radiologists play a critical role in narrowing down the diagnosis, which can govern medical decision making.
- There are several direct and indirect imaging findings of gastrointestinal perforation, which are seen to a varying degree depending on the cause of the perforation.
- Careful evaluation of the bowel wall enhancement pattern, length of the bowel involved, degree of the wall thickening, and the site of injury can provide important clues that can help identify the cause of the perforation.

INTRODUCTION

Gastrointestinal (GI) tract perforation involving the stomach, duodenum, small intestine, or the large bowel occurs as a result of full-thickness GI wall injury with release of intraluminal content into the peritoneal or retroperitoneal cavity. Injury can occur via variety of causes, including ulcers, trauma, ischemia, iatrogenic, neoplasms, and infectious and inflammatory processes. Clinical presentation consequently varies by the location, extent, and the cause of the injury and can range from subacute mild to acute severe abdominal pain with or without sepsis.[1–3] A patient's physiologic state can also affect the severity because immunosuppressed states, for example, can impair inflammatory response and increase the risk of free perforation.[3,4] The incidences and risk factors for GI perforation from different causes are discussed later.

Given the wide range of different causes and clinical presentations, thorough history, physical examination, and laboratory findings can provide important clues that raise clinical suspicion for specific causes. Often, imaging studies, such as computed tomography (CT), are necessary for

Disclosure: The authors have nothing to disclose.
[a] Department of Radiology, Boston University Medical Center, 715 Albany Street, FGH-3007, Boston, MA 02118, USA; [b] Section of Gastroenterology, Department of Medicine, Boston University Medical Center, 650 Albany Street, Boston, MA 02118, USA
* Corresponding author. Department of Radiology, Boston University Medical Center, Boston University School of Medicine, 820 Harrison Avenue, FGH Building, 3rd Floor, Boston, MA 02118.
E-mail address: donghoon.shin@bmc.org

Radiol Clin N Am 58 (2020) 19–44
https://doi.org/10.1016/j.rcl.2019.08.004

proper evaluation because many patients with GI perforation require emergent surgery.[2,3] These cases are associated with high mortality (30%–50%) and require routine use of broad-spectrum antibiotics and aggressive resuscitative measures.[2,4] More recently, some clinicians have advocated initial conservative management in clinically stable patients with contained perforations.[5–7] Therefore, it is important for radiologists to recognize and identify the underlying cause and adequately describe the extent of the injury because these can affect management decisions.[2,8] This article reviews different imaging modalities and findings that may affect management options of GI perforations from various causes.

RELEVANT ANATOMY

Although the esophagus is a part of the GI tract, this article focuses on intraperitoneal and retroperitoneal structures. Retroperitoneal structures include the second, third, and fourth duodenal segments, and the ascending and descending colon. The stomach, first segment of the duodenum, ileum, jejunum, cecum, transverse colon, and the sigmoid colon are intraperitoneal structures. The upper two-thirds of the rectum are intraperitoneal, whereas the remainder is extraperitoneal. Thus, the location of leaked intraluminal content (intraperitoneal vs retroperitoneal) can help localize the perforation site.

Some disorders preferentially affect specific parts of the GI tract. For example, the transition points between the peritoneum and the retroperitoneum along the GI tract tend to be fixed by ligaments and are prone to shear injuries in trauma. Additional disorders associated with different sites are summarized in **Table 1**.

Throughout the GI tract, the intraluminal content also varies, which can affect patient presentation. For example, perforation of the stomach, duodenum, or the large bowel may be accompanied by abundant extraluminal air and a variable amount of fluid. Small bowel perforations are generally associated with a paucity of extraluminal air with a larger amount of fluid, except in the presence of obstruction.

Regarding vascular anatomy, the stomach receives arterial supply from the branches of the celiac trunk. The duodenum receives arterial supply from both the celiac and the superior mesenteric artery (SMA) branches. The SMA also supplies the jejunum and the ileum. The ascending and transverse colon, for the most part, receive arterial supply from the SMA branches, whereas the descending and the sigmoid colon are

Table 1 Differential diagnosis by perforation site	
Site	Differential Diagnosis
Stomach/ duodenum	Peptic ulcer disease Necrotic/ulcerated malignancies Iatrogenic (eg, marginal ulcers, biopsy/endoscopy complication) Ingested foreign body Blunt trauma
Small intestine	Small bowel obstruction Ischemia Crohn disease Iatrogenic (eg, intraoperative) Penetrating trauma Malignancy Chemotherapy/radiation therapy Ingested foreign body Gallstone/enteroliths Infectious (typhoid/ tuberculosis/schistosomiasis)
Large intestine	Appendicitis (right) Diverticulitis (left)[a] Ischemia Inflammatory bowel disease Malignancy Iatrogenic (eg, colonoscopy complication) Trauma

[a] Can be right sided in Asian populations.

supplied by the inferior mesenteric artery (IMA). Note that the marginal artery of Drummond provides important collateral flow between the SMA and the IMA for the colon. However, at the splenic flexure, the anastomoses between the 2 vascular territories are weak or absent and constitute a watershed area prone to ischemia or infarction.

COMMON IMAGING PROTOCOL AND FINDINGS
Radiograph

Clinical presentation of GI perforation can be nonspecific. Plain radiographs are quick, inexpensive, and can help evaluate for different causes of abdominal pain, including pneumoperitoneum, which suggests GI perforation. The sensitivity of upright chest or abdomen and the lateral decubitus radiograph for large pneumoperitoneum is 50% to 90%.[9,10] Supine abdominal radiographs have lower sensitivity, but some patients only tolerate this position. On upright radiographs, pneumoperitoneum is most commonly seen as a crescentic lucency under the diaphragm (**Fig. 1**A). Other

A   **B**

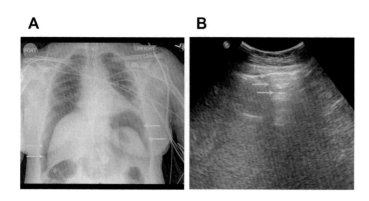

Fig. 1. Pneumoperitoneum on radiograph and ultrasonography (US). A 72-year-old woman after colonoscopy complicated by perforation. Upright chest radiograph (A) showed a large amount of free air under the diaphragm (*yellow arrows*). US (B) of the same patient showed echogenic reflectors with reverberation artifact (*yellow arrows*) not localized to the intraluminal space, consistent with known pneumoperitoneum.

radiographic signs of pneumoperitoneum are described in **Table 2**. Pneumoretroperitoneum can be seen as air outlining the borders of the kidneys or the iliopsoas muscle.

Shortcomings of radiographs include its inability to accurately localize the injury site and low sensitivity for small amounts of air. In addition, false-positive findings can be seen with extension of air from other injury sites, such as the lungs, mediastinum, and the genitourinary system.

Computed Tomography

CT of the abdomen and pelvis is the primary imaging study for evaluating GI perforation because it

Table 2
Radiographic signs of pneumoperitoneum

Finding/Sign	View	Description
Subdiaphragmatic free gas	Upright	Diaphragm outlined by the lung superiorly and by free intraperitoneal air inferiorly
Double bubble sign	Upright	Normal gas in the gastric fundus under the subdiaphragmatic free air
Decubitus abdomen sign	Lateral decubitus	Abdominal wall outlined by air
Rigler sign (double wall sign) (Fig. 2A, B)	Any	Bowel wall outlined by luminal and extraluminal air
Cupola sign	Supine	Lateral borders of the thoracic vertebral bodies projecting below the diaphragm outlined by the intraperitoneal air accumulating under the central tendon of the diaphragm
Lucent liver sign	Supine	Liver appears more radiolucent more medially because the free air collects in the anterior abdomen above the liver
Hepatic edge sign	Supine	Cigar-shaped pocket of air seen under the liver in the right upper quadrant
Doge cap sign	Supine	Triangular lucency in the right upper quadrant as the air collects in the Morison pouch
Football sign	Supine, pediatric	Abdominal wall outlined by air
Telltale triangle sign	Supine	Lucent triangle of air outlined by loops of bowel and abdominal wall
Falciform ligament sign (silver sign)	Supine	Falciform ligament outlined by air
Lateral umbilical ligament sign (inverted V sign)	Supine	Lateral umbilical ligaments outlined by air seen as a line coursing inferolaterally from the umbilicus in the pelvis
Urachus sign	Supine	Median umbilical ligament outlined by air seen as a midline vertical line in the pelvis

Table 3
Common computed tomography protocols by cause

Protocol	Ulcer	Blunt Trauma	Penetrating Trauma	Ischemia	Iatrogenic	Neoplasm	Infection or Inflammatory
CT without contrast	May be appropriate	May be appropriate	May be appropriate	Usually appropriate	May be appropriate	May be appropriate	Not routinely obtained
CT with IV contrast (arterial)*	Not routinely obtained	Usually appropriate	Usually appropriate	Usually appropriate	Usually appropriate	Not routinely obtained	Not routinely obtained
CT with IV contrast (PV)ˆ	Usually appropriate	Usually appropriate	Usually appropriate	Usually appropriate	Usually appropriate	Usually appropriate	Usually appropriate
CT with IV contrast (delayed)˘	Not routinely obtained	May be appropriate	May be appropriate	Not routinely obtained	May be appropriate	Not routinely obtained	Not routinely obtained
CT with IV and PO contrast	Not routinely obtained	Not routinely obtained	May be appropriate	May be appropriate	May be appropriate	Not routinely obtained	Not routinely obtained

* Usually in the late arterial phase about 30 seconds after IV contrast injection
ˆ Portal venous phase about 70-80 seconds after IV contrast injection
˘ 5-10 minutes after IV contrast injection

has the highest diagnostic yield, with an 82% to 90% accuracy.[11,12] However, because most patients present with nonspecific complaints and physical examination, the initial evaluation often involves CT of the abdomen and pelvis with intravenous (IV) contrast in the portal venous phase (PV). If there is suspicion for a more specific cause for the patient's presentation, a more focused CT protocol can be pursued (Table 3).

In general, the entire abdomen and pelvis from the dome of the diaphragm to the pelvic floor are imaged with contiguous axial sections (1.25–5 mm). Multiplanar reformats are helpful in localizing and troubleshooting equivocal findings

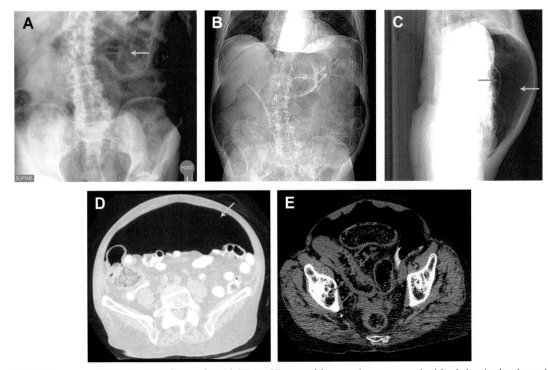

Fig. 2. Pneumoperitoneum on radiograph and CT. An 87-year-old man who presented with abdominal pain and distention. On initial kidney-ureter-bladder radiograph (A), dilated small bowel loops in the left upper quadrant with free air outlining both sides of the bowel wall (*yellow and red arrows*) are seen, consistent with a Rigler sign. The Rigler sign is seen again on the scout images from the CT (B, C). On axial CT, extensive pneumoperitoneum (D, *yellow arrow*) is seen. Diffuse thickening of the sigmoid (E, *red arrows*) with possible pneumatosis is also noted.

on axial images. Although not necessary to detect pneumoperitoneum, IV contrast is almost always helpful because it increases the diagnostic accuracy for other CT findings.[13,14] Patients with equivocal CT findings who are amenable to clinical monitoring may benefit from a repeat CT scan at a later time point (**Fig. 3**). Dual energy CT may help in the detection of abnormally enhancing lesions or bowel wall by increasing the conspicuity of the iodine. Dual energy CT can also increase radiologists' confidence in findings given the availability of iodine maps, spectral curves, iodine quantification, and virtual noncontrast images[10,15,16] (**Fig. 4**).

When GI perforation is suspected, water-soluble oral contrast agent is recommended because barium can cause inflammation and granulomas in the peritoneum. The use of oral or rectal contrast in the acute setting has fallen out of favor in the past decade, because several studies have shown no significant added diagnostic value and that it potentially delays diagnosis and management.[11,12,17,18] The use of oral contrast also exposes patients to aspiration risk.[11,12,17,18]

There are several direct and indirect signs of GI perforation on CT, with varying sensitivities and specificities depending on the cause; **Table 4** summarizes CT findings of bowel and mesenteric injury for trauma as an example.

Because GI perforation requires a full-thickness wall injury, the most direct finding for perforation is bowel wall discontinuity.[19,20] Wall discontinuity may be seen as a low attenuating cleft that is oriented perpendicular to the bowel wall[11] (**Fig. 5B**). However, wall discontinuity is not always detected because the injury site may be small or seal

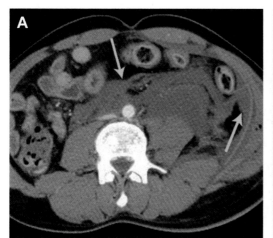
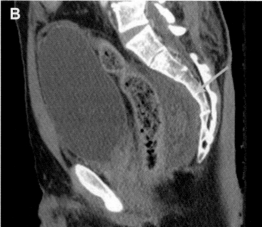
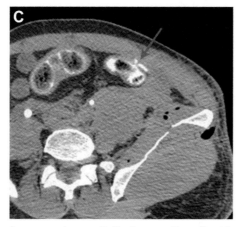

Fig. 3. The value of second look on repeat scans. Patient presenting after blunt trauma was found to have free fluid and pelvic fracture on CT. Initial axial (*A*) and sagittal (*B*) CT show free fluid (*yellow arrows*) without definite evidence of bowel perforation. Repeat imaging at a later time point with oral contrast (*C*) shows extraluminal contrast, consistent with bowel perforation (*red arrow*).

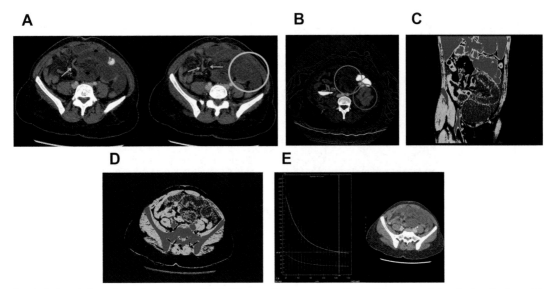

Fig. 4. Ischemic bowel on dual energy CT. A 32-year-old man presenting with acute abdominal pain found to have closed loop small bowel obstruction with ischemia. On axial images of contrast-enhanced CT (CECT) (*A*), 2 adjacent transition points are marked by yellow arrows, along with hypoenhancing dilated loops of small bowel in the left hemiabdomen (*yellow circle*). Axial iodine map (*B*) shows more clearly that the dilated loops of bowel are not enhancing (*blue circle*) compared with normal bowel loops (*red circle*). Coronal and axial Z-effective maps (*C, D*) also show the ischemic small bowel loops in blue compared with adjacent normally enhancing structures. Spectral hounsfield unit (HU) curves (*E*) can be used to assess enhancing pattern, with the blue curve showing the spectral HU of normally enhancing bowel versus yellow curve representing the ischemic small bowel.

spontaneously. Extraluminal oral contrast or air is also highly specific for perforation, with near-100% specificity[19] (**Fig.** 2D; see **Fig.** 3C). Often, the specific site of perforation can be identified by tracking the air bubbles or the extraluminal oral contrast.[11,12]

On supine patients, free air collects antidependently, often found in the anterior abdomen or under the diaphragm. Bone or lung windows can also help increase the conspicuity of air in the abdomen. However, these direct findings tend to have low sensitivity and are seen in less than 55% of these cases.[11,12,19,21,22]

Therefore, the diagnosis of GI perforation often depends on recognizing indirect signs that are more sensitive but less specific. These signs include bowel wall thickening, abnormal wall enhancement patterns, mesenteric fat infiltration, and presence of free fluid. Bowel wall thickening can be caused by edema, hemorrhage, or inflammation, and it is generally defined as wall thickness greater than 3 mm or disproportionately thickened wall compared with adjacent normal bowel[19,23,24] (**Fig.** 2E). Abnormal bowel wall enhancement includes increased and decreased/ absent enhancement compared with the background bowel loops[20,21,25–27] (**Figs.** 6 and 7). Mesenteric infiltration (fat stranding) is characterized by increased attenuation and a hazy appearance of the mesentery caused by edema and hyperemia. These findings are often helpful in identifying the injured segment of the bowel. Although sensitive for bowel injury, free peritoneal fluid does not differentiate acute versus chronic

Table 4
Sensitivity and specificity of computed tomography for bowel and mesenteric injury in trauma

CT Sign	Sensitivity (%)	Specificity (%)
Bowel wall discontinuity	5–34	100
Extraluminal air	20–30	95–99
Abnormal bowel wall enhancement	8–15	90
Focal bowel wall thickening	18–55	76–97
Free intraperitoneal fluid	90–100	15–26
Mesenteric infiltration	55–77	40–90
Extravasation from mesenteric vessel	17–36	99–100

Data from Refs.[20–27,35,39,120]

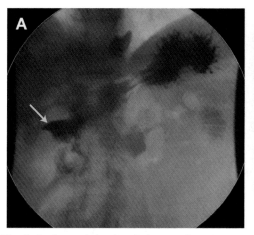
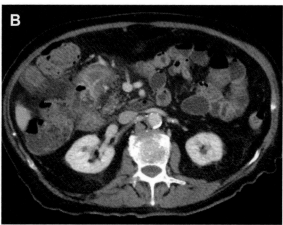

Fig. 5. Perforated duodenal ulcer on fluoroscopy and CT. An 83-year-old man presenting with abdominal pain. On the upper GI study (A), an area of contrast outpouching from the second portion of the duodenum was noted (*yellow arrow*), which remained fixed in morphology throughout the study. On CT (B), there was an air and fluid collection (*red arrow*) adjacent to the duodenum and duodenal wall discontinuity, consistent with perforated duodenal ulcer (*red circle*).

or severe versus mild injuries and can also be a normal physiologic finding.[28] However, attention to the amount of free fluid and its attenuation can be helpful in its assessment.

Mastery of the direct and indirect findings of bowel and mesenteric injury is imperative because a delay in diagnosis portends worse patient outcome. These signs of perforation in combination with the CT findings associated with specific causes, discussed individually later, are crucial in arriving at the correct diagnosis.

Sonography

Ultrasonography (US) is a fast and cost-effective imaging modality that can provide real-time dynamic information that does not use ionizing radiation.[29] It can help provide definitive diagnosis or narrow the differential diagnosis in variety of abdominal disorders.[29]

Pneumoperitoneum can be seen as echogenic reflectors with reverberation artifact that is not localized to the intraluminal space and changes with patient movement[1,29] (Fig. 1B). Reported sensitivity and specificity of US for pneumoperitoneum range from 68% to 96% depending on the operator experience.[29] Localization of perforation is often difficult. However, in certain cases the underlying causes, such as appendicitis, may be found.[29] Patient body habitus, variability of bowel position, and dirty shadowing from intraluminal gas can confound the evaluation of GI perforation on US.

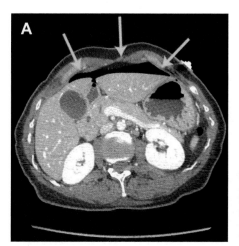
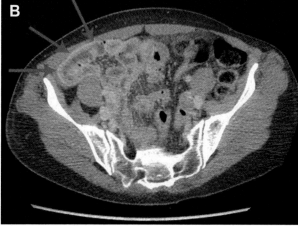

Fig. 6. Hyperenhancing bowel wall on CT. A 52-year-old woman after blunt trauma found to have pneumoperitoneum (A, *yellow arrows*) and a segment of small bowel with bowel wall thickening and mucosal hyperenhancement, suggestive of the site of injury (B, *red arrows*).

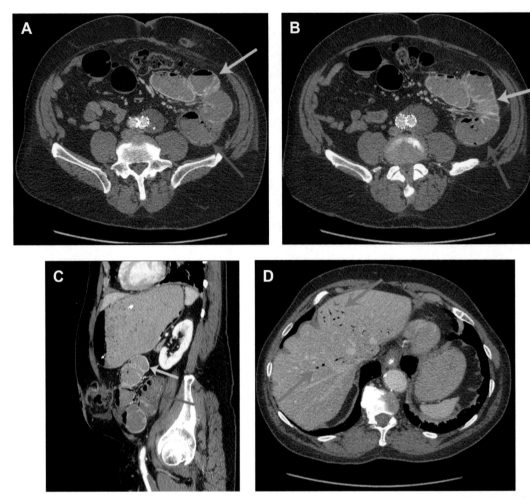

Fig. 7. Small bowel obstruction with ischemic bowel on CT. A 71-year-old man with history of abdominal surgeries who presents with nausea and vomiting found to have an ischemic segment of small bowel shown on CT (*A–C*) as hypoenhancing bowel wall (*red arrows*) compared with normally enhancing adjacent small bowel (*yellow arrows*). Portal venous gas is also found on this patient (*D, blue arrows*).

Acute bowel wall injury on US may be shown by bowel wall thickening, which can be seen as concentric prominence of the bowel wall layers causing targetoid appearance. Reactive inflammatory changes in the surrounding mesenteric fat can also be appreciated as increased echogenicity of the fat as well as free fluid in the peritoneum. Inflamed edematous bowel may be seen as hypoechoic muscularis propria on gray-scale images. Mesenteric or bowel wall hyperemia can be appreciated on Doppler images[29](**Fig. 8**).

ULCERS
Overview

Peptic ulcer disease (PUD) is a common condition with a lifetime prevalence of 5% to 10%, accounting for nearly 150,000 hospitalization in the United States annually.[30] It is most often caused by *Helicobacter pylori* infection or nonsteroidal antiinflammatory drug (NSAID) use, although other less common causes exist.[31,32] *H pylori* causes mucosal injury by bacterial factors in combination with the host's inflammatory response. NSAIDs cause mucosal injury by disrupting cyclooxygenase (COX)-1–derived prostaglandins, which are important in the maintenance of mucosal integrity.[5] This mucosal injury exposes the epithelium to gastric acid, leading to ulceration and extension into the submucosal layers.[5] However, up to70% of the patients with PUD are asymptomatic.[5,30] Symptomatic patients report nonspecific complaints of mild dyspepsia that can be associated with food intake.[5] Common complications of PUD include GI bleeding,

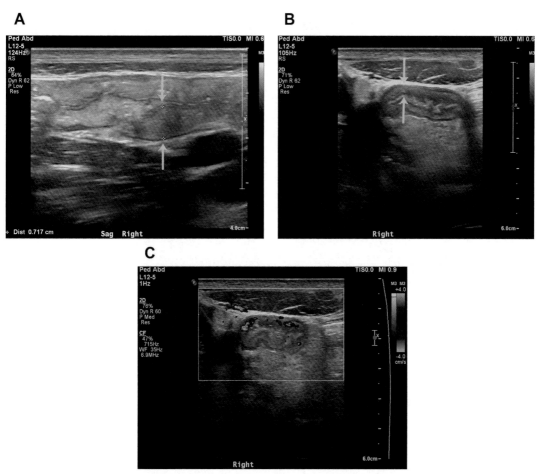

Fig. 8. Active Crohn disease on US. A 16-year-old boy with a history of active Crohn disease presenting with abdominal pain. On the gray-scale US, both longitudinal (*A*) and transverse (*B*) views show marked terminal ileal wall thickening (*yellow arrows*). On color Doppler US (*C*), the terminal ileum shows hyperemia.

perforation, and gastric outlet obstruction. Those patients who are smokers, consume alcohol, and are older than 60 years of age are more likely to have PUD complications.[5]

Perforation occurs in 2% to 10% of patients with PUD, with an incidence of 4 to 14 per 100,000.[5,30,31] It is one of the most serious complications, with a high mortality (24%–30%).[6] Patients with perforated peptic ulcers may complain of sudden-onset severe epigastric pain that may lessen after couple of hours, but becomes generalized over time, often leading to guarding and rigid abdomen. Associated GI bleeding is common, as are shock and sepsis.[6] Treatment of perforated peptic ulcer is most often surgical repair, which can involve peritoneal lavage, suture closure, and omental patch, along with nasogastric tube placement, IV proton pump inhibitors, and broad-spectrum antibiotics.[5,6] However, in certain patients who are stable, initial conservative medical management may be pursued, especially if there is evidence of spontaneous sealing or contained perforation.[5–7] Thus, it is imperative for radiologists to identify and characterize imaging findings that may lead to differential management of patients presenting with perforated ulcers.

Imaging Findings

Upper endoscopy is the study of choice for diagnosing PUD owing to its high sensitivity (>90%) and ability to biopsy suspicious lesions[5] (**Fig. 9**). Fluoroscopic examinations such as upper GI series have fallen out of favor because of their inferior sensitivity and the availability of endoscopy in many institutions. Ulcers on fluoroscopic studies (**Fig. 5**A) with oral contrast agent show a round or oval pocket of contrast surrounded by the smooth mound of edema and gastric folds radiating away from the ulcer.[33] Sometimes, the Hampton line, a radiolucent line separating the

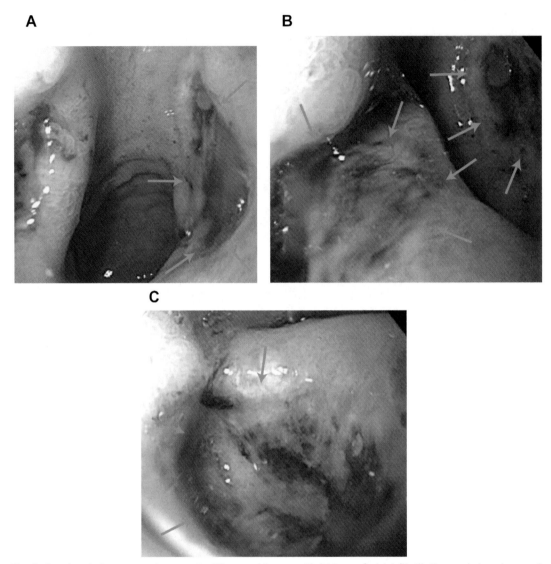

Fig. 9. Duodenal ulcers on endoscopy. An 86-year-old man with history of atrial fibrillation and chronic anemia found to have acute upper GI bleeding after starting warfarin for atrial fibrillation. Endoscopic images show 2 deeply cratered, almost confluent duodenal ulcers with stigmata of recent bleeding (*blue arrows*).

oral contrast in the gastric lumen from the contrast in the ulcer crater, can be seen.[33]

If the initial radiograph or US is unrevealing, CT is the imaging study with the highest yield when perforation is suspected. CT has low sensitivity for detecting uncomplicated mucosal ulcerations, less than 20%.[34] CT rarely shows the ulcer as an outpouching along the gastric or duodenal wall, but more commonly shows indirect signs such as focal wall thickening and local mesenteric fat infiltration. In contrast, CT is exquisitely sensitive for evaluating for pneumoperitoneum and can effectively evaluate for complications of PUD.[34] Note that ulcers on the posterior wall of the stomach are more likely to be associated with

contained perforation because of close proximity of the adjacent soft tissues.[34] Patients with remote abdominal surgeries are also more likely to have contained perforation because of formation of fibrous adhesions from prior surgery.[34]

TRAUMA
Overview

Traumatic injuries to the bowel and mesentery are uncommon, occurring in approximately 1% to 5% and 17% of patients with blunt and penetrating trauma, respectively.[18,20,35,36] Clinical evaluation of patients with trauma can be confounded by concomitant head trauma, intoxication, or distracting injuries, which render the history and physical examination unreliable. Therefore, detecting the presence of bowel and mesenteric injury on CT remains a critical task for radiologists because delays in diagnosis as short as 6 to 8 hours can cause increased morbidity and mortality because of bowel ischemia or necrosis.[36] Most bowel injuries become clinically evident within 72 hours, manifesting with any combination of fever, tachycardia, leukocytosis, abdominal pain, or sepsis.

Three mechanisms have been proposed in the setting of blunt bowel and mesenteric injury: shear, crush, and burst.[35] Shear injuries are caused by differential deceleration at sites of fixation, such as the ligament of Treitz or the ileocecal valve. Crush injuries result from compression of the mesentery or bowel between the abdominal wall and a fixed structure such as the spine. Burst injuries are caused by sudden increases in luminal pressures, often in the setting of abnormal underlying bowel such as ileus, obstruction, or inflammatory bowel disease. In penetrating trauma, it is imperative to follow the track of the penetrating object using multiplanar CT reformations to detect injuries and to assess whether there has been peritoneal violation. Importantly, stab wound tracks are typically narrow, whereas gunshot wounds have a broader trajectory caused by the transmission of shock waves.[37]

Imaging Findings

Although radiographs and US are often used to quickly screen for disorders that may suggest the patient requires urgent surgical interventions, CT is the primary imaging modality for trauma evaluation, with the highest diagnostic yield.

In penetrating trauma, pneumoperitoneum or pneumoretroperitoneum can be an expected finding and is not useful in the detection of GI perforation. It is also important to keep in mind that there can be pseudopneumoperitoneum from chest sources, interventions, or even bladder rupture with Foley catheter placement[38] (Fig. 10). Thus, the GI tract should be carefully evaluated for other signs of bowel injury, such as abnormal thickness, enhancement, or discontinuity of the bowel wall. The presence of free fluid in a patient with trauma without solid organ injury is concerning for bowel and mesenteric injury, with reported specificity of 15% to 26% and sensitivity of 90% to 100%.[20–22,26,35] Extravasation of IV contrast material indicates active mesenteric vessel bleeding, which typically warrants urgent intervention[39] (Fig. 11). These mesenteric injuries place the associated bowel at risk for ischemia, necrosis, and perforation. Bowel wall injury from trauma is usually focal, whereas diffuse bowel wall thickening (>10 mm) can be seen in shock bowel (Fig. 12). Additional injuries associated with bowel

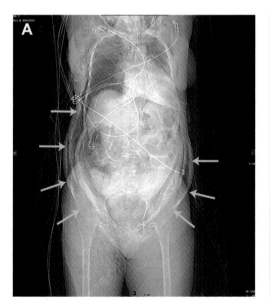 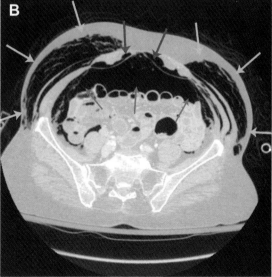

Fig. 10. Pseudopneumoperitoneum and pneumoperitoneum on CT. A 40-year-old woman after blunt trauma. Subcutaneous emphysema tracks along the subcutaneous tissue overlying the anterior abdominal wall can mimic pneumoperitoneum on radiograph, as shown on the scout image (*A, yellow arrows*). There is also soft tissue air tracking just external to the peritoneal lining on axial CT (*B, red arrows*), consistent with pseudopneumoperitoneum. True pneumoperitoneum is concurrently seen in this patient as shown by air beneath the peritoneal lining and outside the bowel (*B, blue arrows*).

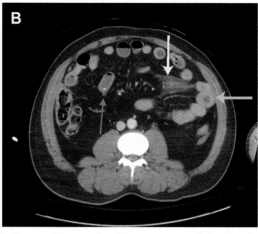
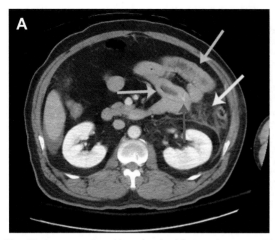

Fig. 11. Intramural and intraluminal hemorrhage on CT. A 43-year-old man after blunt trauma. Axial CT images show small bowel wall thickening (*A, B, yellow arrows*) with intramural hemorrhage (*A, red arrow*) as well as intraluminal hemorrhage (*B, blue arrow*). Mesenteric fat stranding is marked by white arrows.

and mesenteric injury include the so-called seatbelt sign, anterior and lateral traumatic hernias, Chance fractures, multiple abdominal visceral injuries, and pancreatic injuries.[21,27,40,41]

ISCHEMIA

Bowel ischemia is a life-threatening emergency that accounts for approximately 1% of patients presenting with acute abdomen.[42,43] Early recognition and intervention are essential for favorable clinical outcome because mortalities can be as high as 50% to 90% depending on the extent and duration of the insult.[43–45] Intestinal ischemia can be divided into 3 broad categories by cause: arterial, venous, and nonocclusive. Arterial thrombosis or embolization accounts for 60% to 70% of acute bowel ischemia, whereas

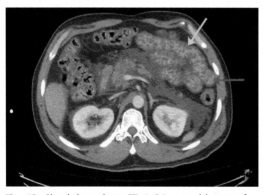

Fig. 12. Shock bowel on CT. A 24-year-old man after blunt trauma found to have shock bowel with bowel wall thickening characterized by submucosal edema (*yellow arrow*) and hyperenhancing mucosa (*red arrow*).

venous thrombosis and nonocclusive causes account for 5% to 10% and 20% to 30%, respectively.[15,46–49]

Mesenteric artery occlusion is most frequently caused by an acute cardioembolic event (40%–50%), but can also be caused by atherosclerosis, aortic/mesenteric artery dissection, cholesterol embolization, iatrogenic events (eg, aortic stenting), trauma, malignant invasion, or vasculitis.[15,46,47,49,50] The SMA is preferentially affected by emboli because of its acute take-off angle.[44,47] Note that some proximal occlusions are well compensated by collateral flow.[46]

Mesenteric venous occlusion can result from bowel strangulation (closed loop obstruction, volvulus), malignant infiltration, external compression, inflammatory/infectious, hypercoagulable state, or vasculitis.[15,44,47] In stercoral colitis, ischemic ulceration and perforation can also occur because of increased intraluminal wall pressure from impacted stool (**Fig. 13**). Nonocclusive mesenteric ischemia can result from a variety of conditions, including hypovolemic shock, severe heart failure, medications (eg, antihypertensives), and drugs (cocaine, heroin).[44,47,50]

In early stages of ischemia, the most common presenting symptom is abdominal pain out of proportion to physical examination, along with other nonspecific symptoms, such as nausea, vomiting, diarrhea, and tachycardia. Sometimes, the abdominal pain can be associated with GI bleeding, prompting endoscopic evaluation (**Fig. 14**). Because of the nonspecific physical examination and laboratory findings, CT imaging remains the primary imaging modality for the detection of bowel ischemia.[47]

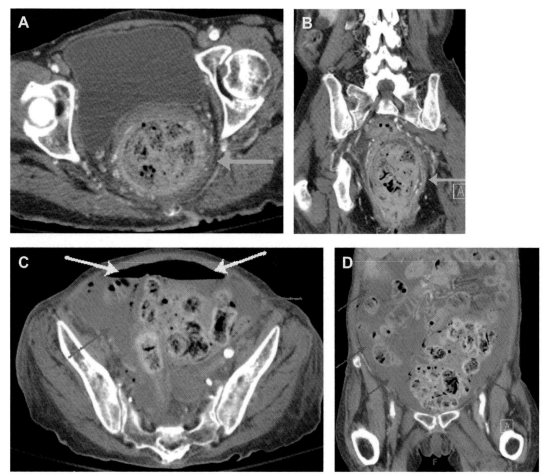

Fig. 13. Perforated stercoral colitis. Axial and coronal CT images show distended rectosigmoid colon with fecal impaction along with surrounding fat stranding (*A, B, yellow arrows*) consistent with stercoral colitis. Axial and coronal CT images obtained 1 week later show evidence of perforation with free air and free fecal material in the peritoneum (*C, D, white and blue arrows*).

Imaging Findings

GI perforation is more common in arterial occlusions. On unenhanced CT, the burden of atherosclerotic disease can be appreciated and hemorrhagic infarction can be seen as hyperattenuating bowel.[15,47,50] On contrast-enhanced CT (CECT), the absence of bowel wall enhancement is the most specific finding of ischemia.[50,51] Filling defects in mesenteric arteries or veins on CECT are also specific for embolic or thrombotic lesions (**Fig. 15**). Pneumatosis intestinalis is associated with bowel ischemia in only about 30% of cases[51] and can be seen in a variety of nonischemic conditions, including infection, asthma, malignancy, or inflammatory bowel disease.[46] In addition, pneumatosis intestinalis needs to be distinguished from pneumatosis cystoides intestinalis, a rare benign condition characterized by multiple gasfilled cysts in the intestinal wall[15,46,51] (**Fig. 16**).

IATROGENIC
Overview

Iatrogenic complications are adverse events that occur from diagnostic or therapeutic procedures. Although advances in medical procedures and surgeries have improved patient outcomes, their increasing availability has contributed to the concurrent increase in the number of iatrogenic complications, which contribute up to 36% of admissions.[52,53] Iatrogenic bowel complications can be broadly categorized by the mechanism of injury: penetrating, burst, and anastomotic leak.

Penetrating iatrogenic injuries are commonly caused by instrumentation. For example, during colectomy, the prevalence of intraoperative complications is approximately 5.4%, with the most common complication being bleeding, followed by bowel injuries, including bowel perforation.[54] Hysterectomy   and   other   obstetric   and

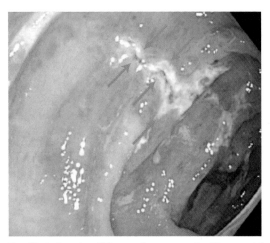

Fig. 14. Ischemic colitis on colonoscopy. An 82-year-old woman with history of diabetes, hypertension, and diverticulosis who presented with acute-onset lower GI bleeding. Colonoscopy revealed diffuse erythema and friability of the mucosa consistent with moderate to severe inflammation and serpentine ulceration (*blue arrows*) in the descending and sigmoid colon.

gynecologic surgeries are most commonly associated with genitourinary tract injuries, but injury to the GI tract can occur.[55,56] During paracentesis or laparoscopic surgeries, penetrating injury from the needle or the trocar while gaining access to the peritoneum can also occur as a rare complication.

Burst iatrogenic injury, such as colonic perforation during colonoscopy, is a rare but morbid complication with prevalence ranging from 0.03% to 0.3%. The risk is almost 2 times higher in cases in which biopsies are performed.[57,58] Other risk factors include dilation of Crohn stricture, age more than 75 years, and previous surgery.[58,59]

Anastomotic leaks are dreaded postoperative complications seen in intra-abdominal surgeries such as colectomy and gastric bypass (**Figs. 17 and 18**). These leaks are associated with more severe postoperative complications and higher rates of reoperations and mortality, with 30-day mortality nearly 3 times that without anastomotic leaks.[60,61] For example, the prevalence of anastomotic leak in colectomy ranges from 2.9% to 15.3%.[54,61,62]

The examples described earlier are just a few of the iatrogenic injuries that can lead to GI tract injuries. Clinical suspicion and patient history can help radiologists in determining whether an iatrogenic injury exists.

Imaging Findings

The detection of GI perforation on CT during the perioperative period may be confounded by expected postoperative changes, such as pneumoperitoneum, intra-abdominal free fluid, fat stranding, and bowel wall thickening. Bowel wall discontinuity is diagnostic when seen, but it is not sensitive.[11] Therefore, in postsurgical cases, if anastomotic leak or GI perforation is suspected, CT studies can be performed with intraluminal, water-soluble contrast because extraluminal oral or rectal contrast indicates a leak.[63] Also, different procedures preferentially involve the parts of the GI tract in close proximity to the surgical sites and can aid in localization of the injury site. For example, hysterectomy and colonoscopy are associated with injuries involving the sigmoid and rectum,[55,56] whereas laparoscopic procedures are more frequently associated with small bowel injuries.

NEOPLASM
Overview

GI perforation is a common bowel related emergency in patients with cancer, along with obstruction, ischemia, and intussusception.[64] Perforation of the colon is a presenting feature in 1.2% to 10% of colorectal cancers[65,66] and is associated with older age (>65 years old) and more advanced stages of the cancer.[65–68] Patients presenting with perforations also have higher mortality, increased local recurrence rate, and risk of peritoneal carcinomatosis.[65,69,70]

Some malignancies, such as adenocarcinoma, lymphoma, and GI stromal tumors, can ulcerate and cause perforations in the stomach or in the small intestine.[64,66,71] Others, such as colon carcinomas and metastatic disease, are more likely to cause chronic obstruction and dilatation of the bowel, which may lead to chronic ischemic changes in the bowel wall in up to 7% of patients.[64] Chronic ischemic changes can result in wall weakening that cause perforation.[64] Malignancies may also result in vascular occlusion and bowel ischemia by direct invasion of the vessels, mechanical obstruction, or by inducing hypercoagulable states.[49,64] Ironically, effective treatment of malignancy can also augment the risk of GI perforation. For example, it has been reported that when lymphoma involving the GI tract is effectively treated by chemotherapy, the tumor may undergo necrosis and weaken the bowel wall, leading to perforation.[71–73]

In addition to tumors causing bowel wall injury, certain therapies for cancer are associated with GI perforations. Many chemotherapeutic and biologic agents target pathways that are essential for rapidly proliferating cells in tumors, but these pathways are also essential in maintaining the

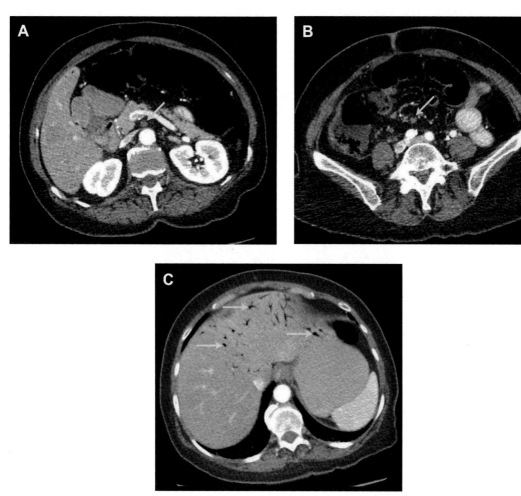

Fig. 15. Mesenteric arterial thrombosis on CT. A 62-year-old woman with history of mesenteric ischemia presenting with worsening abdominal pain. Axial CT images show SMA occlusion (*A, yellow arrow*) along with evidence of ischemic bowel with air in the mesenteric vein (*B, yellow arrow*) and in the hepatic portal veins (*C, yellow arrows*).

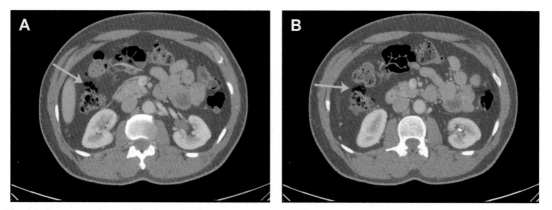

Fig. 16. Pneumatosis cystoides intestinalis on CT. A 58-year-old man with nodular-appearing ascending colon on colonoscopy of unclear cause. On CT, intramural air-filled cysts within the hepatic flexure are seen (*yellow arrows*), which are consistent with pneumatosis cystoides intestinalis.

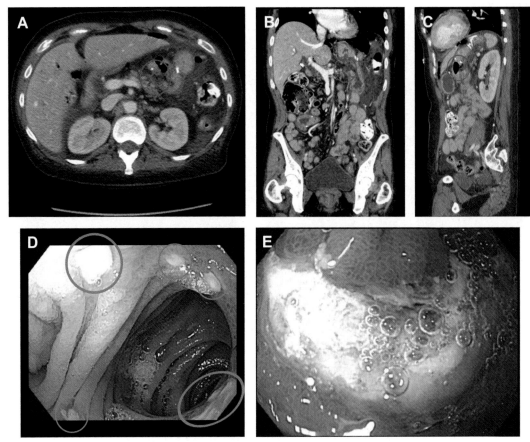

Fig. 17. Marginal ulcers on CT and endoscopy. A 53-year-old woman after Roux-en-Y gastric bypass surgery presenting with abdominal pain. Axial (*A*), coronal (*B*), and sagittal (*C*) CECT show a marginal ulcer at the gastrojejunal anastomosis with an adjacent fluid and air collection (*red circles*) consistent with marginal ulcer perforation at the anastomosis site. Endoscopic images (*D*, *E*) from a different patient after Roux-en-Y gastric bypass who presented with abdominal pain and acute upper GI bleeding show an intact gastrojejunal anastomosis with 4 clean-based marginal ulcers (*blue circles*) without stigmata of bleeding.

integrity of the GI lumen.[74] For example, bevacizumab, a monoclonal antibody against vascular endothelial growth factor, used in treatment of colorectal, lung, ovarian, and breast cancers, is associated with spontaneous intestinal perforation with an incidence of 0.9% to 3.2%.[75–78] Other agents, such as taxols, fluorouracil, cisplatin, mitomycin, interleukin-2, and ipilimumab, are all associated with enteritis or colitis and bowel perforation to varying degrees.[74–76,79,80] Radiation therapy also targets rapidly proliferating cells and may cause radiation-induced enteritis or obliterative endarteritis, both of which may be complicated by GI perforation at doses ranging from 5 to 20 Gy.[74,81,82]

Overall, patients with GI cancer can present with variety of disorders and complications, only 1 of which is perforation. Thus, a broad differential and careful history can aid in arriving at the correct diagnosis.

Imaging Findings

Malignant lesions may be seen as masslike lesions with nodular or diffuse wall thickening associated with lymphadenopathy along the GI tract and in the mesentery (**Fig. 19**). Malignancy-associated bowel wall thickening tends to involve a focal segment of the GI tract.[77] Perforation is more common in the primary site compared with metastatic sites or other nontumor sites: 69% versus 31%, respectively.[77]

GI perforation resulting from chemotherapy or biologic therapy involve more diffuse segments of the GI tract because these agents are systemic.[74] On CECT, diffuse mucosal and serosal hyperenhancement with circumferential wall thickening can be appreciated. There may be focal ulcers and pneumatosis.[74] Perforation from radiation-induced enteritis, in contrast, shows more focal wall enhancement and thickening near the radiation-affected regions of the GI tract.[74,81,82]

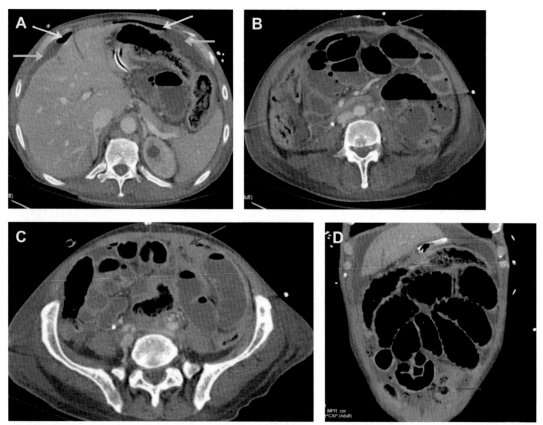

Fig. 18. Colostomy dehiscence. Axial CT images show free air and fluid in the peritoneum (*A, white and yellow arrows*), which are associated with empty skin site (*B, blue arrows*) and retracted end colostomy (*C, D, red arrows*).

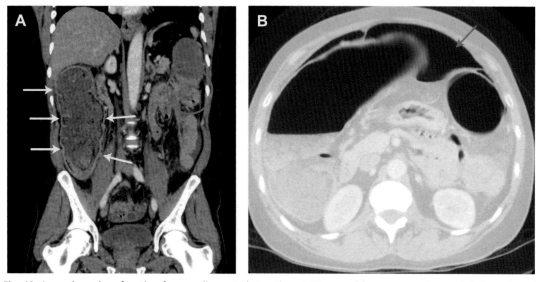

Fig. 19. Large bowel perforation from malignant obstruction. A 50-year-old man presenting with 5 days of gradually worsening abdominal pain, nausea, and emesis along with intractable hiccups. On coronal CT (*A*), he was found to have a large bowel obstruction with massive dilatation of the colon (*white arrows*) and circumferential focal thickening of the mid-descending colon (*red circle*), which was found to be a malignant obstruction. Extensive pneumoperitoneum is shown on the axial CT (*B, red arrow*), consistent with perforation from large bowel obstruction secondary to colon cancer.

INFECTIOUS

Overview

In developing countries, GI perforation from infection is associated with high morality, 10% to 43%,[83-86] and can occur as a result of typhoid, tuberculous, schistosomiasis, or amebic infection. Typhoid infection, in particular, affects children and young adults preferentially and is the most common infectious cause of bowel perforation, with perforation rates ranging from 1% to 33%.[83-87] The pathophysiology leading to GI perforations is different for each organism, but generally involves initial wall injury from the infection or the host's inflammatory response leading to ulcers and eventually necrosis and/or perforation.[84,85]

In developed countries where antibiotic use is common, *Clostridioides difficile* (*Clostridium difficile*) infections (CDIs) may rarely present with bowel perforations (0.1%).[88] In the United States, the burden of CDI is estimated to be about 500,000 cases and is associated with 15,000 to 30,000 deaths annually.[89] Toxic megacolon from CDI may cause perforation in some cases,

whereas CDI colitis may itself cause perforations in high-risk patients (elderly, predisposing conditions such as cancer, inflammatory bowel disease [IBD], and so forth).[88,89]

Imaging findings of infection-associated GI complications may not be distinct from other causes. Therefore, thorough history (travel, prior CDI, recent antibiotic use, and so forth), which may increase the clinical suspicion for infection-associated GI complication, is critical for accurate diagnoses.

Imaging Findings

Knowledge of the underlying pathologic organism can be helpful because different organisms may cause disorders along different sites of the GI tract, which can help narrow the search pattern and the differential diagnosis. For example, *Salmonella* spp have a tendency to involve the Peyer patches in the terminal ileum, where most of the perforations are seen,[83] and *Clostridioides* causes infection in the colon with extension to the small bowel only in rare cases[88] (Fig. 20). Tuberculosis

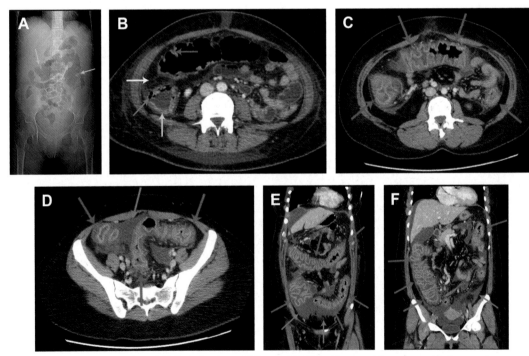

Fig. 20. Three patients with *C difficile* infection colitis on CT. (*A*) A 47-year-old woman with human immunodeficiency virus and recent antibiotic use presenting with fever and diarrhea found to have *C difficile* colitis. The colonic wall thickening is well shown as thumbprinting sign on the scout image (*A*, *yellow arrows*). (*B*) A 25-year-old woman with profuse diarrhea and worsening bandemia found to have *C difficile*–positive pancolitis. CT shows bowel wall thickening (*yellow arrow*), mucosal hyperenhancement (*red arrow*), pneumatosis (*blue arrow*), and pericolonic fat stranding (*white arrow*). (*C–F*) A 42-year-old woman with leukocytosis and worsening abdominal pain, found to have *C difficile* colitis. Axial (*C*, *D*) and coronal (*E*, *F*) CECT images show severe concentric diffuse colonic wall thickening with submucosal edema and mucosal hyperenhancement (*red arrows*) as well as free fluid (*blue arrows*).

can involve any site along the GI tract, but tends to cause diffuse lymphadenopathy, which can be mistaken for malignancy. On imaging, enteritis and colitis show hyperenhancement of the bowel wall and circumferential bowel wall thickening, which can be focal or diffuse depending on the severity of the infection and can mimic IBD.

ACUTE INFLAMMATORY DISORDER: COMPLICATED APPENDICITIS AND DIVERTICULITIS
Overview

Acute appendicitis is the most common abdominal surgical emergency in the world, with an incidence of 11.6 million causing 50,000 deaths annually.[90,91] Prevalence is higher in younger populations and highest in the second decade of life.[91] Perforation is a major concern when the symptoms have lasted longer than 24 hours, and about 13% to 20% of patients present with perforation.[92,93] The risk of perforation is higher in men, young children, and the elderly.[92] Although, in the pediatric population, free perforation is commonly seen owing to underdeveloped omentum, in adults, perforation is more likely to be contained.[94,95]

With respect to acute diverticulitis, approximately 4% of patients with diverticulosis develop diverticulitis.[96,97] Diverticulosis is an extremely common abnormality, usually in the left colon, with prevalence greater than 65% in patients aged more than 65 years.[98] Perforation is a complication of acute diverticulitis seen in about 1% to 2% of cases, but with high mortality of up to 20%.[99,100] In the Asian population, diverticulosis can be seen in the right colon, and diverticulitis is the most common cause of right-sided colonic perforation.[70]

Both disorders are thought to develop with initial obstruction causing stasis of fecal contents within the appendix or the diverticular sac, leading to bacterial proliferation. This process results in increased luminal pressure along with toxin and gas production that leads to bowel wall injury.[98]

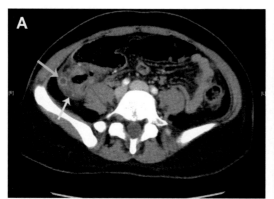
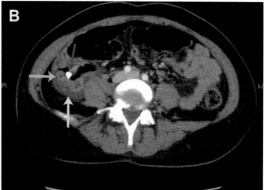
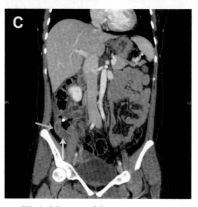

Fig. 21. Perforated appendicitis on CT. A 36-year-old woman presenting with acute abdominal pain found to have perforated appendicitis. On axial CT (*A, B*), a dilated, fluid-filled, enhancing appendix is seen in the right lower quadrant (*yellow arrow*) with surrounding fat stranding (*white arrow*). Appendicolith (*red arrow*) is seen outside the lumen of the GI tract and associated with free air (*blue arrow*), consistent with perforation. Coronal CT (*C*) shows the dilated, fluid-filled, enhancing appendix (*yellow arrow*) with the appendicolith (*red arrow*) and air outside the lumen (*blue arrow*).

Overall, the management of complicated appendicitis or diverticulitis is surgery. The modified Hinchey classification is often used for risk stratification in perforated diverticulitis.[101] Some clinicians have argued for delayed appendectomy or colonic resection with initial conservative medical therapy in stable patients with contained perforations.[102] Ultimately, the decision falls on the surgeon based on clinical and imaging findings. Therefore, it is critical for radiologists to relay relevant imaging findings that may guide medical and surgical decisions.

Imaging Findings

For the general population, CT is preferred to US because of decreased visualization of appendix or diverticuli in the North American population, interoperator variability, and its inability to adequately characterize complications of appendicitis or diverticulitis, such as bowel perforation.[103,104] CT has the added benefit of accurately identifying alternative diagnosis that have similar clinical presentation.[105]

With respect to acute appendicitis, appendix diameter greater than 6 mm, wall thickening (>3 mm), hyperenhancing wall, periappendiceal fat stranding, and fluid are seen on CT (**Fig. 21**). In adults, perforations of acute appendicitis are often contained,[94,95] and may present with periappendiceal abscess shown as fluid collection with peripherally enhancing wall around the appendix. Free appendicolith in the peritoneum is diagnostic of perforated appendicitis. Additional findings of perforated appendicitis are summarized in **Table 5**.

In children and pregnant women, US is often pursued initially for appendicitis, followed by MR imaging to reduce radiation exposure.[103,105–107] MR imaging has high sensitivity and specificity for acute appendicitis (90%–97% for both). MR imaging protocols vary among different institutions but may include multiple orthogonal planes of T_2-weighted fast spin echo with and without fat saturation, precontrast/postcontrast T_1-weighted three-dimensional, gradient echo, and diffusion-weighted imaging (DWI) sequences.[106,107] Perforation should be considered when a large volume of T_2-hyperintense periappendiceal fluid is seen. Free air within the peritoneum may be hard to detect on MR imaging but can be seen as blooming artifact on gradient echo. Appendicolith in the peritoneum may also be identified as blooming artifact on gradient echo sequences. Abscess can be detected as T_2-hyperintense collection with hypointense wall that shows rim enhancement. DWI may also help in identification of abscess.[103,107]

With respect to acute diverticulitis, diagnosis is most often established on CT, showing localized pericolonic fat stranding and edema centered around preexisting colonic diverticulosis (**Fig. 22**). As with acute appendicitis, perforation tends to be contained and may present with pericolonic abscess.

INFLAMMATORY BOWEL DISEASE: ULCERATIVE COLITIS AND CROHN DISEASE
Overview

The 2 main types of idiopathic IBD are ulcerative colitis (UC) and Crohn disease (CD). Although the

	Sensitivity	Specificity
CT Sign	(%)	(%)
Extraluminal air	30	99
Extraluminal appendicolith	14	100
Abscess	38	99
Appendiceal wall enhancement defect	59	96
Fat stranding	94	40
Periappendiceal fluid	42	79
Appendiceal dilatation (>6 mm)	94	9

Table 5
Computed tomography findings related to perforated appendicitis

Data from Kim HY, Park JH, Lee YJ, Lee SS, Jeon J-J, Lee KH. Systematic Review and Meta-Analysis of CT Features for Differentiating Complicated and Uncomplicated Appendicitis. *Radiology.* 2017;287(1):104-115. https://doi.org/10.1148/radiol.2017171260.

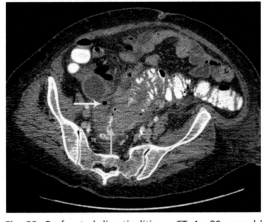

Fig. 22. Perforated diverticulitis on CT. An 80-year-old woman presenting with diffuse abdominal pain and decompensating vital signs found to have perforated diverticulitis. Multiple fluid collections within the pelvis and several small extraluminal foci of air (*white arrow*) are seen. There is also intramural sinus tract with contrast (*yellow arrow*) and air (*red arrow*) seen dissecting into the wall of the inflamed sigmoid colon.

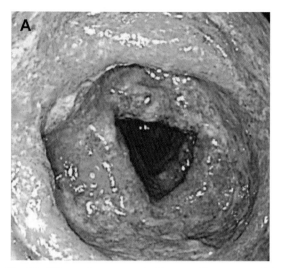
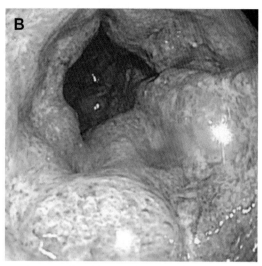

Fig. 23. UC on colonoscopy. A 66-year-old woman with known history of UC (failed infliximab and certolizumab) who presents with ongoing diarrhea and abdominal discomfort. Colonoscopy images show evidence of diffuse circumferential, severely erythematous, hemorrhagic, and inflamed plaque consistent with severe, active UC.

cause of IBD is unknown, evidence is mounting that it relates to an inappropriate inflammatory response to the intestinal environment in patients with genetic susceptibilities.[108] The incidence of IBD in North America is estimated to be 319 and 249 cases per 100,000 persons, respectively,

and both have a bimodal distribution for the initial diagnosis (20–30 years old and 60–80 years old).[109–111]

UC is a mucosal and submucosal inflammatory disease that typically originates in the rectum and may extend proximally in a continuous

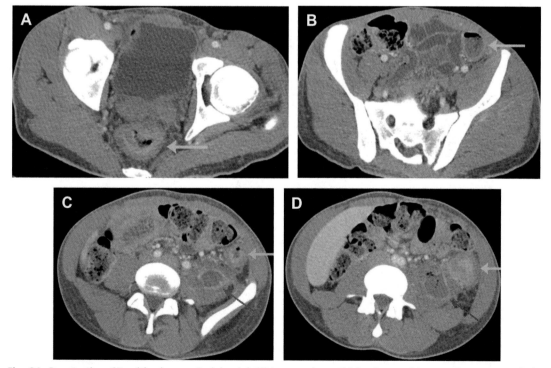

Fig. 24. Penetrating CD with abscess. Serial axial CT images show thickening and hyperenhancement of the bowel wall in the descending colon (yellow arrows), with penetrating component into the left psoas muscle causing an abscess (C, D, red arrows).

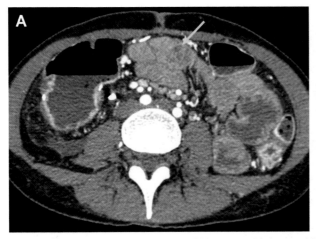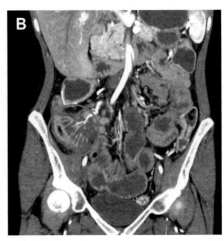

Fig. 25. Active Crohn on CT. A 40-year-old woman with known history of CD after ileocecectomy presenting with acute abdominal pain. On CT, there is a short segment of distal ileal bowel wall thickening (A, *yellow arrow*) along with adjacent mesenteric fat stranding and engorged vasa recta (comb sign; B, *red circle*), which are consistent with active CD.

manner.[112,113] Initially, UC is associated with mucosal edema, which blunts the colonic haustra. An inflammatory infiltrate collects at the bases of crypts, leading to abscesses and ulcers, which can extend into the submucosa (Fig. 23). As these ulcers coalesce and leave islands of spared mucosa, pseudopolyps form. In severe cases, transmural extension can occur, as can superficial inflammatory changes in the ileum, also known as backwash ileitis.[113] Over time, the affected colon can become thickened, narrowed, shortened, and featureless.[114]

CD is a chronic transmural inflammatory disease of the bowel, and most commonly affects the terminal ileum. As the disease progresses, it may form skip lesions anywhere along the GI tract. Chronic inflammation of the bowel eventually causes strictures, upstream dilatation, and bowel wall weakening, which increase the risk of abscess formations and perforations, which occur in 1% to 4% of cases.[74,115]

Free bowel perforation along with toxic megacolon are two of the most serious, potentially lethal complications of IBD.[115] Given the high morbidity and mortality of these complications, emergent surgery is often warranted.[116] In penetrating disease, intra-abdominal abscesses can also form (Fig. 24). These abscesses are often managed with antibiotics, along with percutaneous or surgical drainage initially, and may be followed by surgical resection after the resolution of the abscess to prevent recurrence.[117,118]

Imaging Findings

On CT, UC can manifest as inflamed and thickened colonic wall with hyperenhancement and, if large

enough, pseudopolyps can be seen within the distended colonic lumen. Of note, CT is insensitive to early mucosal disease in UC. Chronic UC can result in bowel shortening, luminal narrowing, submucosal fat deposition (particularly in the rectum), and extramural perirectal fat deposition. Complications of UC, including perforation, abscess, and colorectal carcinoma, can be identified.[119]

On CT, CD is characterized by stratified wall thickening in discontinuous small bowel segments.[74] Target or double halo sign can be seen in acute flares caused by the hyperenhancing mucosa, low-density or edematous submucosa, and dense muscularis propria and serosa. Comb sign is another classic finding seen in CD, representing engorged vasa recta (Fig. 25). Chronic findings of the disease may also be present concurrently, such as strictures, abscesses, fistulas, sinus tracts, and diffuse mildly enlarged mesenteric lymph nodes. These findings may help differentiate perforation from CD from other causes.

SUMMARY

The causes of GI tract perforation occurring in the abdomen in hospitalized patients are varied. Clinical presentations may be nonspecific and similar for many cases, and, in severely ill patients, history and physical examination may not be reliable. Therefore, imaging studies are crucial in early detection of bowel perforation and can provide important information with regard to the site and the extent of the injury. CT is the primary imaging study in this setting, and careful evaluation of the enhancement pattern of the bowel wall, length of the bowel involved, degree of the wall thickening, and the site of injury provide important clues that can narrow the differential diagnoses.

REFERENCES

1. Stoker J, van Randen A, Laméris W, et al. Imaging patients with acute abdominal pain. Radiology 2009;253(1):31–46.
2. Langell JT, Mulvihill SJ. Gastrointestinal perforation and the acute abdomen. Med Clin North Am 2008; 92(3):599–625.
3. Espinoza R, Rodriguez A. Traumatic and nontraumatic perforation of the hollow viscera. Surg Clin North Am 1997;77(6):1291–304.
4. Ismael H, Horst M, Farooq M, et al. Adverse effects of preoperative steroid use on surgical outcomes. Am J Surg 2011;201(3):305–9.
5. Stern E, Journey JD. Peptic ulcer perforated. Treasure Island (FL): StatPearls; 2019. Available at: http://www.ncbi.nlm.nih.gov/pubmed/30855910.
6. Søreide K, Thorsen K, Harrison EM, et al. Perforated peptic ulcer. Lancet 2015;386(10000): 1288–98.
7. Crofts TJ, Park KG, Steele RJ, et al. A randomized trial of nonoperative treatment for perforated peptic ulcer. N Engl J Med 1989;320(15):970–3.
8. Guarner F. Enteric flora in health and disease. Digestion 2006;73(SUPPL. 1):5–12.
9. Gans SL, Stoker J, Boermeester MA. Plain abdominal radiography in acute abdominal pain; past, present, and future. Int J Gen Med 2012;5:525–33.
10. Murray N, Kathryn Darras FE, Frances Walstra FE, et al. Dual-energy CT in evaluation of the acute abdomen. Radiographics 2019;39(7):264–86.
11. Kim SH, Shin SS, Jeong YY, et al. Gastrointestinal tract perforation: MDCT findings according to the perforation sites. Korean J Radiol 2009;10(1):63.
12. Kim HC, Shin HC, Park SJ, et al. Traumatic bowel perforation: analysis of CT findings according to the perforation site and the elapsed time since accident. Clin Imaging 2004;28(5):334–9.
13. Hill BC, Johnson SC, Owens EK, et al. CT scan for suspected acute abdominal process: impact of combinations of IV, oral, and rectal contrast. World J Surg 2010;34(4):699–703.
14. Gore RM, Miller FH, Pereles FS, et al. Helical CT in the evaluation of the acute abdomen. AJR Am J Roentgenol 2000;174(4):901–13.
15. Moschetta M. Multi-detector CT features of acute intestinal ischemia and their prognostic correlations. World J Radiol 2014;6(5):130.
16. Vlahos I, Chung R, Nair A, et al. Dual-energy CT: vascular applications. AJR Am J Roentgenol 2012;199(5_supplement):S87–97.
17. Razavi SA, Johnson J-O, Kassin MT, et al. The impact of introducing a no oral contrast abdominopelvic CT examination (NOCAPE) pathway on radiology turn around times, emergency department length of stay, and patient safety. Emerg Radiol 2014;21(6):605–13.
18. Stuhlfaut JW, Soto JA, Lucey BC, et al. Blunt abdominal trauma: performance of CT without oral contrast material. Radiology 2004;233(3): 689–94.
19. Brody JM, Leighton DB, Murphy BL, et al. CT of blunt trauma bowel and mesenteric injury: typical findings and pitfalls in diagnosis. Radiographics 2013;20(6):1525–36.
20. Soto JA, Anderson SW. Multidetector CT of blunt abdominal trauma. Radiology 2012;265(3):678–93.
21. Brofman N, Atri M, Hanson JM, et al. Evaluation of bowel and mesenteric blunt trauma with multidetector CT. Radiographics 2008;26(4):1119–31.
22. Atri M, Hanson JM, Grinblat L, et al. Surgically important bowel and/or mesenteric injury in blunt trauma: accuracy of multidetector CT for evaluation. Radiology 2008;249(2):524–33.
23. Dowe MF, Shanmuganathan K, Mirvis SE, et al. CT findings of mesenteric injury after blunt trauma: implications for surgical intervention. AJR Am J Roentgenol 1997;168(2):425–8.
24. Breen DJ, Janzen DL, Zwirewich CV, et al. Blunt bowel and mesenteric injury: diagnostic performance of CT signs. J Comput Assist Tomogr 1997;21(5):706–12.
25. Yu J, Fulcher AS, Turner MA, et al. Blunt bowel and mesenteric injury: MDCT diagnosis. Abdom Imaging 2011;36(1):50–61.
26. LeBedis CA, Anderson SW, Bates DDB, et al. CT imaging signs of surgically proven bowel trauma. Emerg Radiol 2016;23(3):213–9.
27. Faget C, Taourel P, Charbit J, et al. Value of CT to predict surgically important bowel and/or mesenteric injury in blunt trauma: performance of a preliminary scoring system. Eur Radiol 2015;25(12):3620–8.
28. Drasin TE, Anderson SW, Asandra A, et al. MDCT evaluation of blunt abdominal trauma: clinical significance of free intraperitoneal fluid in males with absence of identifiable injury. AJR Am J Roentgenol 2008;191(6):1821–6.
29. Joshi G, Crawford KA, Hanna TN, et al. US of right upper quadrant pain in the emergency department: diagnosing beyond gallbladder and biliary disease—erratum. Radiographics 2018;38(5):1590.
30. Lau JY, Sung J, Hill C, et al. Systematic review of the epidemiology of complicated peptic ulcer disease: incidence, recurrence, risk factors and mortality. Digestion 2011;84(2):102–13.
31. Lanas A, Chan FKL. Peptic ulcer disease. Lancet 2017;390(10094):613–24.
32. Kavitt RT, Lipowska AM, Anyane-Yeboa A, et al. Diagnosis and treatment of peptic ulcer disease. Am J Med 2019;132(4):447–56.

33. Levine MS, Rubesin SE. The Helicobacter pylori revolution: radiologic perspective. Radiology 1995;195(3):593–6.

34. Jacobs JM, Hill MC, Steinberg WM. Peptic ulcer disease: CT evaluation. Radiology 1991;178(3):745–8.

35. Bates DDB, Wasserman M, Malek A, et al. Multidetector CT of surgically proven blunt bowel and mesenteric injury. Radiographics 2017;37(2): 613–25.

36. Ahmed I, Ahmed N, Bell DJ, et al. The role of computed tomography in the diagnosis and management of clinically occult post-traumatic small bowel perforation. Radiography 2009;15(3): 228–32.

37. Bennett AE, Levenson RB, Dorfman JD. Multidetector CT imaging of bowel and mesenteric injury: review of key signs. Semin Ultrasound CT MR 2018;39(4):363–73.

38. Hamilton P, Rizoli S, McLellan B, et al. Significance of intra-abdominal extraluminal air detected by CT scan in blunt abdominal trauma. J Trauma 1995; 39(2):331–3. Available at: http://www.ncbi.nlm.nih. gov/pubmed/7674403.

39. Steenburg SD, Petersen MJ, Shen C, et al. Multi-detector CT of blunt mesenteric injuries: usefulness of imaging findings for predicting surgically significant bowel injuries. Abdom Imaging 2015;40(5):1026–33.

40. LeBedis CA, Anderson SW, Soto JA. CT imaging of blunt traumatic bowel and mesenteric injuries. Radiol Clin North Am 2012;50(1):123–36.

41. Gupta A, Stuhlfaut JW, Fleming KW, et al. Blunt trauma of the pancreas and biliary tract: a multimodality imaging approach to diagnosis. Radiographics 2004;24(5):1381–95.

42. Gore RM, Yaghmai V, Thakrar KH, et al. Imaging in intestinal ischemic disorders. Radiol Clin North Am 2008;46(5):845–75.

43. Reginelli A, Genovese E, Cappabianca S, et al. Intestinal ischemia: US-CT findings correlations. Crit Ultrasound J 2013;5(S1):S7.

44. Florim S, Almeida A, Rocha D, et al. Acute mesenteric ischaemia: a pictorial review. Insights Imaging 2018;9(5):673–82.

45. Scholz FJ. Ischemic bowel disease. Radiol Clin North Am 1993;31(6):1197–218. Available at: http:// www.ncbi.nlm.nih.gov/pubmed/8210346.

46. Wiesner W, Khurana B, Ji H, et al. CT of acute bowel ischemia. Radiology 2003;226(3):635–50.

47. Dhatt HS, Behr SC, Miracle A, et al. Radiological evaluation of bowel ischemia. Radiol Clin North Am 2015;53(6):1241–54.

48. Angelelli G, Scardapane A, Memeo M, et al. Acute bowel ischemia: CT findings. Eur J Radiol 2004; 50(1):37–47.

49. Rha SE, Ha HK, Lee SH, et al. CT and MR imaging findings of bowel ischemia from various primary causes. Radiographics 2000;20(1):29–42.

50. Kanasaki S, Furukawa A, Fumoto K, et al. Acute mesenteric ischemia: multidetector CT findings and endovascular management. Radiographics 2018;38(3):945–61.

51. Diamond M, Lee J, LeBedis CA. Small bowel obstruction and ischemia. Radiol Clin North Am 2019;57(4):689–703.

52. Darchy B, Le Mière E, Figuérédo B, et al. Iatrogenic diseases as a reason for admission to the intensive care unit. Arch Intern Med 1999;159(1):71.

53. Steel K, Gertman PM, Crescenzi C, et al. Iatrogenic illness on a general medical service at a university hospital. N Engl J Med 1981;304(11):638–42.

54. Rose J, Schneider C, Yildirim C, et al. Complications in laparoscopic colorectal surgery: results of a multi-centre trial. Tech Coloproctol 2004;8(Suppl 1):s25–8.

55. Mesdaghinia E, Abedzadeh-Kalahroudi M, Hedayati M, et al. Iatrogenic gastrointestinal injuries during obstetrical and gynecological operation. Arch Trauma Res 2013;2(2). https://doi.org/ 10.5812/atr.12088.

56. Tonolini M. Multidetector CT of expected findings and complications after hysterectomy. Insights Imaging 2018;9(3):369–83.

57. Navaneethan U, Parasa S, Venkatesh PGK, et al. Prevalence and risk factors for colonic perforation during colonoscopy in hospitalized inflammatory bowel disease patients. J Crohns Colitis 2011;5(3):189–95.

58. Lohsiriwat V. Colonoscopic perforation: incidence, risk factors, management and outcome. World J Gastroenterol 2010;16(4):425.

59. Lüning TH, Keemers-Gels ME, Barendregt WB, et al. Colonoscopic perforations: a review of 30,366 patients. Surg Endosc 2007;21(6):994–7.

60. Turrentine FE, Denlinger CE, Simpson VB, et al. Morbidity, mortality, cost, and survival estimates of gastrointestinal anastomotic leaks. J Am Coll Surg 2015;220(2):195–206.

61. Park JS, Huh JW, Park YA, et al. Risk factors of anastomotic leakage and long-term survival after colorectal surgery. Medicine (Baltimore) 2016; 95(8):e2890.

62. Kirchhoff P, Clavien P-A, Hahnloser D. Complications in colorectal surgery: risk factors and preventive strategies. Patient Saf Surg 2010;4(1):5.

63. Samji KB, Kielar AZ, Connolly M, et al. Anastomotic leaks after small- and large-bowel surgery: diagnostic performance of ct and the importance of intraluminal contrast administration. AJR Am J Roentgenol 2018;210(6):1259–65.

64. Katabathina VS, Restrepo CS, Betancourt Cuellar SL, et al. Imaging of oncologic emergencies: what every radiologist should know. Radiographics 2013;33(6):1533–53.

65. Abdelrazeq AS, Scott N, Thorn C, et al. The impact of spontaneous tumour perforation on outcome

following colon cancer surgery. Colorectal Dis 2008;10(8):775–80.

66. Mandava N, Kumar S, Pizzi WF, et al. Perforated colorectal carcinomas. Am J Surg 1996;172(3):236–8. Available at: http://www.ncbi.nlm.nih.gov/pubmed/8862074.

67. Kim SW, Kim HC, Yang DM. Perforated tumours in the gastrointestinal tract: CT findings and clinical implications. Br J Radiol 2012;85(1017):1307–13.

68. Guniganti P, Bradenham CH, Raptis C, et al. CT of gastric emergencies. Radiographics 2015;35(7):1909–21.

69. Carraro PG, Segala M, Orlotti C, et al. Outcome of large-bowel perforation in patients with colorectal cancer. Dis Colon Rectum 1998;41(11):1421–6. Available at: http://www.ncbi.nlm.nih.gov/pubmed/9823810.

70. Tan K-K, Zhang J, Liu JZ, et al. Right colonic perforation in an asian population: predictors of morbidity and mortality. J Gastrointest Surg 2009;13(12):2252–9.

71. Ara C, Coban S, Kayaalp C, et al. Spontaneous intestinal perforation due to Non-Hodgkin's lymphoma: evaluation of eight cases. Dig Dis Sci 2007;52(8):1752–6.

72. McDermott EW, Cassidy N, Heffernan SJ. Perforation through undiagnosed small bowel involvement in primary thyroid lymphoma during chemotherapy. Cancer 1992;69(2):572–3. Available at: http://www.ncbi.nlm.nih.gov/pubmed/1728388.

73. Meyers PA, Potter VP, Wollner N, et al. Bowel perforation during initial treatment for childhood non-Hodgkin's lymphoma. Cancer 1985;56(2):259–61. Available at: http://www.ncbi.nlm.nih.gov/pubmed/4005797.

74. Sugi MD, Menias CO, Lubner MG, et al. CT findings of acute small-bowel entities. Radiographics 2018;38(5):1352–69.

75. Birch JC, Khatri G, Watumull LM, et al. Unintended consequences of systemic and ablative oncologic therapy in the abdomen and pelvis. Radiographics 2018;38(4):1158–79.

76. Torrisi JM, Schwartz LH, Gollub MJ, et al. CT findings of chemotherapy-induced toxicity: what radiologists need to know about the clinical and radiologic manifestations of chemotherapy toxicity. Radiology 2011;258(1):41–56.

77. Kang MH, Kim SN, Kim NK, et al. Clinical outcomes and prognostic factors of metastatic gastric carcinoma patients who experience gastrointestinal perforation during palliative chemotherapy. Ann Surg Oncol 2010;17(12):3163–72.

78. Hapani S, Chu D, Wu S. Risk of gastrointestinal perforation in patients with cancer treated with bevacizumab: a meta-analysis. Lancet Oncol 2009;10(6):559–68.

79. Heimann DM, Schwartzentruber DJ. Gastrointestinal perforations associated with interleukin-2 administration. J Immunother 2004;27(3):254–8. Available at: http://www.ncbi.nlm.nih.gov/pubmed/15076143.

80. Cronin CG, O'Connor M, Lohan DG, et al. Imaging of the gastrointestinal complications of systemic chemotherapy. Clin Radiol 2009;64(7):724–33.

81. Capps GW, Fulcher AS, Szucs RA, et al. Imaging features of radiation-induced changes in the abdomen. Radiographics 1997;17(6):1455–73.

82. Maturen KE, Feng MU, Wasnik AP, et al. Imaging effects of radiation therapy in the abdomen and pelvis: evaluating "innocent bystander" tissues. Radiographics 2013;33(2):599–619.

83. Eid HO, Hefny AF, Joshi S, et al. Non-traumatic perforation of the small bowel. Afr Health Sci 2008;8(1):36–9. Available at: http://www.ncbi.nlm.nih.gov/pubmed/19357730.

84. Gedik E, Girgin S, Taçyıldız IH, et al. Risk factors affecting morbidity in typhoid enteric perforation. Langenbecks Arch Surg 2008;393(6):973–7.

85. Athié-Gutiérrez C, Rodea-Rosas H, Guízar-Bermúdez C, et al. Evolution of surgical treatment of amebiasis-associated colon perforation. J Gastrointest Surg 2010;14(1):82–7.

86. Edino ST, Yakubu AA, Mohammed AZ, et al. Prognostic factors in typhoid ileal perforation: a prospective study of 53 cases. J Natl Med Assoc 2007;99(9):1042–5. Available at: http://www.ncbi.nlm.nih.gov/pubmed/17913115%0Ahttp://www.pubmedcentral.nih.gov/articlerender.fcgi?artid=PMC2575870.

87. Sharma D, Gupta A, Jain BK, et al. Tuberculous gastric perforation: report of a case. Surg Today 2004;34(6):537–41.

88. Abou Chakra CN, McGeer A, Labbé A-C, et al. Factors associated with complications of clostridium difficile infection in a multicenter prospective cohort. Clin Infect Dis 2015;61(12):1781–8.

89. McDonald LC, Gerding DN, Johnson S, et al. Clinical practice guidelines for clostridium difficile infection in adults and children: 2017 update by the Infectious Diseases Society of America (IDSA) and Society for Healthcare Epidemiology of America (SHEA). Clin Infect Dis 2018;66(7):e1–48.

90. Vos T, Allen C, Arora M, et al. Global, regional, and national incidence, prevalence, and years lived with disability for 310 diseases and injuries, 1990–2015: a systematic analysis for the Global Burden of Disease Study 2015. Lancet 2016;388(10053):1545–602.

91. Addiss DG, Shaffer N, Fowler BS, et al. The epidemiology of appendicitis and appendectomy in the United States. Am J Epidemiol 1990;132(5):910–25.

92. Andersson RE, Hugander A, Thulin AJ. Diagnostic accuracy and perforation rate in appendicitis: association with age and sex of the patient and with

appendicectomy rate. Eur J Surg 1992;158(1): 37–41. Available at: http://www.ncbi.nlm.nih.gov/pubmed/1348639.

93. Temple CL, Huchcroft SA, Temple WJ. The natural history of appendicitis in adults. A prospective study. Ann Surg 1995;221(3):278–81.

94. Marzuillo P. Appendicitis in children less than five years old: a challenge for the general practitioner. World J Clin Pediatr 2015;4(2):19.

95. Rasmussen OO, Hoffmann J. Assessment of the reliability of the symptoms and signs of acute appendicitis. J R Coll Surg Edinb 1991;36(6): 372–7. Available at: http://www.ncbi.nlm.nih.gov/pubmed/1774704.

96. Parks TG. Natural history of diverticular disease of the colon. A review of 521 cases. Br Med J 1969; 4(5684):639–42.

97. Shahedi K, Fuller G, Bolus R, et al. Long-term risk of acute diverticulitis among patients with incidental diverticulosis found during colonoscopy. Clin Gastroenterol Hepatol 2013;11(12):1609–13.

98. West AB. The pathology of diverticulitis. J Clin Gastroenterol 2008;42(10):1137–8.

99. Constantinides VA, Tekkis PP, Athanasiou T, et al. Primary resection with anastomosis vs. Hartmann's procedure in nonelective surgery for acute colonic diverticulitis: a systematic review. Dis Colon Rectum 2006;49(7):966–81.

100. Kriwanek S, Armbruster C, Beckerhinn P, et al. Prognostic factors for survival in colonic perforation. Int J Colorectal Dis 1994;9(3):158–62. Available at: http://www.ncbi.nlm.nih.gov/pubmed/7814991.

101. Bates DDB, Fernandez MB, Ponchiardi C, et al. Surgical management in acute diverticulitis and its association with multi-detector CT, modified Hinchey classification, and clinical parameters. Abdom Radiol (NY) 2018;43(8):2060–5.

102. Cheng Y, Xiong X, Lu J, et al. Early versus delayed appendicectomy for appendiceal phlegmon or abscess. Cochrane Database Syst Rev 2017;(6): CD011670.

103. Eng KA, Abadeh A, Ligocki C, et al. Acute appendicitis: a meta-analysis of the diagnostic accuracy of US, CT, and MRI as second-line imaging tests after an initial US. Radiology 2018;288(3):717–27.

104. Carpenter JL, Orth RC, Zhang W, et al. Diagnostic performance of US for differentiating perforated from nonperforated pediatric appendicitis: a prospective cohort study. Radiology 2017;282(3): 835–41.

105. Werner A, Diehl SJ, Farag-Soliman M, et al. Multislice spiral CT in routine diagnosis of suspected acute left-sided colonic diverticulitis: a prospective study of 120 patients. Eur Radiol 2003;13(12): 2596–603.

106. Harringa JB, Bracken RL, Davis JC, et al. Prospective evaluation of MRI compared with CT for the etiology of abdominal pain in emergency department patients with concern for appendicitis. J Magn Reson Imaging 2019. https://doi.org/10.1002/jmri.26728.

107. Mervak BM, Wilson SB, Handly BD, et al. MRI of acute appendicitis. J Magn Reson Imaging 2019; 1–10. https://doi.org/10.1002/jmri.26709.

108. Abraham C, Cho JH. Inflammatory bowel disease. N Engl J Med 2009;361(21):2066–78.

109. Molodecky NA, Soon IS, Rabi DM, et al. Increasing incidence and prevalence of the inflammatory bowel diseases with time, based on systematic review. Gastroenterology 2012;142(1):46–54.e42. https://doi.org/10.1053/j.gastro.2011.10.001 [quiz: e30].

110. Wilkins T, Jarvis K, Patel J. Diagnosis and management of Crohn's disease. Am Fam Physician 2011;84(12):1365–75. Available at: http://www.ncbi.nlm.nih.gov/pubmed/22230271.

111. Scholz F, Humphrey P. Crohn's disease. In: Levy A, Mortele K, Yeh B, editors. Gastrointestinal imaging. Oxford (England): Oxford University Press; 2015. p. 136–41.

112. Danese S, Fiocchi C. Ulcerative colitis. N Engl J Med 2011;365(18):1713–25.

113. Gore R, Berlin J, Ivanovic A. Ulcerative and granulomatous colitis: idiopathic inflammatory bowel disease. In: Gore R, Levine M, editors. Textbook of gastrointestinal radiology. 4th edition. Philadelphia: Elsevier; 2015. p. 984–1016.

114. Kaushal P, Somwaru AS, Charabaty A, et al. MR enterography of inflammatory bowel disease with endoscopic correlation. Radiographics 2017; 37(1):116–31.

115. Werbin N, Haddad R, Greenberg R, et al. Free perforation in Crohn's disease. Isr Med Assoc J 2003;5(3):175–7. Available at: http://www.ncbi.nlm.nih.gov/pubmed/12725136.

116. Ausch C, Madoff RD, Gnant M, et al. Aetiology and surgical management of toxic megacolon. Colorectal Dis 2006;8(3):195–201.

117. Fleshman JW. Pyogenic complications of Crohn's disease, evaluation, and management. J Gastrointest Surg 2008;12(12):2160–3.

118. Poritz LS, Koltun WA. Percutaneous drainage and ileocolectomy for spontaneous intraabdominal abscess in Crohn's disease. J Gastrointest Surg 2007;11(2):204–8.

119. Gore RM, Balthazar EJ, Ghahremani GG, et al. CT features of ulcerative colitis and Crohn's disease. AJR Am J Roentgenol 1996;167(1):3–15.

120. Park M-H, Shin BS, Namgung H. Diagnostic performance of 64-MDCT for blunt small bowel perforation. Clin Imaging 2013;37(5):884–8.

Imaging of Acute Hepatobiliary Dysfunction

HeiShun Yu, MD, Jennifer W. Uyeda, MD*

KEYWORDS

- Hepatobiliary dysfunction • Acute cholecystitis • Gallstone

KEY POINTS

- Abdominal pain is a common cause for emergency department visits in the United States, and biliary tract disease is the fifth most common cause of hospital admission.
- Common causes of acute hepatobiliary include gallstones and its associated complications and multiple other hepatobiliary etiologies, including infectious, inflammatory, vascular, and neoplastic causes.
- Postoperative complications of the biliary tract can result in an acute abdomen.
- Imaging of the hepatobiliary tree is integral in the diagnostic evaluation of acute hepatobiliary dysfunction, and imaging of the biliary tree requires a multimodality approach utilizing ultrasound, computed tomography, nuclear medicine, and MR imaging.

INTRODUCTION

Abdominal pain is 1 of the top 5 causes of emergency department visits in the adult population. Within this population, biliary tract disease is the fifth most common cause of hospital admission in the 18 year old to 44 year old age group.[1] Common causes of acute hepatobiliary include gallstones and its associated complications. There are many additional hepatobiliary etiologies, however, including infectious, inflammatory, vascular, and neoplastic causes.[2,3] Postoperative complications of the biliary tract also may be seen in the setting of an acute abdomen.[4] In addition to a comprehensive history and physical along with appropriate laboratory tests, imaging is an integral part of the diagnostic evaluation of acute hepatobiliary dysfunction,[2] and imaging of the biliary tree often entails a multimodality approach, including any combination of ultrasound (US), computed tomography (CT), nuclear medicine, and MR imaging.

IMAGING MODALITIES

Ultrasound

In the setting of biliary disease, US is often the imaging modality of choice.[5] It is an excellent modality for detection of gallstones, in particular those that are radiolucent on CT. US can be used for the assessment for ductal dilatation or presence of fluid collection. US often is limited, however, in its ability to identify a cause for these findings. Doppler US also can be useful for assessment of hepatic vasculature. This is of particular importance in the post-transplant patient.

Computed Tomography

CT is the most commonly utilized imaging modality to assess acute abdominal pain and plays a major role in the evaluation of acute hepatobiliary disease. It is best performed after administration of intravenous contrast, when possible, and is an excellent modality for assessing hepatic parenchyma and adjacent structures, such as the pancreas, kidney, and stomach. CT also is useful

Department of Radiology, Brigham and Women's Hospital, 75 Francis Street, Boston, MA 02115, USA
* Corresponding author.
E-mail address: juyeda@bwh.harvard.edu

Radiol Clin N Am 58 (2020) 45–58
https://doi.org/10.1016/j.rcl.2019.08.008

radiologic.theclinics.com

for identifying fluid collections, but, as with US, there are limitations, including inability to definitely characterize intraabdominal and pelvic collections and to identify an etiology for the patient's symptoms and potential underestimation of gallstone burden because many stones are radiolucent.

Nuclear Medicine

Hepatobiliary iminodiacetic acid scan (HIDA) scan is performed by administering a technetium Tc 99m iminodiacetic acid analog, which is taken up by hepatocytes and excreted into the biliary tree. It is an excellent modality for the detection of cystic duct obstruction in the setting of acute cholecystitis. False-positive results may occur in the settings of severe liver disease, prior sphincterotomy, prolonged fasting, and prior administration of cholecystokinin.[4] HIDA scan also may offer complementary information to US or CT, in the postoperative setting for diagnosis of biliary leak.

MR Imaging

As with CT, MR imaging offers excellent soft tissue characterization, specifically in evaluating hepatic parenchyma as well as the adjacent organs. Unlike CT, it also is sensitive for detecting gallstones. MR cholangiopancreatography (MRCP) also may be performed, taking advantage of heavily T2-weighted images, to evaluate the biliary tree (Fig. 1). In the postcholecystectomy patient, administration of a hepatobiliary agent may offer functional and anatomic information, including assessing the anatomy and detecting a biliary leak. Patients with normal liver function excrete contrast into the common bile duct in approximately 20 minutes after administration of gadoxetate. This also offers anatomic information because excreted contrast delineates the biliary tree and in the presence of a leak can localize the site of injury.

INFLAMMATION/INFECTION
Acute Cholecystitis

Cholelithiasis is present in 10% to 15% of the American population.[6] Approximately 2% to 4% of patients with gallstones develop symptoms, most commonly biliary colic. Acute cholecystitis should be suspected in the setting of fever and is caused by cystic duct obstruction with secondary irritation of the gallbladder by bile salts.[7]

US is the preferred imaging modality for detection of cholelithiasis. Because cystic duct obstruction cannot always be assessed on US, acute cholecystitis also must be identified based on secondary signs, such as cholelithiasis, gallbladder wall thickening, wall edema, and pericholecystic fluid (Fig. 2A, B).[8,9] A distinct advantage of US is its ability to elicit a sonographic Murphy sign.[9] Despite being rapid and effective, sonographic findings often are difficult to interpret given that gallbladder wall abnormalities are nonspecific and also can be seen in the setting of liver, heart or renal disease.[8,9]

CT may offer complementary information and can diagnose acute cholecystitis by identifying a distended gallbladder with wall thickening, wall edema, pericholecystic fluid, and pericholecystic stranding (Fig. 2C). Gallstones may or may not be seen on CT.[10] Use of dual-energy CT, however, with creation of monochromatic low or high kiloelectron volt images, has been shown to increase conspicuity of stones (Fig. 3).[11] MR/MRCP may show similar findings to CT with the added benefit of the T2-weighted sequence, which has a higher sensitivity for stone detection (Fig. 2D). Review of diffusion-weighted images also has been shown helpful for differentiation of acute from chronic cholecystitis.[12,13]

Equivocal cases can be further evaluated with HIDA. On HIDA scan, acute cholecystitis can demonstrate cystic duct obstruction by showing radiotracer excretion into small bowel without accumulation in the gallbladder.[9,14] Morphine administration can be attempted to increase muscle tone in the sphincter of Oddi and promote gallbladder filling. In cases of chronic cholecystitis, the cystic duct is patent and radiotracer can accumulate in the gallbladder. These cases may demonstrate delayed gallbladder filling or delayed transit to small bowel. Administration of cholecystokinin and evaluation for an impaired ejection fraction can be helpful in these cases.[14]

Acute Acalculous Cholecystitis

Acute acalculous cholecystitis (AAC) is characterized by gallbladder inflammation without obstruction from gallstones. It often affects critically ill patients particularly after surgery, trauma, burn injury and cardiac arrest. Diabetes, abdominal vasculitis, and congestive heart failure also have been associated with AAC.[15] AAC in critically ill patients tends to have a worse prognosis with a mortality rate of up to 50% and these patients also are more likely to develop complications of cholecystitis, such as gangrene and perforation. As such, it is of critical importance to diagnose and treat these patients in a timely manner. Early imaging is necessary for these patients and demonstrates similar findings to acute calculous cholecystitis, including gallbladder distention, wall thickening, and pericholecystic fluid without the

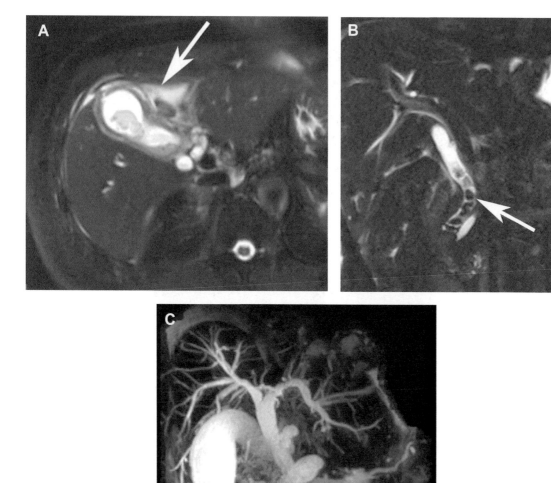

Fig. 1. A 45-year-old woman with right upper quadrant pain. Axial T2-weighted fat-saturated MR imaging (*A*) shows an inflamed gallbladder with wall thickening and pericholecystic fluid (*arrow*) and intraluminal gallstones. Coronal thin MRCP (*B*) and 3-dimensional maximum intensity projection MRCP (*C*) images show choledocholithiasis with multiple gallstones in the common bile duct (*arrows*). Note that the individual gallstones are better visualized on the thin MRCP image compared with and 3-dimensional MIP image.

presence of gallstones. The sonographic Murphy sign generally is unreliable in these cases because the patients are too ill and may be medicated.[16]

Complications of Acute Cholecystitis

Acute cholecystitis can be complicated by secondary infection of the inflamed gallbladder, which can lead to emphysematous cholecystitis and gangrenous cholecystitis. Emphysematous cholecystitis is the result of superinfection of

the gallbladder by a gas-forming organism and commonly affects diabetics, men more than women, and patients 40 years old to 60 years old. On imaging, it is readily identified on CT with intramural gas involving the gallbladder. US can be difficult because gas in the gallbladder wall can obscure the gallbladder or be mistaken for bowel gas. Early diagnosis is important because these patients are prone to develop gangrene, perforation (**Fig. 4**) and abscess.[10]

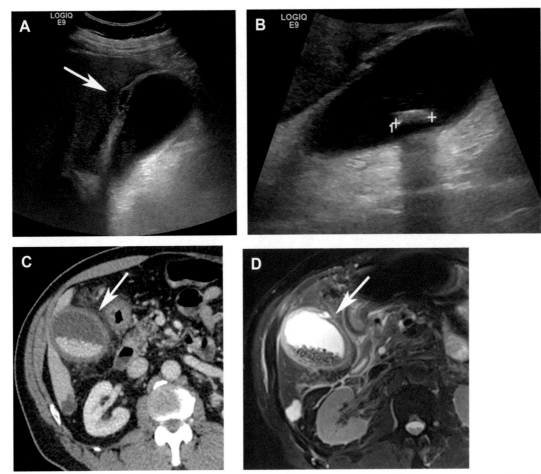

Fig. 2. A 54-year-old man with acute calculous cholecystitis. Longitudinal US images demonstrate gallbladder wall thickening up to 11 mm and pericholecystic edema (*A* [*arrow*]) as well as a gallstone (*B*). A 47-year-old man with acute calculous cholecystitis illustrates layering dependent calcified gallstones on axial CT (*C*) with gallbladder wall thickening and pericholecystic inflammation (*arrow*) with similar findings on axial T2-weighted MR image (*D* [*arrow*]).

Gangrenous cholecystitis is associated with increased morbidity and mortality. It is characterized by the presence of intramural hemorrhage, necrosis, and development of microabscesses. On imaging, mural irregularity, sloughed intraluminal membranes, and intraluminal debris suggest the presence of gangrenous cholecystitis.[17,18] In these cases, evidence of perforation as evidenced by focal wall discontinuity, extraluminal gallstones, and pericholecystic abscesses also may be detected.[18] Dual-energy CT images may be helpful because the gallbladder wall may demonstrate areas of absent iodine uptake.

Xanthogranulomatous Cholecystitis

Xanthogranulomatous cholecystitis (XGC) is a rare and chronic form of cholecystitis characterized by a destructive inflammatory process with features of perforation, abscess formation, fistula, and invasion of adjacent structures, and which often is difficult to differentiate from gallbladder carcinoma.[19] Radiologic findings include diffuse or focal gallbladder wall thickening with hypoattenuating intramural nodules, heterogeneous wall enhancement, infiltration of the liver and adjacent pericholecystic fat, and continuity of the enhancing gallbladder mucosa (**Fig. 5**).[18] Similar findings are demonstrated on MR imaging, noting high T2 signal corresponding to hypoattenuating intramural nodules on CT, which represent xanthogranulomas. This finding has been suggested to be a discriminating feature from gallbladder carcinoma; however, cholecystectomy is often performed to confirm the diagnosis and plan definitive treatment.

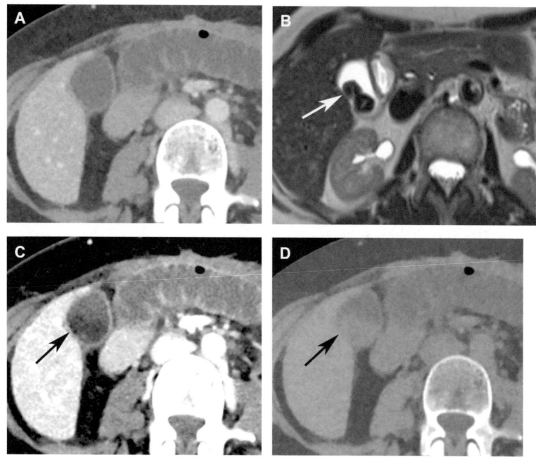

Fig. 3. A 38-year-old woman with noncalcified gallstones, which are isoattenuating to bile at 70 keV (*A*) and confirmed on T2-weighted single-shot fast spin-echo MR imaging (*B*) (*arrow*) performed 21 days after the dual-energy CT. The stones decrease in attenuation using virtual monochromatic imaging at 40 keV (*C*) (*arrow*) and increase in attenuation at 190 keV (*D*) (*arrow*), with corresponding increase in conspicuity relative to surrounding bile.

Acute Ascending Cholangitis

Acute cholangitis occurs in the setting of common biliary obstruction. The most common cause for cholangitis is choledocholithiasis, but other causes include malignant obstruction or prior biliary manipulation. The diagnosis of cholangitis is made clinically by the presence of Charcot triad of fever, jaundice, and right upper quadrant pain. Reynolds pentad also includes hypotension and altered mental status.[3,4,6,20] Imaging with US may detect the presence of ductal dilatation.[4] CT evaluation of the biliary tree may demonstrate choledocholithiasis, periductal inflammation, ductal wall thickening and mural enhancement.[21] MRCP shows similar findings but may also show parenchymal changes related to cholangitis, specifically wedge-shaped or peribiliary regions of T2 hyperintensity or enhancement.[3] Unless stones

are impacted, choledocholithiasis on both CT and MR imaging often are dependent in position. On CT, stones commonly are angulated and lamellated with an anterior crescent of fluid or gas. MRCP may have a higher sensitivity for detecting radiolucent stones but CT is a better modality for differentiating pneumobilia from choledocholithiasis.[5]

Mirizzi Syndrome

Mirizzi syndrome is defined by common hepatic duct obstruction from extrinsic compression due to stone in the gallbladder infundibulum or cystic duct.[22,23] As with other acute biliary disease, patients present with fever, jaundice, and/or right upper quadrant pain. Anatomically, a parallel configuration of the cystic and common hepatic ducts along with a long, low inserting cystic duct

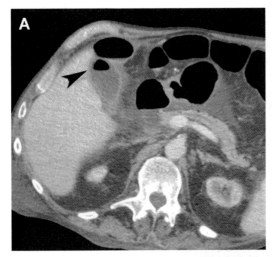
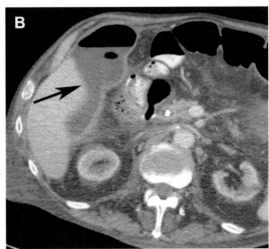
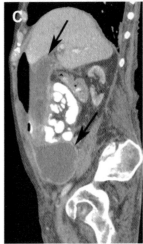

Fig. 4. A 61-year-old man with history of gallstone pancreatitis presents with abdominal pain. Axial CT images (*A*, *B*) and sagittal CT image (*C*) show air within the gallbladder fundus (*arrowhead*) and a large bilobed peripherally enhancing collection extending from the gallbladder into the right paracolic gutter (*arrows*). The perforated gallbladder with subsequent abscess development required multiple percutaneous drainages.

predisposes patients to this entity.[23] On imaging, US may detect an ectatic common hepatic duct. CT may show a similar finding and also may demonstrate periportal inflammation. MRCP is the preferred imaging modality given its ability to delineate ductal anatomy. On heavily T2-weighted images, MRCP may demonstrate a stone impacted in the cystic duct or gallbladder infundibulum compressing the common hepatic duct, which is dilated proximal to the level of the stone. Distally, the common bile duct is normal in caliber.[18,23]

Gallstone Ileus

A rare complication of gallstones is gallstone ileus, which is characterized by mechanical obstruction of the gastrointestinal tract secondary to an impacted gallstone. Large stones (>2 cm) within

the gallbladder can pass into the gastrointestinal tract by eroding into an adjacent bowel loop. It then can cause obstruction at sites of decreased luminal diameter, most commonly the terminal ileum and ileocecal valve. Rarely, the gallstone can migrate proximally causing gastric outlet obstruction, a phenomenon known as Bouveret syndrome.[2] Cases of gallstones ileus are best diagnosed on CT, which demonstrate dilated bowel loops to the level an ectopic gallstone, pneumobilia as well as a fistulous connection between the gallbladder and adjacent bowel loop (**Fig. 6**).[2,18]

Primary Sclerosing Cholangitis

Primary sclerosing cholangitis (PSC) is characterized by chronic inflammation and fibrosis of both intrahepatic and extrahepatic bile ducts. Etiology

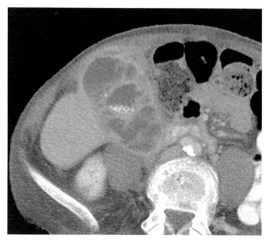

Fig. 5. Axial CT image demonstrates XGC with a distended gallbladder containing calcified gallstones with multiple hypoattenuating intramural nodules.

is unknown but likely autoimmune. The disease is commonly seen with inflammatory bowel disease, most often ulcerative colitis, and patients carry an increased risk of cholangiocarcinoma.[3,24] In the acute setting, patients may present with abdominal pain, pruritis and jaundice. The most common acute complication in these patients is recurrent bouts of cholangitis, discussed previously.[25] MRCP is best imaging modality for evaluation of PSC and may demonstrate a multifocal beaded appearance of the biliary tree with areas of ductal dilatation.[24]

Recurrent Pyogenic Cholangitis

Recurrent pyogenic cholangitis (RPC) is characterized by repeated bouts of cholangitis.

Associations have been made with infestations of *Clonorchis sinensis*, *Ascaris lumbricoides*, and *Opisthorchis viverrini* although the exact pathogenesis has yet to be determined. As with PSC, patients are subject to repeated bouts of bacterial cholangitis. Patients may present acutely with abdominal pain, fever, and jaundice. Complications include portal venous thrombosis, abscesses, and strictures.[3,26] Portal venous thrombosis and abscess are readily diagnosed on CT or MR imaging whereas strictures are best characterized on MRCP or transhepatic cholangiogram. In patients with these presenting symptoms, MR imaging has an added benefit of being able to assess hepatic parenchymal enhancement, which may suggest active inflammation or infection, and periductal inflammation.[26]

Parasitic Infection

Several parasitic infections may affect the biliary tree. Clinical manifestations of these infections are variable and may be indistinguishable from ascending cholangitis. Work-up of these patients requires eliciting a history of travel to endemic regions as well as laboratory tests, including serology, stool examination, and detection of eosinophilia. Imaging is included in the work-up, particularly in the setting of *Echinococcus granulosus*.[26,27] Echinococcal infections occur in stages, which can be differentiated on imaging. Depending on the stage of infection, treatment options can differ ranging from medical management to drainage to resection. Left untreated, echinococcal infections can fistulize into the bile ducts, resulting in cholangitis. Alternatively, it can rupture

A
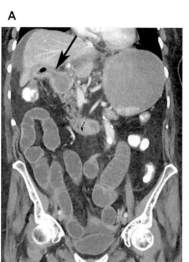
B
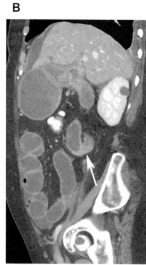

Fig. 6. An 81-year-old woman with abdominal pain. Coronal CT image (*A*) shows a choledochoduodenal fistula (*arrow*) and small bowel obstruction with a transition point in the right lower quadrant (*arrow*) is seen on the sagittal CT image (*B*).

into the peritoneum causing peritonitis or anaphylaxis.[26] A grading system has been created by the World Health Organization for classification of these lesions on US. On US, an early (active) stage of infection may demonstrate a simple appearing cyst. This also may be seen on CT. Occasionally, punctate echogenic foci can be seen within the cyst representing hydatid sand, which is a combination of fluid and protoscolices. Active disease also may present as a multivesicular cyst, with multiple daughter cysts within a larger cyst in a spoke-wheel appearance. As the parasite dies, the cyst enters a transitional stage where an endocyst may detach from the pericyst, as demonstrated by a floating membranes appearance. Progression of this finding can be seen as the multiple wavy lines, also known as the water lily sign. As the cyst progresses into the inactive stage, the cyst takes on a more solid appearance and may calcify.[27] Biliary involvement of echinococcal infection can be identified on imaging as intrahepatic ductal dilatation extending to the periphery, cystobiliary fistulas and extension of daughter cysts or hydatid membranes into the biliary tree.[26]

Immunocompromised Patients

Opportunistic infections of the biliary tract are commonly seen in the immunocompromised patients. With regard to human immunodeficiency virus (HIV) patients, the biliary tract tends to be affected as CD4 count falls below $100/mm^3$. Clinical findings are nonspecific and may include right upper quadrant pain and fever. Abnormal liver function tests may also be seen although this may be related to hepatitis or drug reaction. As such, imaging plays an important role in evaluation of these patients.[26] Biliary disease in the setting of HIV includes a spectrum of disease that is grouped as acquired immunodeficiency syndrome (AIDS) cholangiopathy. This group of diseases includes acalculous cholecystitis, sclerosing cholangitis, papillary stenosis, lymphoma, and Kaposi sarcoma, among others.[28] Several pathogens have been identified as possible causative agents for AIDS cholangiopathy, including cytomegalovirus, herpes simplex virus, *Cryptosporidium parvum*, and *Mycobacterium avium complex*.[26] The pathogen, however, is not always identified.[28]

Imaging of patients with HIV may demonstrate hepatic and pancreatic parenchymal as well as biliary abnormalities. Imaging with CT and US may demonstrate hepatic and pancreatic findings, including hepatomegaly, periportal lymphadenopathy and acalculous cholecystitis. Findings of acute or chronic pancreatitis can be identified on CT. CT and MR imaging may demonstrate patchy arterial enhancement in the setting of hepatitis, although abnormal hepatic parenchymal enhancement also may be seen in the setting of opportunistic infection, hepatosteatosis or Kaposi sarcoma.[28] Biliary findings are best characterized on MRCP where bile duct and gallbladder walls are commonly thickened. Findings of the biliary tree are similar to PSC, including intrahepatic and extrahepatic stenoses and ductal dilatation as well as pruning of peripheral ducts.[26,28] One feature that may help distinguish the 2 processes is the presence of long segment extrahepatic strictures, which is seen in AIDS cholangiopathy.[28]

Acute Hepatitis

Viral hepatitis can occur in acute and chronic forms. Acute viral hepatitis usually is caused by hepatitis A virus, hepatitis B virus, hepatitis C virus, HBV-associated delta agent/hepatitis D virus, or hepatitis E virus, and symptoms are variable ranging from asymptomatic to fulminant and fatal illness. Chronic hepatitis results from inflammation and necrosis occur for greater than 6 months and complications include ascites, varices and bleeding, encephalopathy, and hepatocellular carcinoma.[29]

Acute viral hepatitis is diagnosed on serology and clinical findings rather than imaging because the imaging findings are nonspecific. On US, there usually is hepatomegaly with increased echogenicity of the portal triad resulting in the starry night pattern.[29] On CT and MR, hepatomegaly and periportal edema may be seen, which appears as low attenuation around the portal triads on CT and high signal areas on T2-weighted images on MR.[29] Extrahepatic findings include diffuse gallbladder wall thickening and possible ascites.[29] A normal-appearing liver on imaging does not exclude acute hepatitis.

VASCULAR
Budd-Chiari Syndrome

Budd-Chiari syndrome comprises several disorders that can cause venous outflow obstruction of the liver, with the most common cause a clotting disorder. Malignant causes also are possible and typically involve invasion of the hepatic veins and/or inferior vena cava (IVC) (**Fig. 7**). Obstruction may occur at the level of the hepatic veins, IVC, or right atrium. Partial or complete obstruction may occur, resulting in increased sinusoidal pressure leading to portal hypertension, hepatic congestion, and reduced perfusion.[30] Budd-Chiari syndrome has a variable presentation depending on

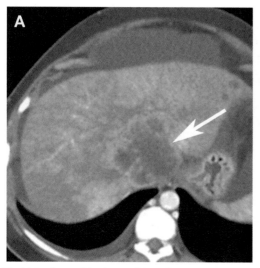 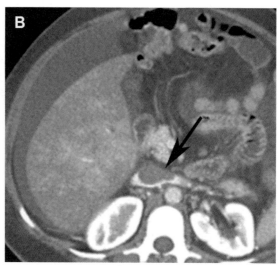

Fig. 7. Patient with elevated liver function tests and abdominal pain found to have Budd-Chiari syndrome. Axial CT images show a heterogeneously enhancing intrahepatic mass (*A* [*arrow*]) compressing the hepatic veins with resulting thrombus formation in the infrahepatic IVC (*B* [*arrow*]). Note the heterogeneous enhancement with diffuse edema of the hepatic parenchyma.

whether it is acute, subacute, or chronic. In the acute form, patients may present with jaundice and encephalopathy.[30]

Imaging of Budd-Chiari syndrome may reveal many different findings. On US, Doppler may be obtained to assess the hepatic veins for the presence and direction of flow. Gray-scale sonography also may demonstrate changes in hepatic echotexture and caudate lobe enlargement.[30] In the acute form, CT may demonstrate findings of hepatomegaly, suggesting congestion, and decreased attenuation, which may be secondary to edema.[30] Hypoattenuating thrombus also may be seen in the hepatic veins.[30] The corresponding MR imaging shows T1 signal loss with T2 hyperintensity, particularly in the periphery, where edema is most significant. Administration of contrast may reveal a similar distribution of decreased peripheral enhancement, where edema and congestion is most severe, with maintained central enhancement.[30] Contrast-enhanced images also may demonstrate compensatory hypertrophy and enhancement of the caudate lobe due to preservation of its veins, which directly drain into the IVC.[30]

Portal Vein Thrombosis

Although rare in the healthy population, portal venous thrombosis is not uncommon in cirrhotic patients. This is due mainly to factors, such as hypercoagulability and reduced portal venous flow, in these patients. Thrombus can occur in the portal vein exclusively or extend into the superior mesenteric and splenic veins.[31,32]

Portal venous thrombosis can be asymptomatic. Symptomatic patients may present with abdominal pain, nausea, vomiting diarrhea, gastrointestinal hemorrhage, and fever.[31] In the acute setting, work-up of these patients may begin with US, which may demonstrate thrombus within the portal vein. Application of Doppler US may also show absence of flow. Contrast-enhanced CT or MR imaging is often obtained after an US in order to determine extent of thrombosis. CT also may offer the added benefit of assessing bowel for ischemia in the presence of extensive superior mesenteric venous thrombosis.[31,32]

Portal vein thrombophlebitis usually is secondary to an ascending infection, usually originating from a gastrointestinal source, including diverticulitis, cholangitis, pancreatitis, appendicitis, and inflammatory bowel disease.[32] Patients may present with abdominal pain. Portal vein thrombophlebitis has a mortality rate up to 50%, given the associated complications, including bowel ischemia, hepatic abscess formation, and sepsis.[32] Imaging findings include thrombus in the portal vein on contrast-enhanced CT or MR as well as hepatic abscesses (**Fig. 8**).

NEOPLASM

Malignancy as a cause of acute hepatobiliary dysfunction presents with symptoms of biliary obstruction or hepatic congestion. Tumors may be primary, most commonly hepatocellular

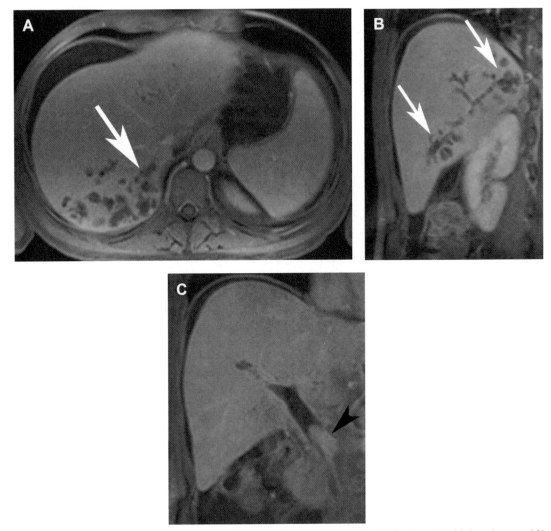

Fig. 8. Patient presenting with abdominal pain found to have gastrointestinal infection. Axial (*A*) and coronal (*B, C*) MR postgadolinium images with fat-saturation images show portal vein thrombophlebitis with a thrombus in the portal vein (*arrowhead*) with multiple intrahepatic abscesses (*arrows*).

carcinoma or cholangiocarcinoma, metastatic, or directly extend from an adjacent organ. The role of imaging in these cases is to identify the tumor, assess involvement of the biliary tree, and detect the patency of the hepatic vasculature.[30,33]

Extrahepatic tumors, such as cholangiocarcinoma, pancreatic adenocarcinoma, and ampullary carcinoma, can present with painless jaundice, pruritis, and weight loss. These tumors infiltrate or directly compress the common duct causing upstream ductal dilatation, which can be seen on US, CT, or MRCP. Tumors that are located very distally in the biliary tree also can cause obstruction and dilatation of the pancreatic duct creating the appearance of a double duct sign.[21] Klatskin tumors are more proximal and are located at the confluence of the left and right hepatic ducts. Tumors at this level cause intrahepatic ductal dilatation whereas the common duct remains normal in caliber.[34] As with biliary obstruction from gallstone disease, complications, such as cholangitis, cholecystitis, and pancreatitis, also can result from these tumors. In these patients, symptoms also may include fever and pain.

Intrahepatic tumors, such as hepatocellular carcinoma and metastases, can present with milder symptoms, such as dull pain, jaundice, and encephalopathy, to liver failure.[30,34] These tumors can cause obstruction of venous outflow by direct invasion of the hepatic veins, leading to hepatic congestion. Elevated pressure in the sinusoids can result in decreased hepatocyte perfusion and ultimately necrosis. Similarly, primary tumors in adjacent organs, such the kidney, adrenal, and heart, also may invade the IVC or hepatic veins and cause symptoms through a similar mechanism.[30]

POSTOPERATIVE/POSTPROCEDURAL COMPLICATIONS
Cholecystectomy

Cholecystectomy can be performed using a laparoscopic or open approach. Although the open approach is associated with a lower postoperative complication rate, the laparoscopic approach is favored given improved cosmesis, faster recover times, and patient comfort.[35] Complications of either approach include bile leak, dropped stones, retained stones, bleeding, and abscesses (**Fig. 9**).[2,35] Given that imaging is required for identification of injury and treatment planning, work-up often entails a multimodality approach.[36]

Many imaging options are available for detection of postoperative complications. HIDA scan is a highly accurate modality for detection of bile leak but is limited by low spatial resolution and, therefore, poor localization of injury. CT and US are excellent for identification of fluid collections and assessment of ductal dilatation. When collections are identified, neither modality can prove the presence of a bile leak given that they may alternative represent hematoma, abscess, or postoperative seroma. CT has the added benefit of being able to detect vascular injury and to identify dropped calcified gallstones (**Fig. 10**). MRCP can

identify fluid collections and with the administration of intravenous contrast allows for the evaluation of vascular injury. If a hepatobiliary agent is used, an excretory phase of imaging may also be obtained for detection and localization of biliary leak.[36] MRCP also may be used to assess for retained stones in the biliary tree.[2]

Transarterial Chemoembolization

Transarterial chemoembolization (TACE) involves administration of a chemotherapeutic agent and thrombogenic material into select branches of the hepatic artery that supply tumors. Although this method of drug delivery is very effective against tumors, it also may cause ischemia of the biliary tree, given that the peribiliary capillary plexus also arises from branches of the hepatic artery.[37,38]

Ischemia of the biliary tree results in necrosis of biliary epithelium, allowing bile to leak and form bilomas. Bilomas are the most common post-TACE complication and may present emergently if they become superinfected by enteric flora and form abscesses. Abscesses may also form when enteric flora superinfects necrotic tumor.[37] In either scenario, CT or MR imaging may be required for diagnosis. Another complication that may result from biliary ischemia is formation of strictures. These strictures tend to form after repeated TACE procedures and typically involve large bile ducts. Patients with post-TACE strictures may present with jaundice although prolonged biliary stasis from these strictures also may result in cholangitis.[37,38]

Transplant

Liver transplantation is first-line treatment of end-stage liver disease. Complications after liver transplantation include rejection, vascular, and biliary complications. Other complications, which may be seen with any surgery, include hematoma, infection, and abscess.[39,40] Rejection, which is the most common complication, is a clinical diagnosis and does not require imaging. Imaging may be obtained, however, to rule out complications that may simulate rejection.[39,41]

Assessment of vascular and biliary complications requires a multimodality approach. Initial investigation should be performed with US. Doppler evaluation of the hepatic vasculature should be performed.[39,40] The hepatic artery thrombosis is the most common post-transplantation vascular complication, accounting for more than half of the post-transplant vascular complications.[39,41] Hepatic artery stenosis occurs in 10% of liver transplants and the

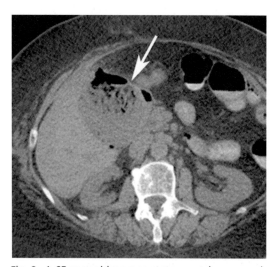

Fig. 9. A 65-year-old woman status post–laparoscopic cholecystectomy. Axial CT image shows a large complex fluid and air collection in the gallbladder fossa (*arrow*), which developed 11 days after surgery. The collection was successfully drained percutaneously.

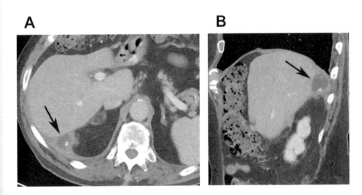

Fig. 10. An 82-year-old man status post–laparoscopic cholecystectomy with dropped gallstones. Axial (A) and sagittal (B) CT images show a peripherally enhancing fluid collection along the posterior inferior margin of the liver containing a calcified gallstone (arrows).

stenosis occurs most commonly at the anastomosis (**Fig. 11**).[39,41] The hepatic artery should be assessed for thrombosis, stenosis, and pseudoaneurysm. Hepatic artery thrombosis should raise concern for biliary ischemia and necrosis, which can subsequently lead to biloma and abscess formation, as discussed previously. Intrahepatic pseudoaneurysms may rupture and/or cause fistulas with the portal vein or biliary tree.[39] Complications of the portal veins, hepatic veins and IVC

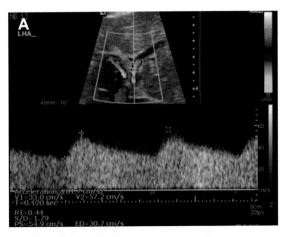

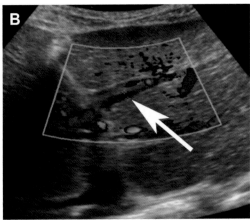

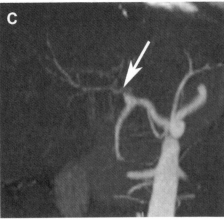

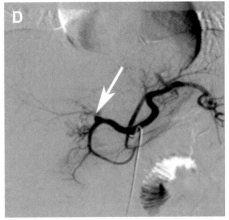

Fig. 11. Abnormal liver function tests in a transplant recipient. Spectral waveforms (A) demonstrate a tardus parvus waveform with a high velocity of 201 cm/s^2 (normal <200 cm/s^2) and US with color Doppler (B) shows decreased flow in the heaptic artery (arrow). CT angiography maximum intensity projection image (C) illustrates a focal stenosis of the hepatic artery at the anastomosis (arrow), which was confirmed and dilated on angiography (D [arrow]).

include stenosis and thrombosis.[39–41] Cases of hepatic venous or IVC thrombosis can be complicated by Budd-Chiari, discussed previously. Any abnormality on US should be confirmed with CT or MR imaging because it is more accurate for detection of thrombus and may detect parenchymal abnormalities.[39,41]

Biliary complications of liver transplant include biliary obstruction and bile leak.[40] US can be performed to assess for biliary ductal dilation, biliary obstruction, presence of a fluid collection, and presence of a biliary leak. Biliary obstruction may be due to either choledocholithiasis or biliary strictures. Strictures forming at the anastomosis are due to fibrosis and are the most common cause of biliary obstruction. Nonanastomotic strictures may also form as a result of ischemia. In all cases of biliary obstruction, MRCP should be performed for definitive diagnosis. Biliary leak commonly occurs at the anastomosis and may be difficult to differentiate from other postoperative fluid collections on US or CT. Definitive diagnosis may require MRCP with hepatobiliary contrast or HIDA scan.[39,41]

SUMMARY

Acute hepatobiliary dysfunction typically presents with right upper quadrant pain, fever, and occasionally jaundice. It has a broad differential consisting of infectious, inflammatory, vascular, and neoplastic etiologies. Additional considerations include immune status and recent procedures or surgery. Irrespective of etiology, work-up often requires a multimodality approach beginning with US. US is an excellent screening tool to assess for biliary ductal dilatation, cholelithiasis, and fluid collections. Depending on clinical presentation and US findings, CT, MR imaging, and HIDA can be considered for further evaluation. CT is an excellent modality for assessing hepatic parenchyma whereas MR imaging can offer complementary information. CT angiography and MR angiography can be considered when trying to assess for vascular complications. MRCP is the best noninvasive modality for delineation of the biliary tree. HIDA scan may be performed when US and CT are equivocal for cholecystitis or when there is suspicion for bile leak.

REFERENCES

1. Weiss AJ, Wier LM, Stocks C, et al. Overview of emergency department visits in the United States, 2011: Statistical Brief #174. Healthcare Cost and Utilization Project (HCUP) Statistical Briefs [Internet]. Rockville (MD): Agency for Healthcare Research and Quality (US); 2006–2014.
2. Chung AYA, Duke MC. Acute biliary disease. Surg Clin North Am 2018;98(5):877–94.
3. Walshe TM, Bao MBB, Rcsi FFR, et al. Infection, inflammation and infiltration. Appl Radiol 2016;4: 20–6.
4. Moparty B, Carr-Locke DL. Biliary emergencies. In: Tham T, Collins J, Soetikno R, editors. Gastrointestinal emergencies. 2nd edition. Blackwell Publishing; 2009. p. 134–40.
5. O'Connor OJ, O'Neill S, Maher MM. Imaging of Biliary Tract Disease Owen. Am J Roentgenol 2011;197(4):W551–8.
6. Wilkins T, Agabin E, Varghese J, et al. Gallbladder dysfunction: cholecystitis, choledocholithiasis, cholangitis, and biliary dyskinesia. Prim Care 2017; 44(4):575–97.
7. Gurusamy K. Gallstones. Br Med J 2014;348:1–6.
8. Ralls PW, Colletti PM, Lapin SA, et al. Real-time sonography in suspected acute cholecystitis. Prospective evaluation of primary and secondary signs. Radiology 1985;155(3):767–71.
9. O'Connor OJ, Maher MM. Imaging of cholecystitis. Am J Roentgenol 2011;196(4):W367–74.
10. Shakespear JS, Shaaban AM, Rezvani M. CT findings of acute cholecystitis and its complications. Am J Roentgenol 2010;194(6):1523–9.
11. Chen A, Liu A, Wang S, et al. Detection of gallbladder stones by dual-energy spectral computed tomography imaging. World J Gastroenterol 2015; 21(34):9993–8.
12. Gupta A, LeBedis CA, Uyeda J, et al. Diffusion-weighted imaging of the pericholecystic hepatic parenchyma for distinguishing acute and chronic cholecystitis. Emerg Radiol 2018;25(1):7–11.
13. Wang A, Shanbhogue AK, Dunst D, et al. Utility of diffusion-weighted MRI for differentiating acute from chronic cholecystitis. J Magn Reson Imaging 2016;44(1):89–97.
14. Chamarthy M, Freeman LM. Hepatobiliary scan findings in chronic cholecystitis. Clin Nucl Med 2010; 35(4):244–51.
15. Barie PS, Eachempati SR. Acute calculous cholecystitis. Gastroenterol Clin North Am 2010;39(2): 343–57.
16. Treinen C, Lomelin D, Krause C, et al. Acute acalculous cholecystitis in the critically ill: risk factors and surgical strategies. Langenbecks Arch Surg 2015; 400(4):421–7.
17. Jeffrey R, Laing F, Wong W, et al. Gangrenous cholecystitis: diagnosis by ultrasound. Radiology 1983; 148:219–21.
18. Ratanaprasatporn L, Uyeda JW, Wortman JR, et al. Multimodality imaging, including dual-energy CT, in the evaluation of gallbladder disease. Radiographics 2018;38(1):75–89.

19. Kang T, Kim S, Park H, et al. Differentiating xanthogranulomatous cholecystitis from wall-thickening type of gallbladder cancer: added value of diffusion-weighted MRI. Clin Radiol 2013;68(10):992–1001.

20. Attasaranya S, Fogel EL, Lehman GA. Choledocholithiasis, ascending cholangitis, and gallstone pancreatitis. Med Clin North Am 2008;92(4):925–60.

21. Yeh BM, Liu PS, Soto JA, et al. MR imaging and CT of the biliary tract. RadioGraphics 2009;29(6): 1669–88.

22. Yu HS, Gupta A, Soto JA, et al. Emergency abdominal MRI: current uses and trends. Br J Radiol 2016; 89(1061):20150804.

23. Chen H, Siwo E, Khu M, et al. Current trends in the management of Mirizzi syndrome. Medicine (Baltimore) 2018;97(4):1–7.

24. Bali MA, Pezzullo M, Pace E, et al. Benign biliary diseases. Eur J Radiol 2017;93(May 2017):217–28.

25. Silveira MG, Lindor KD. Primary sclerosing cholangitis. Can J Gastroenterol 2008;22(8):689–98.

26. Catalano OA, Sahani DV, Forcione DG, et al. Biliary infections: spectrum of imaging findings and management. Radiographics 2009;29(7): 2059–80.

27. Pakala T, Molina M, Wu GY. Hepatic echinococcal cysts: a review. J Clin Transl Hepatol 2016;4(1): 39–46.

28. Bilgin M, Balci NC, Erdogan A, et al. Hepatobiliary and pancreatic MRI and MRCP findings in patients with HIV infection. Am J Roentgenol 2008;191(1): 228–32.

29. Mortele KJ, Segatto E, Ros PR. The infected liver: radiologic-pathologic correlation. Radiographics 2004;24:937–55.

30. Brancatelli G, Vilgrain V, Federle MP, et al. Budd-Chiari syndrome: spectrum of imaging findings. Am J Roentgenol 2007;188(2):168–76.

31. Von Kockritz L, De Gottardi A, Trebicka J, et al. Portal vein thrombosis in patients with cirrhosis. Gastroenterol Rep (Oxf) 2017;5:148–56.

32. Jha RC, Khera SS, Kalaria AD. Portal vein thrombosis: imaging the spectrum of disease with an emphasis on MRI features. Am J Roentgenol 2018; 211:14–24.

33. Watanabe Y, Nagayama M, Okumura A, et al. MR Imaging of acute biliary disorders. Radiographics 2007;27:477–95.

34. Anderson C, Pinson C, Berlin J, et al. Diagnosis and treatment of cholangiocarcinoma. Oncologist 2004; 9:43–57.

35. Vollmer C, Callery M. Biliary injury following laparoscopic cholecystectomy: why still a problem? Gastroenterology 2007;133(3):1039–45.

36. Thompson CM, Saad NE, Quazi RR, et al. Management of iatrogenic bile duct injuries: role of the interventional radiologist. Radiographics 2013;33(1): 117–34.

37. Clark T. Complications of hepatic chemoembolization. Semin Intervent Radiol 2006;23(2):119–25.

38. Kim HK, Chung YH, Song BC, et al. Ischemic bile duct injury as a serious complication after transarterial chemoembolization in patients with hepatocellular carcinoma. J Clin Gastroenterol 2001;32(5): 423–7.

39. Singh AK, Nachiappan AC, Verma HA, et al. Postoperative imaging in liver transplantation: what radiologists should know. Radiographics 2010;30(2): 339–51.

40. Moreno R, Berenguer M. Post-liver transplantation medical complications. Ann Hepatol 2006;5(2): 77–85.

41. Caiado A, Blasbalg R, Marcelino A, et al. Complications of liver transplantation: multimodality imaging approach. Radiographics 2007;27:1401–17.

Imaging of Acute Renal Failure in the Hospital Setting

Mostafa Alabousi, MD[a], Abdullah Alabousi, MD, FRCPC[b],
Michael N. Patlas, MD, FRCPC, FCAR, FSAR[c],*

KEYWORDS

- Acute kidney injury • Ultrasonography • Tomography • X-ray computed • MR imaging
- Nuclear medicine

KEY POINTS

- Acute kidney injury affects up to 20% of hospitalized patients, and is even more common among intensive care unit admissions.
- Ultrasonography serves as the first-choice imaging modality for renal assessment, and can provide valuable information, including differentiating acute from chronic kidney injury.
- Computed tomography is the second-choice imaging modality, because it can identify obstructive, infectious, and ischemic causes of acute kidney injury, as well as delineate disease chronicity.
- Magnetic resonance imaging may be useful in pregnant and young patients, because it can provide much of the same information as computed tomography without radiation exposure.
- Ultrasonography and nuclear medicine imaging can help evaluate acute kidney injury in transplant recipients and identify causes, including rejection, acute tubular necrosis, and drug nephrotoxicity.

INTRODUCTION

Acute kidney injury (AKI), previously known as acute renal failure, is a condition characterized by a decline in the glomerular filtration rate (GFR) over a short course (hours to days) resulting in azotemia.[1–4] Although debated, multiple definitions have emerged from groups such as the Acute Dialysis Initiative, the Acute Kidney Injury Network, and the Kidney Disease: Improving Global Outcomes group.[1,5,6] However, the clinical presentation generally consists of an increase in creatinine level and, in some cases, oliguria or anuria.[1–4] AKI usually occurs in the setting of acute and chronic diseases, and is common in the hospital setting, affecting up to 20% of hospitalized patients, as well as up to 36% to 60% of admissions to the intensive care unit (ICU).[1,2,7–9]

The causes of AKI are often divided into prerenal, renal, and postrenal categories.[3] Prerenal causes of AKI are the result of hypoperfusion or hypovolemia, including decreased intake, vomiting, diarrhea, blood loss, heart failure, hepatorenal syndrome, sepsis, and less commonly renal artery stenosis and thrombosis.[2,3,10] The most common renal or intrinsic cause of AKI is acute tubular necrosis (ATN).[10] However, other renal causes include glomerular, interstitial, and small-vessel diseases, which may be secondary to vasculitis, infection, or drug reaction, among other causes.[3] Postrenal causes of AKI are obstructive, such as nephrolithiasis, malignancy, and benign prostatic

Disclosure: Dr M.N. Patlas received an honorarium from Springer. The other authors have nothing to disclose.
[a] Department of Radiology, McMaster University, 1200 Main St W, Hamilton, ON L8S 4L8, Canada;
[b] Department of Radiology, St. Joseph's Healthcare Hamilton, McMaster University, Hamilton, 50 Charlton Ave E, Hamilton, ON L8N 4A6, Canada; [c] Department of Radiology, McMaster University, Hamilton General Hospital, 237 Barton St E, Hamilton, ON L8L 2X2, Canada
* Corresponding author.
E-mail address: patlas@hhsc.ca

Radiol Clin N Am 58 (2020) 59–71
https://doi.org/10.1016/j.rcl.2019.08.001
0033-8389/20/© 2019 Elsevier Inc. All rights reserved.

hyperplasia.[1–3] Regardless of the cause, AKI may lead to complications caused by uremia (encephalopathy, neuropathy, pericarditis), volume overload (dyspnea, pulmonary edema), and electrolyte disturbances (hyperkalemia).[1,10] These complications are associated with increased mortality in patients who develop AKI.[11] Furthermore, some patients never fully recover their baseline renal function, and may ultimately need long-term dialysis.[12] Of course, this common entity has a great impact on patient outcomes, length of hospital stay, and cost of care.[1,2,10]

Although an acute increase in creatinine level is key to the diagnosis of AKI, imaging of the kidneys can provide valuable information for the work-up and management of AKI. Different imaging modalities can be used to evaluate renal anatomy, evaluate renal perfusion, rule out urinary tract obstruction, as well as assess for signs of renal inflammation and edema.[4,11] This article discusses the utility of the different imaging modalities in characterizing AKI in adults, including ultrasonography (US), computed tomography (CT), magnetic resonance (MR) imaging, and nuclear medicine imaging.

ULTRASONOGRAPHY

The first-choice imaging modality for the kidneys in the context of AKI is US, specifically two-dimensional (2D) gray-scale US, given its ease of use, noninvasiveness, accessibility, low cost, and excellent safety profile.[13,14] Advances in imaging technology have further improved visualization of the kidneys with US.[13,14] Furthermore, portable US provides an advantage for imaging critically ill patients in the ICU.[4,13] Although only approximately 10% of renal US examinations show abnormal findings related to AKI, these can have a significant impact on guiding patient management. A normal US also helps guide management by excluding major structural abnormalities.[13]

Size

Kidney size can help differentiate acute from chronic kidney disease (CKD).[3,13,14] Small or atrophic kidneys are often seen with CKD, in which case the patient's renal function is unlikely to fully recover (Fig. 1).[3,13,15] Enlarged kidneys may suggest an infiltrative disease process, including lymphoma and monoclonal gammopathies.[3,15] Other causes of enlarged kidneys in the setting of AKI include pyelonephritis, ATN, acute interstitial nephritis, and acute proliferative glomerulonephritis (GN).[13,15] A rarer cause of an enlarged kidney is renal vein thrombosis.[3,13] In renal transplant patients, an enlarged kidney may be seen in the setting of acute rejection (sensitivity and specificity >80%).[3,13,16]

Echogenicity

Parenchymal echogenicity of the kidneys is compared with the adjacent liver and spleen and can also help characterize AKI. Markedly increased renal cortical echogenicity is seen in CKD (see Fig. 1). Infiltrative diseases, such as ATN, monoclonal gammopathy, as well as proliferative and crescentic GN, show increased renal cortical echogenicity and loss of the normal corticomedullary differentiation (Fig. 2).[17,18] In contrast, renal parenchymal edema appears hypoechoic on US. Pyelonephritis can be seen as decreased renal cortical echogenicity with loss of the corticomedullary differentiation, but may also appear as a focus of masslike enlargement or increased echogenicity as well.[13,19] More focal hypoechoic foci/fluid collections in the context of suspected pyelonephritis can be seen in the setting of abscess formation (Fig. 3).[19] The presence of a hypoechoic band surrounding the kidney may be seen in the setting of acute cortical necrosis.[13]

Cortical Thickness

Cortical thickness can also help differentiate AKI from CKD, whereby the latter should result in decreased cortical thickness (see Fig. 1).[13] Increased cortical thickness is generally seen with edema or infiltrative diseases, including ATN, acute GN, and acute interstitial nephritis.[17] However, given that there is no established normal cutoff for cortical thickness, a baseline US scan is required to adequately detect disorder and assess for changes in patients with declining renal function.

Obstruction

US can be used to detect signs of obstruction involving the renal collecting system, ureters, or bladder. This is one of the most important causes of AKI to diagnose by imaging because the treatment is typically centered on relieving the obstruction by catheter placement, stenting, or urinary diversion. Hydronephrosis, manifested with calyceal dilatation on US, can be seen in the context of nephrolithiasis (Fig. 4), or a urinary outlet obstruction caused by an intrinsic or extrinsic cause such as a mass.[10,20,21] Calyceal dilatation may also be secondary to urinary tract infection, physiologic dilatation in pregnancy, and in patients with diabetes insipidus.[22,23] Doppler imaging may also be used to assess for obstruction, with the unilateral absence of a ureteric jet suggesting obstruction.[3,21]

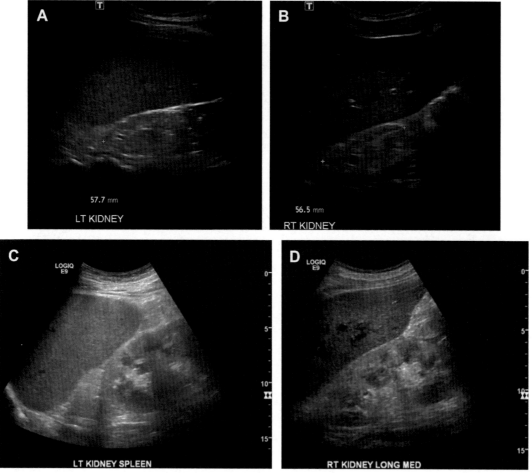

Fig. 1. US findings of CKD, including bilateral decreased kidney size and cortical thickness, on longitudinal images of the left (*A*) and right (*B*) kidneys. In another patient, US findings of chronic kidney disease, including markedly increased cortical echogenicity and cortical thinning on longitudinal images of the left (*C*) and right (*D*) kidneys. ([*C, D*] *Courtesy of* Vincent M. Mellnick, MD, Mallinckrodt Institute of Radiology, St.Louis, MO, USA.)

Renal Doppler

Doppler US can provide valuable information on renal blood flow. Doppler US can determine the resistive index (RI) (peak systolic velocity – peak diastolic velocity/peak systolic velocity) within the main renal arteries and smaller branches.[24] Although some studies have found a higher RI is associated with intrarenal causes of AKI, such as ATN and vasculitis, variability caused by body habitus and an increasing RI with the patient's age makes this measure less reliable.[25] For example, 1 study comparing patients with ATN and prerenal AKI found that 96% of patients with ATN had an RI greater than 0.70. However, there were several false-negative examinations in patients with nephrotoxic drug-induced ATN.[26] More recent studies have found an association between an increased RI (>0.74) in sepsis-associated AKI[27] and post–cardiac surgery AKI,[28] as well as persistent AKI in the ICU (RI>0.795).[24] These findings may set the foundation for using the RI as a predictor for critical care patients at high risk for AKI.[29] Color Doppler may also be useful in evaluating the renal

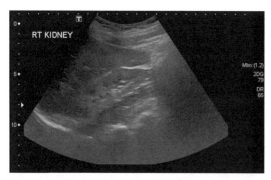

Fig. 2. US findings of increased renal echogenicity, which may be seen in ATN, monoclonal gammopathy, as well as proliferative and crescentic GN.

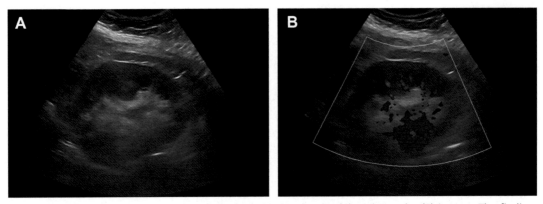

Fig. 3. US findings of pyelonephritis in a transplanted kidney on 2D (*A*) and Doppler (*B*) images. The findings, including decreased cortical echogenicity, echogenic renal sinus fat, and increased Doppler flow, are seen in the context of infection.

parenchyma. For example, pyelonephritis typically presents with decreased color flow in the affected portions of the kidney. Urolithiasis, either in the renal parenchyma or more distally in the urinary tract, may be more conspicuous with color Doppler imaging as well because of so-called twinkling artifact (see **Fig. 4**).

Contrast

US contrast agents have been found to be safe for use even in patients with increased creatinine level and AKI/CKD. They essentially behave like red blood cells, allowing assessment of the renal vasculature.[20,30] Contrast-enhanced US (CEUS) can provide an estimate of red blood cell velocity, as well as regional changes in renal blood flow to aid in the work-up of AKI.[20,29,31] Studies in healthy patients have found CEUS to be promising in quantifying renal blood flow and assessing changes in flow, and thus may play a future role

in characterizing AKI.[32–34] Furthermore, a more recent study has found CEUS allows dynamic assessment of renal perfusion impairment, which may serve as a predictor of progression from AKI to CKD.[31]

Renal Transplant

US is generally the first-line imaging test for assessment of renal transplant patients, particularly in the context of a increasing creatinine level.[35] A diminished renal function may be the result of hyperacute, acute (**Fig. 5**), or chronic rejection (**Fig. 6**), among other causes that may also occur in the native kidney, such as ATN and drug nephrotoxicity.[35] US may show a variety of different findings in the context of AKI, including increased size of the kidney, increased or decreased cortical echogenicity, loss of corticomedullary differentiation, prominent pyramids, thickening of the collecting system, and

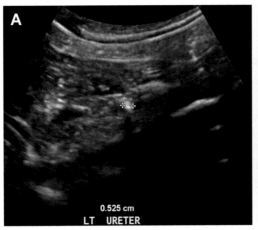

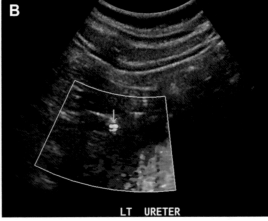

Fig. 4. US findings of a midureteric renal calculus on 2D (*A*) and Doppler (*B*) images. The stone seems echogenic with posterior shadowing on the 2D-image, with twinkle artifact (*arrow*) evident on Doppler.

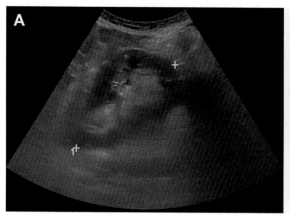

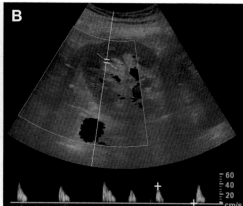

Fig. 5. US findings of acute renal transplant rejection (postoperative day 10) on 2D (*A*) and Doppler (*B*) images showing an increasing RI (R = 1.00) with high-resistance systolic flow and loss of diastolic flow.

effacement of the central sinus echo complex.[35] In the setting of chronic transplant rejection, thinning of the renal cortex and mild hydronephrosis may be seen.[35] Furthermore, Doppler US may be used for assessment of renal transplants, with an RI greater than 0.8 being a nonspecific indicator of renal transplant dysfunction.[3,29,35] Reversal of diastolic flow may also be seen with chronic rejection, but is much less common.[35]

COMPUTED TOMOGRAPHY

Abdominal and pelvic CT can serve as a valuable second-line imaging test for assessing patients with AKI when the initial US is inconclusive. Although the topic is much debated, the use of intravenous (IV) contrast for a CT scan is avoided whenever possible in the setting of AKI.[36,37] The findings of both unenhanced CT (UECT) and contrast-enhanced CT (CECT) are discussed, because contrast administration can provide rele-vant additional information on the renal paren-chyma and corticomedullary differentiation.

Size

Similar to US, renal size can help differentiate AKI and CKD, as well as provide useful information related to infiltrative disease, pyelonephritis, ATN, renal vein thrombosis, and acute rejection in transplant patients, as described earlier.

Obstruction

An unenhanced CT scan of the abdomen and pelvis can detect nephrolithiasis leading to obstructive AKI.[21] This finding is especially impor-tant in the setting of a solitary kidney or bilateral obstructive nephrolithiasis (**Fig. 7**). A CT scan can also show findings of hydronephrosis, hydro-ureter, as well as perinephric and periureteric stranding in the context of nephrolithiasis, even after a stone has passed.[21,38,39] This finding may

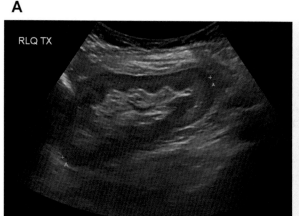

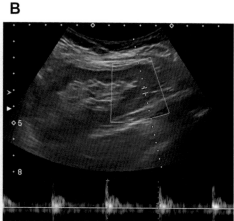

Fig. 6. US findings of chronic renal transplant rejection (5 years posttransplant) with gradually increased renal cortical echogenicity and atrophy on 2D images (*A*), and an increasing RI (R = 0.84) on Doppler images (*B*).

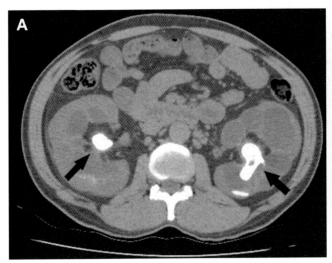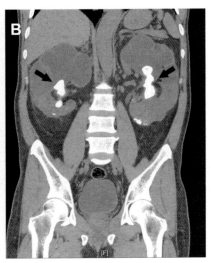

Fig. 7. UECT shows bilateral obstructive staghorn calculi (*arrows*) on axial (*A*) and coronal (*B*) images with resulting bilateral hydronephrosis and increased renal size.

be particularly useful in the context of a negative or inconclusive/nondiagnostic initial renal US scan; for example, one that shows hydronephrosis but no definite obstructive stone.[21,38,39]

Nearly every type of renal calculus can be detected on CT, with the exception of indinavir-associated stones.[13] However, although determining renal calculus composition was previously only possible following stone extraction, the introduction of dual-energy CT (DECT) has provided an alternative, reliable, noninvasive method for this.[40] DECT uses the differences in attenuation produced by 2 different x-ray energy levels to determine stone composition; for example, whether a stone is composed of uric acid or not.[40,41] This information can help guide patient management, but may be limited by pitfalls, such as stone size (<3 mm).[40]

Other potential causes of obstruction may be further downstream in the renal collecting system. Urothelial malignancy or strictures may result in AKI. Alternatively, a malignant process either intrinsic or extrinsic to the bladder may invade and occlude the ureteric insertion sites into the bladder, resulting in hydronephrosis and AKI (Fig. 8).[40,41] Common examples include transitional cell carcinoma as well as direct extension of gynecologic tumors.

Infection

If IV contrast is used, it may provide additional information related to the cause of AKI. For instance, CECT is preferred to US in assessing for pyelonephritis in patients who are diabetic, elderly, immunocompromised, or who fail to respond to antibiotics within 72 hours.[42] Infection within the kidney can result in tubular obstruction secondary to luminal debris, interstitial edema, and vasospasm.[19] This finding is reflected on the nephrographic phase of CECT by 1 or more wedge-shaped areas extending from the renal papilla to the cortex showing decreased enhancement relative to the normal renal parenchyma.[19] The alternating bands of decreased and normal parenchymal enhancement are known as the striated nephrogram (Fig. 9), also a classic feature of pyelonephritis.[19] Other signs to look for include perinephric stranding, thickening of Gerota fascia, and abscess formation.[42] The typical appearance for abscess is a rim-enhancing round collection with a fluid-filled center.[19] The additional presence of gas locules within renal parenchyma, on the background of infectious features, indicates emphysematous pyelonephritis, which needs prompt intervention, because it is rapidly progressive with a high associated mortality.[19] Emphysematous pyelitis is a less severe form, because it is an infectious process focused in the collecting system with sparing of the renal parenchyma (Fig. 10).[19] Thus, gas locules or gas-fluid levels are isolated to the collecting system.[19] The management of emphysematous pyelitis depends on whether or not ureteral obstruction is present and may warrant urgent decompression.

Ischemia

A UECT study of the abdomen and pelvis may be completely unremarkable with normal renal parenchyma and no obvious abnormality in the setting of ATN.[43] However, a persistent nephrogram may be visualized in some of those cases on CECT up to 24 hours after the contrast administration.[43] Renal

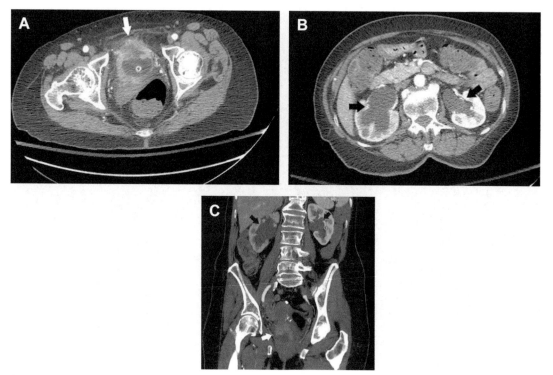

Fig. 8. CECT shows a bladder mass (*white arrows*) on axial (*A*) and coronal (*C*) images resulting in bilateral obstruction and hydronephrosis (*black arrows*) (*A, B*). Pathologic findings indicated transitional cell carcinoma.

infarction results from interrupted vascular flow, which may be secondary to trauma, shock, thromboembolic disease, among other causes.[44] Renal infarcts on CECT are classically wedge-shaped nonenhancing, peripheral lesions with an enhancing cortical rim (**Fig. 11**).[44] Acute cortical necrosis is a rare cause of AKI involving ischemic injury to the renal cortex caused by arterial insufficiency.[43] A UECT can show hyperattenuation of the renal cortex with hypoattenuation of the renal medulla.[43] Meanwhile, CECT shows hypoattenuation of the renal cortex with normally enhancing renal medulla, and potentially a subcapsular rim of normally enhancing tissue.[43] Patients with renal

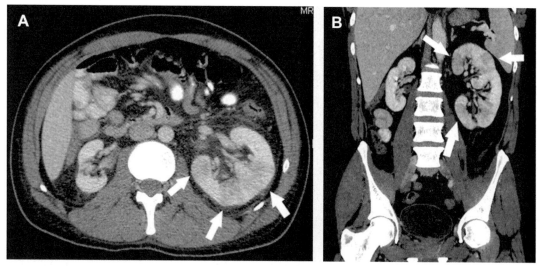

Fig. 9. CECT shows pyelonephritis in the left kidney on axial (*A*) and coronal (*B*) images with findings of a striated nephrogram (*arrows*), as well as an enlarged kidney.

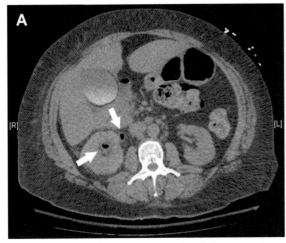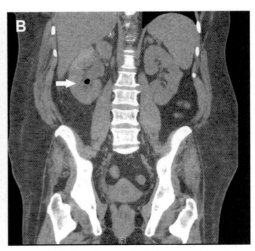

Fig. 10. UECT shows emphysematous pyelitis in the right kidney on axial (*A*) and coronal (*B*) images with findings of gas locules (*arrows*) within the collecting system.

papillary necrosis, which results from ischemia of the renal papilla, may also present with AKI.[43,45] UECT is often normal in those cases, whereas CECT shows areas of decreased enhancement at the medullary tip.[43,45] The delayed phase on a CT urogram may show a filling defect within the renal pelvis, corresponding with sloughed papilla, as well as extracalyceal contrast in the renal medulla with clubbed calyces.[43,45]

Other Considerations

An unenhanced abdominopelvic CT scan may identify other potential culprits leading to AKI, such as a leaking abdominal aortic aneurysm, or an infectious/inflammatory intra-abdominal process.[13] However, CECT improves diagnostic

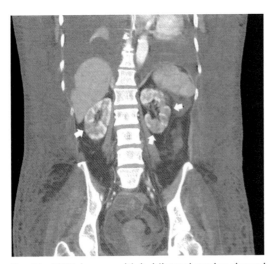

Fig. 11. CECT shows multiple bilateral wedge-shaped foci of hypoattenuation (*arrow*) in keeping with renal infarction on a coronal reconstruction.

accuracy for these, and is necessary to detect other causes of AKI, including malignancy, renal parenchymal disease, renal artery stenosis, and renal vein thrombosis.[13]

MAGNETIC RESONANCE IMAGING

Currently used MR imaging contrast agents are gadolinium based, which poses a rare potential risk of nephrogenic systemic fibrosis (NSF) if used in patients with AKI.[46] However, unenhanced MR imaging sequences can provide valuable information in the work-up for AKI. They may be particularly useful for patients who are pregnant, young, or for whom iodinated contrast is contraindicated.

Obstruction

Magnetic resonance urography with T2-weighted imaging (T2-WI) may be used in characterizing obstructive causes of AKI. Given that fluid appears bright on the T2-WI, hydronephrosis and hydroureter can be detected with high sensitivity (**Fig. 12**).[47] Although T2-WI is less sensitive than CT for identifying renal calculi, it can effectively detect secondary signs of obstruction.[47] A calcified renal or ureteric stone appears as a region of low T2 signal or signal void (**Fig. 13**), which suggests an obstructive stone when combined with findings of hydronephrosis and/or hydroureter proximally.[47,48] Furthermore, the presence of perinephric and/or periureteric edema also supports these findings.[48] Clinicians must be careful not to confuse findings of hydronephrosis with the physiologic appearance of the renal collecting system during pregnancy (**Fig. 14**).[47,48] In addition to stones, an alternative cause of obstructive AKI is external compression of any component of the

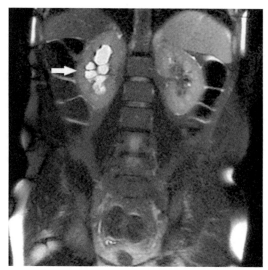

Fig. 12. T2-WI in a pregnant patient shows right-sided hydronephrosis (*arrow*) on a coronal image. The collecting system appears hyperintense on the T2WI sequence.

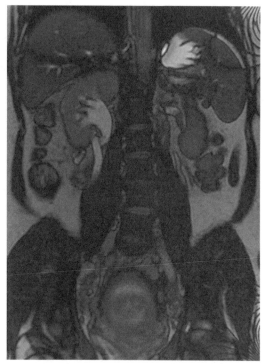

Fig. 14. T2-WI MR imaging shows the physiologic dilatation of the collecting system in a pregnant patient.

collecting system. For example, **Fig. 15** shows a large subserosal uterine fibroid that directly compresses the ureter, resulting in hydronephrosis.

Infection

MR imaging findings of pyelonephritis are similar to those of CT, and they include renal enlargement, edema, and potentially renal parenchymal abscess formation and perinephric collections.[19] Findings of inflammation and fluid collections

appear hyperintense on T2-WI and hypointense on T1-weighted imaging (T1-WI). Diffusion-weighted imaging (DWI) may also be useful in assessing for pyelonephritis, because a striated pattern of restricted diffusion is expected in the renal parenchyma.[47] Moreover, a renal abscess is represented by a fluid-filled cavity that shows restricted diffusion on DWI, as opposed to a renal cyst, for example (**Fig. 16**).[47] If a gadolinium-based contrast agent is administered, decreased enhancement in the regions of tubular obstruction and edema is expected, analogous to CT findings.[19,47] As a result, the affected regions have less of a signal decrease and appear hyperintense compared with the normal background of renal parenchyma.[19,47]

Ischemia and Other Causes

On MR imaging, acute cortical necrosis may show hypointensity of the renal cortex and columns of Bertin on both T1-WI and T2-WI.[43] Furthermore, a thin rim of subcapsular hyperintensity may also be seen on T2-WI.[43]

Future Applications in Magnetic Resonance Imaging

New iron-based contrast agents, including iron oxide, are being tested and have currently

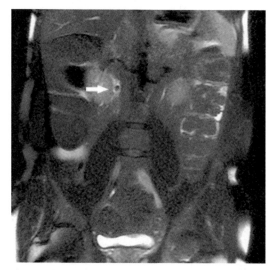

Fig. 13. T2-WI in a pregnant patient shows a right proximal ureteric stone (*arrow*) on a coronal image as a flow void artifact.

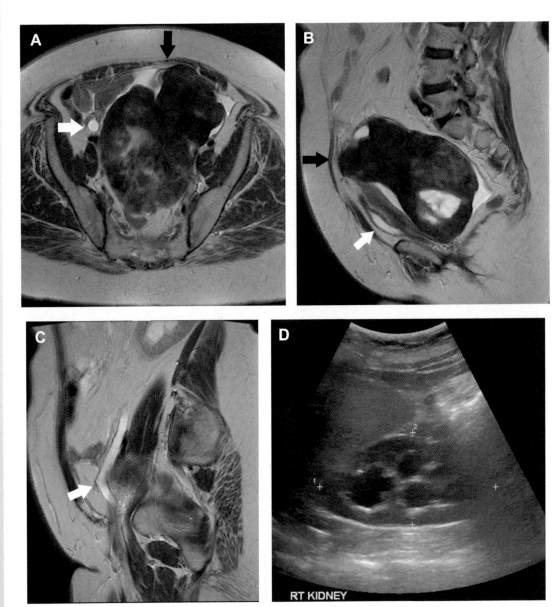

Fig. 15. T2-WI shows a large subserosal fibroid (*black arrow*) resulting in hydroureter (*white arrow*) on axial (*A*) and sagittal (*B, C*) images, as well as right-sided hydronephrosis on US (*D*).

shown safety while behaving similarly to gadolinium-based agents.[49,50] Studies have found that increased uptake of these new contrast agents can indicate inflammation, and this has been found in cases of GN and acute cellular rejection in renal transplants.[49,50] In addition, early studies have been performed investigating the utility of functional MR imaging in AKI: blood oxygen level–dependent, arterial spin labeling, dynamic contrast-enhanced, diffusion-weighted, intravoxel incoherent motion, diffusion tensor, and diffusion kurtosis imaging.[51,52] These techniques may play a future role in the characterization of AKI.

NUCLEAR MEDICINE

Nuclear medicine imaging is not commonly used to assess for AKI. Technetium-99m is most effective given its low radiation dose, with technetium-labeled mercaptoacetyltriglycine (MAG3) and diethylenetriamine pentaacetic acid (DTPA) used to assess renal blood flow and GFR, respectively.[13] Renal uptake of MAG3 is reduced in the first 1 to 2 minutes for intrarenal causes of AKI compared with prerenal causes.[13] After 20 minutes, renal uptake of MAG3 is expected to be normal for ATN, vascular, and prerenal AKI, but reduced in parenchymal disease and postrenal/obstructive AKI.[13]

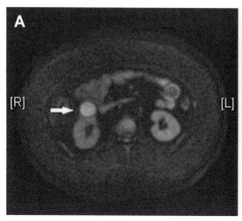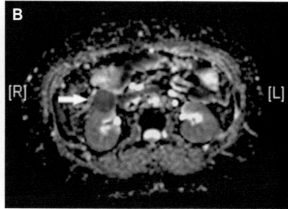

Fig. 16. Renal abscess in the right kidney (*arrows*), which is hyperintense on DWI (*A*) and shows diffusion restriction on apparent diffusion coefficient (*B*).

MAG3 excretion is reduced in all forms of AKI.[13] DTPA may help differentiate acute from chronic kidney injury. Given that GFR is more affected than renal blood flow in AKI, DTPA accumulation should be decreased in AKI.[3] Assessment of renal function using PET is not currently part of the standard practice, but is undergoing early clinical trials, and may play a future role in renal imaging.[53,54]

In the setting of renal transplant, nuclear medicine imaging may play a role in identifying causes of diminished renal function, such as ATN, rejection, and drug nephrotoxicity. Findings of ATN include delayed transit of MAG3, delayed time to maximal activity, and radionuclide retention within the parenchyma.[35] Similar to ATN, diminished flow is also seen in acute transplant rejection with radionuclide imaging, with the timing of these findings being the differentiating factor between the two.[35] Although ATN is the most common cause of delayed graft function requiring dialysis in the first week after transplant, acute transplant rejection rarely develops within the first few days after transplant.[35] A baseline scan is key for assessment of acute transplant rejection, because this manifests over serial radionuclide studies.[35] In the case of chronic transplant rejection, diminished radionuclide uptake is expected with normal parenchymal transit and minimal or absent retention within the cortex.[35] Advanced chronic transplant rejection may show radiotracer parenchymal retention.[35] Cyclosporine toxicity is similar in appearance to transplant rejection in both the acute and chronic stages, and these findings should be correlated with cyclosporine levels.[35]

SUMMARY

AKI commonly affects hospitalized patients, and ICU patients in particular, showing a significant burden on the health care system. It can lead to a higher morbidity and mortality in patients, if not treated appropriately and in a timely manner. This article discusses the role and value of imaging in patients with AKI. US is the imaging workhorse for the initial assessment of the kidneys, and can help differentiate AKI from CKD, as well as help further characterize the cause, especially in identifying postrenal causes and in renal transplant patients. UECT plays a more specific role in identifying nephrolithiasis in addition to signs of obstructive uropathy, whereas CECT can provide additional information in the context of infection, ischemia, and renal parenchymal disease, taking into account the risks of contrast administration. Meanwhile, MR imaging may be useful when initial US is negative for patients who are pregnant, or with a contraindication to iodinated contrast. Early trials using CEUS, MR imaging, and nuclear medicine imaging show promise and may play an important future role in imaging for AKI.

REFERENCES

1. Bellomo R, Kellum JA, Ronco C. Acute kidney injury. Lancet 2012;380(9843):756–66.
2. Levey AS, James MT. Acute kidney injury. Ann Intern Med 2017;167(9):ITC66.
3. Remer EM, Papanicolaou N, Casalino DD, et al. ACR appropriateness criteria® on renal failure. Am J Med 2014;127(11):1041–8.e1.
4. Pakula AM, Skinner RA. Acute kidney injury in the critically ill patient. J Intensive Care Med 2016; 31(5):319–24.
5. Bellomo R, Ronco C, Kellum JA, et al, Acute Dialysis Quality Initiative Workgroup. Acute renal failure - definition, outcome measures, animal models, fluid therapy and information technology needs: the Second International Consensus Conference of the

Acute Dialysis Quality Initiative (ADQI) Group. Crit Care 2004;8(4):R204–12.

6. The Kidney Disease Improving Global Outcomes (KDIGO) Working Group. Definition and classification of acute kidney injury. Kidney Int 2012;(suppl 2):19–36.

7. Kellum JA, Lameire N, Aspelin P, KDIGO (KDIGO) AKIWG. KDIGO clinical practice guideline for acute kidney injury. Kidney Int 2012;suppl 1:1–38.

8. Bagshaw SM, George C, Bellomo R, ANZICS Database Management Committee. Early acute kidney injury and sepsis: a multicentre evaluation. Crit Care 2008;12(2):R47.

9. Hoste EA, Clermont G, Kersten A, et al. RIFLE criteria for acute kidney injury are associated with hospital mortality in critically ill patients: a cohort analysis. Crit Care 2006;10(3):R73.

10. Kanagasundaram NS. Pathophysiology of ischaemic acute kidney injury. Ann Clin Biochem 2015; 52(2):193–205.

11. Bagshaw SM. Short- and long-term survival after acute kidney injury. Nephrol Dial Transplant 2008; 23(7):2126–8.

12. Bagshaw SM, George C, Dinu I, et al. A multi-centre evaluation of the RIFLE criteria for early acute kidney injury in critically ill patients. Nephrol Dial Transplant 2007;23(4):1203–10.

13. Kalantarinia K. Novel imaging techniques in acute kidney injury. Curr Drug Targets 2009;10(12): 1184–9. Available at: http://www.ncbi.nlm.nih.gov/pubmed/19715540. Accessed December 31, 2018.

14. Meola M, Nalesso F, Petrucci I, et al. Ultrasound in acute kidney disease. In: Meola M, Petruccil I, Ronco C, editors. Ultrasound Imaging in Acute and Chronic Kidney Disease. Contrib Nephrol, vol. 188. Basel (Switzerland): Karger; 2016. p. 11–20. https://doi.org/10.1159/000445461.

15. Pozzi Mucelli R, Bertolotto M, Quaia E. Imaging techniques in acute renal failure. Contrib Nephrol 2001;132:76–91. Available at: http://www.ncbi.nlm.nih.gov/pubmed/11395914. Accessed January 6, 2019.

16. Nicholson ML, Bell A, Burton PR, et al. Probability of rejection predicted from ultrasonographic measurement of renal transplant swelling. Br J Surg 1993; 80(8):1059–62. Available at: http://www.ncbi.nlm.nih.gov/pubmed/8402067. Accessed January 6, 2019.

17. O'Neill WC. B-mode sonography in acute renal failure. Nephron Clin Pract 2006;103(2):c19–23.

18. Longmaid HE, Rider E, Tymkiw J. Lupus nephritis. New sonographic findings. J Ultrasound Med 1987; 6(2):75–9. Available at: http://www.ncbi.nlm.nih.gov/pubmed/3550130. Accessed January 6, 2019.

19. Craig WD, Wagner BJ, Travis MD. Pyelonephritis: radiologic-pathologic review. Radiographics 2008; 28(1):255–77 [quiz: 327–8].

20. Hull TD, Agarwal A, Hoyt K. New ultrasound techniques promise further advances in AKI and CKD. J Am Soc Nephrol 2017;28(12):3452–60.

21. Alabousi A, Patlas MN, Mellnick VM, et al. Renal colic imaging: myths, recent trends, and controversies. Can Assoc Radiol J 2019. https://doi.org/10.1016/j.carj.2018.09.008.

22. Rajaei Isfahani M, Haghighat M. Measurable changes in hydronephrosis during pregnancy induced by positional changes: ultrasonic assessment and its diagnostic implication. Urol J 2005;2(2): 97–101. Available at: http://www.ncbi.nlm.nih.gov/pubmed/17629879. Accessed January 6, 2019.

23. Stevens S, Brown BD, McGahan JP. Nephrogenic diabetes insipidus: a cause of severe nonobstructive urinary tract dilatation. J Ultrasound Med 1995;14(7):543–5. Available at: http://www.ncbi.nlm.nih.gov/pubmed/7563304. Accessed January 6, 2019.

24. Darmon M, Schortgen F, Vargas F, et al. Diagnostic accuracy of Doppler renal resistive index for reversibility of acute kidney injury in critically ill patients. Intensive Care Med 2011;37(1):68–76.

25. Tublin ME, Bude RO, Platt JF. Review. The resistive index in renal Doppler sonography: where do we stand? AJR Am J Roentgenol 2003; 180(4):885–92.

26. Platt JF, Rubin JM, Ellis JH. Acute renal failure: possible role of duplex Doppler US in distinction between acute prerenal failure and acute tubular necrosis. Radiology 1991;179(2):419–23.

27. Lerolle N, Guérot E, Faisy C, et al. Renal failure in septic shock: predictive value of Doppler-based renal arterial resistive index. Intensive Care Med 2006;32(10):1553–9.

28. Bossard G, Bourgoin P, Corbeau JJ, et al. Early detection of postoperative acute kidney injury by Doppler renal resistive index in cardiac surgery with cardiopulmonary bypass. Br J Anaesth 2011; 107(6):891–8.

29. Le Dorze M, Bouglé A, Deruddre S, et al. Renal Doppler ultrasound. Shock 2012;37(4):360–5.

30. Correas JM, Bridal L, Lesavre A, et al. Ultrasound contrast agents: properties, principles of action, tolerance, and artifacts. Eur Radiol 2001;11(8):1316–28.

31. Cao W, Cui S, Yang L, et al. Contrast-enhanced ultrasound for assessing renal perfusion impairment and predicting acute kidney injury to chronic kidney disease progression. Antioxid Redox Signal 2017; 27(17):1397–411.

32. Kishimoto N, Mori Y, Nishiue T, et al. Renal blood flow measurement with contrast-enhanced harmonic ultrasonography: evaluation of dopamine-induced changes in renal cortical perfusion in humans. Clin Nephrol 2003;59(6):423–8. Available at: http://www.ncbi.nlm.nih.gov/pubmed/12834173. Accessed January 6, 2019.

33. Kalantarinia K, Belcik JT, Patrie JT, et al. Real-time measurement of renal blood flow in healthy subjects using contrast-enhanced ultrasound. Am J Physiol Renal Physiol 2009;297(4):F1129–34.

34. Schwenger V, Korosoglou G, Hinkel U-P, et al. Real-Time contrast-enhanced sonography of renal transplant recipients predicts chronic allograft nephropathy. Am J Transplant 2006;6(3):609–15.

35. Brown ED, Chen MYM, Wolfman NT, et al. Complications of renal transplantation: evaluation with US and radionuclide imaging. Radiographics 2000;20(3):607–22.

36. Hinson JS, Ehmann MR, Fine DM, et al. Risk of acute kidney injury after intravenous contrast media administration. Ann Emerg Med 2017;69(5):577–86.e4.

37. McDonald JS, McDonald RJ, Williamson EE, et al. Post-contrast acute kidney injury in intensive care unit patients: a propensity score-adjusted study. Intensive Care Med 2017;43(6):774–84.

38. Smith-Bindman R, Aubin C, Bailitz J, et al. Ultrasonography versus computed tomography for suspected nephrolithiasis. N Engl J Med 2014;371(12):1100–10.

39. Coursey CA, Casalino DD, Remer EM, et al. ACR appropriateness criteria® acute onset flank pain–suspicion of stone disease. Ultrasound Q 2012;28(3):227–33.

40. Jepperson MA, Cernigliaro JG, Sella D, et al. Dual-energy CT for the evaluation of urinary calculi: image interpretation, pitfalls and stone mimics. Clin Radiol 2013;68(12):e707–14.

41. Ananthakrishnan L, Duan X, Xi Y, et al. Dual-layer spectral detector CT: non-inferiority assessment compared to dual-source dual-energy CT in discriminating uric acid from non-uric acid renal stones ex vivo. Abdom Radiol (N Y) 2018;43(11):3075–81.

42. Goel RH, Unnikrishnan R, Remer EM. Acute urinary tract disorders. Radiol Clin North Am 2015;53(6):1273–92.

43. Curran-Melendez SM, Hartman MS, Heller MT, et al. Sorting the alphabet soup of renal pathology: a review. Curr Probl Diagn Radiol 2018;47(6):417–27.

44. Romano S, Scaglione M, Gatta G, et al. Association of splenic and renal infarctions in acute abdominal emergencies. Eur J Radiol 2004;50(1):48–58.

45. Jung DC, Kim SH, Jung S II, et al. Renal papillary necrosis: review and comparison of findings at multidetector row CT and intravenous urography. Radiographics 2006;26(6):1827–36.

46. Daftari Besheli L, Aran S, Shaqdan K, et al. Current status of nephrogenic systemic fibrosis. Clin Radiol 2014;69(7):661–8.

47. Bisla JK, Saranathan M, Martin DR, et al. MR imaging evaluation of the kidneys in patients with reduced kidney function. Magn Reson Imaging Clin N Am 2019;27(1):45–57.

48. Masselli G, Derme M, Laghi F, et al. Imaging of stone disease in pregnancy. Abdom Imaging 2013;38(6):1409–14.

49. Choyke PL, Kobayashi H. Functional magnetic resonance imaging of the kidney using macromolecular contrast agents. Abdom Imaging 2006;31(2):224–31.

50. Neuwelt EA, Hamilton BE, Varallyay CG, et al. Ultrasmall superparamagnetic iron oxides (USPIOs): a future alternative magnetic resonance (MR) contrast agent for patients at risk for nephrogenic systemic fibrosis (NSF)? Kidney Int 2009;75(5):465–74.

51. Zhou HY, Chen TW, Zhang XM. Functional magnetic resonance imaging in acute kidney injury: present status. Biomed Res Int 2016;2016:1–7. https://doi.org/10.1155/2016/2027370.

52. Thoeny HC, De Keyzer F, Oyen RH, et al. Diffusion-weighted MR imaging of kidneys in healthy volunteers and patients with parenchymal diseases: initial experience. Radiology 2005;235(3):911–7.

53. Wakabayashi H, Werner RA, Hayakawa N, et al. Initial preclinical evaluation of 18F-fluorodeoxysorbitol PET as a novel functional renal imaging agent. J Nucl Med 2016;57(10):1625–8.

54. Werner RA, Wakabayashi H, Chen X, et al. Functional renal imaging with 2-deoxy-2- [18] F-fluorosorbitol PET in rat models of renal disorders. J Nucl Med 2018;59(5):828–32.

Imaging of Abdominal Postoperative Complications

Ryan B. O'Malley, MD[a],*, Jonathan W. Revels, DO[b,1]

KEYWORDS

- Postoperative complications • Abdominal surgery • Postoperative imaging
- Abdominal complications

KEY POINTS

- Postoperative imaging is crucial for detecting and characterizing complications in the abdomen.
- Many complications are common to all types of surgery, but some are specific to the type of operation performed.
- Radiologists must use the type of operation, acuity of presentation, indication for surgery, timing relative to operation, and presence of comorbidities to help identify and characterize complications.
- Radiologists must also be able to distinguish normal or expected postsurgical appearance from a complication.

In the postoperative setting, imaging plays a crucial role in detecting and characterizing complications. Many complications are common to all types of surgery, whereas others are specific to the type of operation performed. Complications vary according to the type of operation, acuity of presentation, indication for surgery, timing relative to operation, and presence of comorbidities. It is also important to distinguish normal or expected postsurgical appearance from a complication. As such, radiologists must be aware of the surgery performed and use the operative report or in-person discussion to clarify uncertainty when appropriate.

This article presents a case-based review of abdominal postoperative complications, organized by the organ system affected, including general, hepatobiliary, pancreatic, gastrointestinal, genitourinary, and vascular complications. Among these categories, specific considerations for certain types of operations are included, as well as potential pitfalls that can be confused with complications. Computed tomography (CT) is the most commonly used modality in the immediate postoperative period and/or for acutely ill hospitalized patients, but other modalities are highlighted for certain situations, including fluoroscopy, ultrasound, MR imaging, and nuclear medicine. Management options are described, highlighting those that require radiologist input or intervention.

GENERAL

Certain complications can occur after all abdominal surgeries and have a similar imaging appearance no matter the type of operation performed. These include surgical site infection, abscess, active bleeding, hematoma, and anastomotic

Disclosure Statement: The authors have nothing to disclose.
[a] Department of Radiology, Abdominal Imaging, University of Washington, 1959 Northeast Pacific Street, Box 357115, Seattle, WA 98195, USA; [b] Department of Radiology, Body and Thoracic Imaging, University of New Mexico, Albuquerque, NM, USA
[1] Prseent address: 1959 Northeast Pacific Street, Box 357115, Seattle, WA 98195.
* Corresponding author.
E-mail address: ryanomal@uw.edu

Radiol Clin N Am 58 (2020) 73–91
https://doi.org/10.1016/j.rcl.2019.08.007

leak (if an anastomosis has been performed). Radiologists should be familiar with the appearance of all of these but also focus their search depending on the surgery that was performed, particularly regarding the type and location of the anastomosis or anastomoses.

Wound complications include surgical site infections, seromas, hematomas, wound dehiscence, and hernias. Approximately 5% to 10% of patients who undergo major abdominal surgery will develop wound infections.[1] Incisional surgical site infections can be superficial or deep, depending on whether the skin or subcutaneous tissue, or fascia or muscle, is infected. Both can occur within 30 days postoperatively and typically manifest with fever, peri-incisional pain, erythema, and/or purulent drainage. Diagnosis is often clinical and can be managed conservatively, but imaging can be performed when there is concern for deeper involvement or to assess for underlying fluid collections.

Soft tissue gas, nonorganized fluid, and fluid collections are common and expected postoperative findings at the incision and throughout the abdomen and pelvis. When seen on postoperative imaging, these should not necessarily be assumed to represent wound infection and should be taken in the context of the type and timing of the operation performed. As such, pneumoperitoneum in the first few days after a major operation is expected but would raise concern if increasing or persisting over time, particularly if near an anastomosis. Hemostatic material in the operative bed or packing material in a superficial wound can also mimic an infected fluid collection (Fig. 1). Moreover, imaging alone cannot include or exclude the presence of infection in a postoperative collection but should be used to document the size and extent.[2] A superficial or intraabdominal collection

that becomes more well-organized, particularly with increasing internal gas and rim enhancement, should be considered highly suspicious for abscess when there are concurrent clinical signs of infection (Fig. 2). When abscess is suspected, percutaneous aspiration and/or drainage should be performed to confirm the diagnosis.

Hematomas are the most common superficial postoperative collection and can occur as a result of incomplete hemostasis and/or bleeding diathesis (Fig. 3). No matter their location, all hematomas have similar imaging findings: high attenuation on CT, heterogeneously echogenic on ultrasound, and high signal on T1-weighted imaging (Fig. 4). On CT, the attenuation will vary depending on the composition of the hematoma. Clotted blood is 45 to 70 HU, whereas unclotted blood is 30 to 45 HU, which can result in the hematocrit effect in which higher attenuation layers along the dependent portion of the hematoma.[3] After laparoscopic procedures, abdominal wall hematomas can occur secondary to trocar insertion and damage to the small vessels in the abdominal wall. Intraabdominal hematomas usually occur in the surgical bed, near the vascular anastomosis (if performed) or in dependent spaces, and normally resolve spontaneously within a few weeks.[4] Multiphase CT can demonstrate active bleeding by showing intravenous contrast extravasation into a hematoma.

Other vascular complications include thrombosis, pseudoaneurysm, stenosis, and infarction, and can be seen after any type of surgery, though the risk is higher with increasing complexity or acuity of the operation. Pseudoaneurysms should be considered whenever there is an apparently cystic structure near an arterial anastomosis. Pseudoaneurysms occurring after biopsy or other percutaneous interventional procedure may also

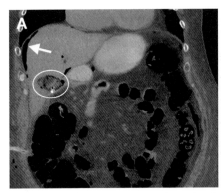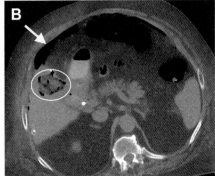

Fig. 1. A 70-year-old man underwent CT 4 days after laparoscopic converted to open subtotal cholecystectomy. Coronal (A) and axial (B) CT images demonstrate expected perihepatic pneumoperitoneum (arrows), as well as hemostatic material in the gallbladder fossa (circles).

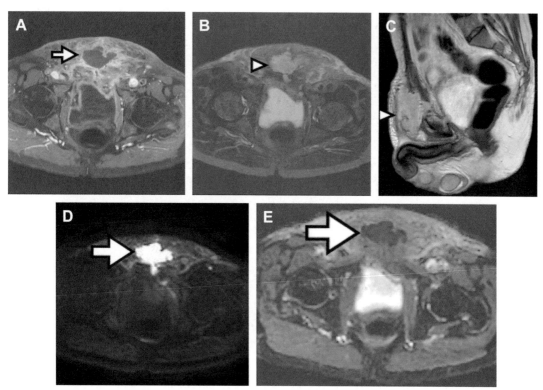

Fig. 2. A 63-year-old man status after cystectomy and neobladder for pT2N1 bladder carcinoma underwent pelvic MR imaging for fevers and cutaneous findings concerning for infection. Postcontrast axial T1-weighted image (*A*) demonstrates thick rim enhancement of the collection (*arrow*) with central fluid signal on T2-weighted axial (*B*) and sagittal (*C*) images (*arrowheads*). The contents also demonstrate restricted diffusion with hyperintense signal on diffusion-weighted imaging (DWI), b-value=800 (*arrow* in *D*) and corresponding hypointense signal on apparent diffusion coefficient (ADC) (*arrow* in *E*).

be seen within the parenchyma.[5] Doppler ultrasound will demonstrate bidirectional flow at the neck, whereas CT or MR angiography will show a saccular lesion enhancing with the blood pool.[4] Embolization and/or stent placement are usually performed to prevent rupture. Biliary or gastrointestinal tract fistulas can also result from pseudoaneurysms.[6]

A thrombosed artery or vein will demonstrate absent flow with an echogenic filling defect on

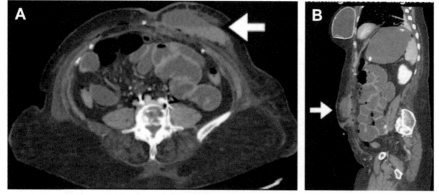

Fig. 3. A 71-year-old woman 3 days status after incisional hernia repair underwent CT of the abdomen and pelvis due to decreasing hematocrit. Axial (*A*) and sagittal (*B*) images demonstrate a large complex hematoma with layering hematocrit (*arrows*) measuring up to 11 cm.

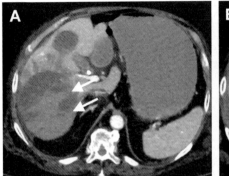
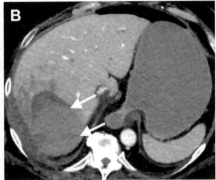

Fig. 4. A 70-year-old man status after open subtotal cholecystectomy underwent CT for increasing postoperative abdominal pain. Axial CT images (A, B) demonstrate a complex perihepatic fluid collection posterior to the right lobe with layering hematocrit levels (arrows) consistent with a hematoma.

ultrasound, whereas CT and MR imaging depict a filling defect. For superficial venous thrombus, lack of compressibility on ultrasound may be the earliest finding as the actual thrombus is isoechoic to blood. Stenosis on ultrasound manifests as focal color aliasing, poststenotic dilation, and manifestations of portal hypertension (for portal vein stenosis).[6] After liver transplant, the normal portal vein commonly has reduced caliber at the anastomosis (reflecting a size discrepancy between donor and recipient) with turbulent flow, but this does not indicate stenosis.

Seromas are superficial or intraabdominal collections of serous fluid that typically have simple fluid attenuation and commonly resolve by resorption. Although most small collections spontaneously resolve, they can predispose to superinfection and wound dehiscence if they persist. As such, any collection can be aspirated or drained

prophylactically to prevent subsequent infection and dehiscence, especially when present in large dead spaces or in high-risk patients. Wound dehiscence can involve a portion or the entire incision. CT findings include separation of the abdominal wall layers, commonly with interspersed fluid or gas (Fig. 5).

Incisional hernias are more common with vertical than horizontal incisions, occurring in 5% to 15% of open procedures and 1% to 3% of minimally invasive procedures.[2,7] Incisional hernias are commonly managed expectantly until there are significant symptoms or concern for incarceration. Imaging can be used to confirm the diagnosis, particularly to distinguish a hernia from diastasis and to assess for concurrent findings of bowel obstruction. Ultrasound can be used to diagnose or confirm small hernias, but CT is most frequently used for preoperative planning. In this

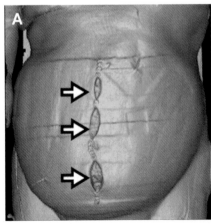
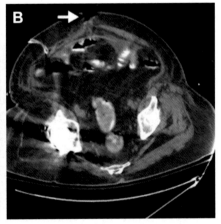

Fig. 5. A 77-year-old woman underwent CT of the abdomen and pelvis 3 days after exploratory laparotomy for pancreatitis complicated by abdominal compartment syndrome. Three-dimensional (3D) reformatted (A) and axial CT image (B) through the vertical midline incision demonstrate 3 distinct areas of separation (arrows), indicating wound dehiscence.

context, radiologists should describe the size, location, and type of the incisional hernia, as well as the presence of fluid collections, mesh, or bowel, within the defect, including specific types of hernias (**Fig. 6**).

Prosthetic mesh is used for most incisional hernia repairs and infection of the mesh is a specific postoperative complication that reportedly occurs in 0.7% to 1.9% of patients.[8,9] Use of concurrent immunosuppression, urgent repair, and postoperative surgical site infection are predictors of mesh infection.[9] Most meshes are synthetic or biologic and can be placed intraperitoneal (between the peritoneum and greater omentum) or retromuscular (between the muscle and its posterior aponeurosis). On CT, the appearance is variable but, often, thin curvilinear structures that are iso-attenuation or high attenuation relative to the adjacent muscle. Infected mesh with abscess is the most feared complication because it almost always requires reoperation with mesh removal, debridement of surrounding tissue, and repair of the abdominal defect (either immediately or in a delayed fashion), which can be a very challenging operation.[10] When infection is suspected on CT, it is important to describe the location of the fluid or fluid collection relative to the mesh and abdominal wall musculature in order to facilitate percutaneous aspiration and surgical planning.

Surgical anastomoses can be vascular, biliary, enteric, or urinary, all of which can be complicated by dehiscence and leaking. Nonorganized fluid, gas, edema, and fat stranding around an anastomosis are common postoperative findings and confirming the presence of a leak often requires visualizing extraluminal contrast in the operative bed. Nondistended bowel loops are common pitfalls that can be mistaken for fluid collections. The different types of anastomoses may be best evaluated with specific types of contrast (eg, enteric, biliary, urinary) and attention to certain locations (see later discussion).

Pitfalls
- Expected postoperative fluid and gas
- Hemostatic material containing gas
- Portal vein size discrepancy between donor and recipient
- Diastasis
- Wound healing by secondary intention (**Fig. 7**)
- Nondistended bowel loops mimicking fluid collection.

HEPATOBILIARY

Hepatobiliary complications most commonly occur after hepatic resection, cholecystectomy, liver transplant, and liver biopsy but can also occur after total and partial gastrectomy due to the proximity of the stomach to the liver. Potential complications include bile duct injury, bile leak, biliary ischemia, thrombosis, arterial stenosis, and hepatic infarct.

Iatrogenic biliary injury is the most feared complication after cholecystectomy, particularly if it involves the common bile duct (CBD). CBD injury is widely reported at 0.4% to 0.6% in laparoscopic cholecystectomy compared with 0.2% to 0.3% after open cholecystectomy, although more recent reports suggest that the rates may be similar as laparoscopic experience becomes more uniform.[11] Of these, cystic duct stump leak is the most common source after laparoscopic cholecystectomy. Bile leaks also complicate 2% to 25% of liver transplants or hepatic resection, often at sites of biliary anastomosis or from the cut liver surface, and are the second-most-common cause of graft dysfunction after liver transplant.[6,12,13] Similarly, CBD injuries are very important to recognize and manage because they have a devastating impact on morbidity and mortality for patients after cholecystectomy, with an 8.8% increase in all-cause mortality compared with patients without CBD injury, and 5-year mortality rates exceeding 20%.[14] The risk of iatrogenic CBD injury significantly increases when patients present with acute cholecystitis or have variant anatomy.[15] If unrecognized intraoperatively, patients with biliary injuries typically present within

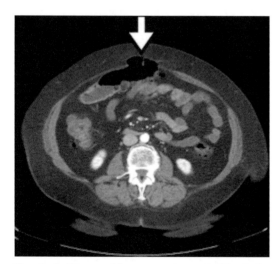

Fig. 6. A 72-year-old man underwent CT of the abdomen and pelvis to evaluate severe abdominal pain. Axial CT image demonstrates anterior abdominal wall hernia along a previous ventral incision site measuring 4.5 cm, which contains the antimesenteric portion of colonic wall, consistent with a Richter hernia (*arrow*).

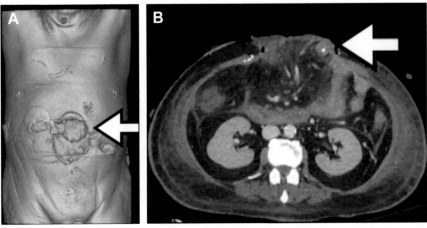

Fig. 7. A 55-year-old man was transferred from Mexico after numerous abdominal surgeries due to small bowel obstructions, which were subsequently complicated by enterocutaneous fistulas. Reportedly, the wound could not be closed at the outside hospital due to infection and was left open to heal by secondary intention. 3D reformatted image (A) and axial CT image (B) of the mid abdomen demonstrate a 12 cm by 15 cm open wound (arrows) with bowel and mesenteric vasculature near the surface.

1 week with symptoms of bile leak or stasis, such as abdominal pain, fever, nausea, and hyperbilirubinemia.

Imaging evaluation can be performed with ultrasound, CT, MR cholangiopancreatography (MRCP), or hepatobiliary iminodiacetic acid (HIDA) scan, with the choice determined by the acuity of presentation and level of suspicion. Ultrasound is useful for documenting the presence of a fluid collection and biliary dilation but is unlikely to identify to site of injury. CT can demonstrate similar findings, as well as the extent of fluid collections or peritoneal inflammation and concomitant vascular injuries. MRCP is very accurate for identifying the exact site of biliary injury and distinguishing between biliary and nonbiliary fluid collections, particularly when a hepatobiliary contrast agent is used (eg, gadoxetic acid [Gd-EOB-DTPA]) (Fig. 8).[12,16] Compared with endoscopic retrograde cholangiopancreatography, MRCP also has the advantage of delineating anatomy proximal and distal to the injury, including discontinuous ducts, as well as the patency of biliary-enteric anastomosis, which is important for treatment planning (Fig. 9). MRCP is also the best imaging modality for assessing for postoperative biliary stricture, including in the setting of biliary-enteric anastomosis (Fig. 10). HIDA is the most sensitive test for detecting a bile leak and can help demonstrate contained versus free leakage. It historically has lacked the spatial resolution to localize the exact site of injury, although single-photon emission CT is now commonly used with improved specificity (Fig. 11).[16] Notably,

postoperative fluid collections and gas are commonly detected and are not specific for a biliary injury.[17]

Biliary injuries can involve the CBD, cystic duct, or ducts of Luschka, with various classification schemes to characterize the injury. Radiologists must localize the injury and, if the CBD is involved, describe the relationship to the primary biliary confluence because this is crucial for determining the biliary repair that may be needed. It is also important to identify coexistent findings that will be used to determine multidisciplinary management, such as the presence of biloma, stricture, or vascular injury. Initially, management is directed at controlling the source of sepsis, so percutaneous drain may be placed in an abscess or biloma, whereas percutaneous biliary drainage can be used to decompress an obstructed biliary tree. Operative repair is ultimately the gold standard, although endoscopic sphincterotomy and stent placement can be effective for injuries that do not result in complete CBD occlusion or transection.[11]

Hepatic vascular injuries depend on the type and extent of operation performed, and can include hematoma, thrombosis, unintentional ligation, or pseudoaneurysm, with or without associated active bleeding. Ultrasound is the best initial test to evaluate the hepatic vasculature for routine surveillance or for potential complications. Vascular complications affect 9% of liver transplants and are the second-most-common cause of graft failure after liver transplant, of which hepatic arterial thrombosis is the most common

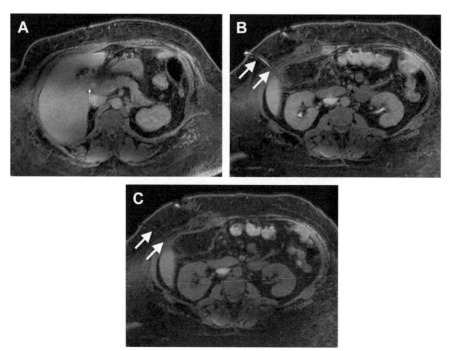

Fig. 8. A 58-year-old woman status after complicated excision of necrotic gallbladder underwent abdominal MR imaging with hepatobiliary contrast (Gd-EOB-DTPA) used to evaluate for bile leak. Axial 20-minute image (*A*) demonstrates a focus of excreted contrast adjacent to the cystic duct remnant (*arrow*), as well as contrast accumulation within a percutaneous drainage catheter (*arrows* in *B*), that terminated in the gallbladder fossa. Precontrast image at the same level for comparison (*C*) indicate lack of contrast in the drain (*arrows*).

vascular complication (2%–12% of cases).[4,6] Hepatic arterial complications are particularly devastating after liver transplant because the hepatic artery is the sole supply for the bile ducts, and thrombosis or stenosis can lead to biliary ischemia, stricture, or biloma (**Fig. 12**).[4] Nonvisualization of the hepatic artery signal on ultrasound is highly predictive of thrombosis (92%), although this often must be confirmed by CT or MR angiography because transient spasm, low cardiac output, and other technical factors can make ultrasound very challenging in the immediate postoperative period.[5] Early diagnosis is crucial to allow for appropriate intervention because the mortality rate

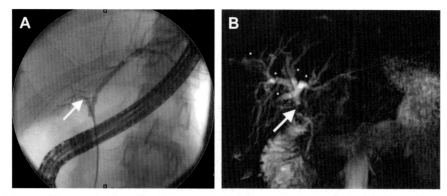

Fig. 9. A 24-year-old woman status after laparoscopic cholecystectomy presented with elevated transaminases. Endoscopic retrograde cholangiopancreatography (ERCP) (*A*) demonstrates abrupt cutoff of the right biliary tree at the level of the surgical clips (*arrow*), but with nonopacification upstream from the cutoff. MRCP (*B*) demonstrates dilated right biliary radicles (*asterisks*) extending to abrupt cutoff (*arrow*) and susceptibility artifact, which corresponded to the surgical clips seen on ERCP, consistent inadvertent iatrogenic clipping of a right hepatic bile duct.

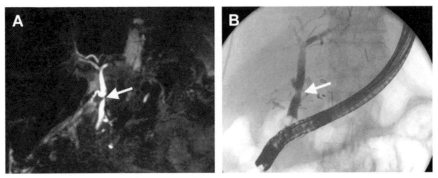

Fig. 10. A 56-year-old man was readmitted 4 weeks after liver transplant for rising liver function tests and rejection not responding to immunosuppression. MRCP was performed and maximum intensity projection image (*A*) demonstrates a focal short segment stricture at the biliary-enteric anastomosis (*arrow*) with associated upstream dilation. ERCP with balloon dilation was performed (*B*), which demonstrates improvement of the stricture (*arrow*).

approaches 30%, even after retransplantation.[6] Hepatic artery stenosis complicates 2% to 11% of liver transplants and typical ultrasound findings include focally increased peak systolic velocity (>200 cm/s) at the stenosis with poststenotic turbulent flow, low resistive indices (<0.5), and tardus-parvus waveforms distal to the stenosis (**Fig. 13**).[4] Stenosis most commonly occurs at the anastomosis and can lead to thrombosis, ischemia, biliary stricture, sepsis, and graft

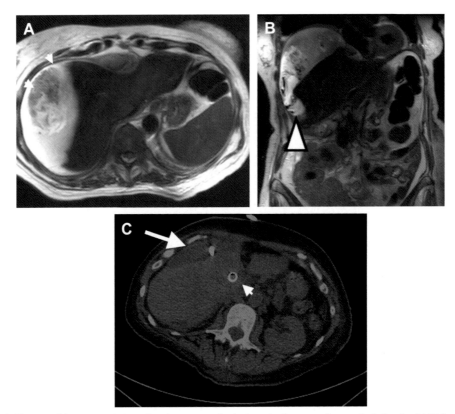

Fig. 11. A 71-year-old woman status after laparoscopic cholecystectomy underwent abdominal MR imaging for concern for bile leak. Axial (*A*) and coronal (*B*) T2-weighted images demonstrate a large complex perihepatic fluid collection with mixed T2 signal (*arrowheads*). HIDA was subsequently performed and an axial single-photon emission CT image (*C*) demonstrates radiotracer activity in both the stented CBD (*arrowhead*) and the perihepatic fluid collection (*arrow*), confirming the bile leak although not localizing the exact site.

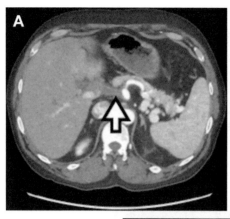
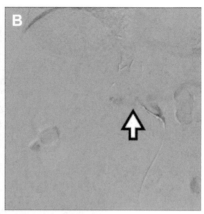
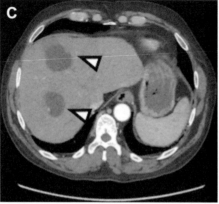

Fig. 12. A 55-year-old man status after liver transplant presented with acute abdominal pain. Axial CT image in arterial phase (*A*), confirmed on angiography (*B*), demonstrates abrupt cutoff of the hepatic artery with complete thrombosis (*arrows*). Axial CT image more superiorly (*C*) demonstrates lentiform intrahepatic collections consistent with bilomas related to biliary necrosis (*arrowheads*).

failure.[6] Notably, ultrasound can be falsely negative in the setting of stenosis or thrombosis if there are periportal arterial collateral vessels.[6] A tortuous hepatic artery can also mistakenly result in falsely elevated systolic velocity if the sample volume angle is incorrect.[4] In the immediate postoperative period (<72 hours), elevated resistive indices (>0.8) are common and usually return to normal within a few days.[6]

Bile duct ischemia and hepatic infarction occur after liver transplants due to hepatic arterial stenosis or thrombosis.[6] Hepatic infarcts are also rarely described after a Whipple procedure, typically when there is an underlying mesenteric vascular abnormality (eg, severe atherosclerosis, vasculitis) or intraoperative arterial injury.[18] Infarcts manifest as geographic or wedge-shaped areas of hypoenhancement but must be distinguished from perfusional hypoenhancement by the lack of enhancement on all phases of a multiphase examinations. Infarcts also tend to undergo liquefaction, which can result in abscess, often in the setting of biliary stricture, arterial insufficiency, or immunosuppression.[4]

Pitfalls
- Transient spasm or low cardiac output resulting in nonvisualization of hepatic artery
- Periportal arterial collateral vessels
- Tortuous hepatic artery resulting in falsely elevated systolic velocity
- Transient elevated resistive indices (>0.8)
- Perfusional hepatic enhancement.

PANCREATIC

Pancreatic surgeries are typically performed for resection of neoplasms or management of the sequelae of acute or chronic pancreatitis. Procedures include pancreatoduodenectomy (Whipple procedure), central pancreatectomy, distal pancreatectomy, total pancreatectomy, Berger procedure, Puestow procedure, Frey procedure, necrosectomy, and pseudocyst derivation.[19] CT is the most useful imaging modality in the immediate postoperative period and early complications on imaging include gastric outlet obstruction, pancreatic fistulas, pancreatitis, abscess, hemorrhage, thrombosis, pseudoaneurysm, splenic infarction, and

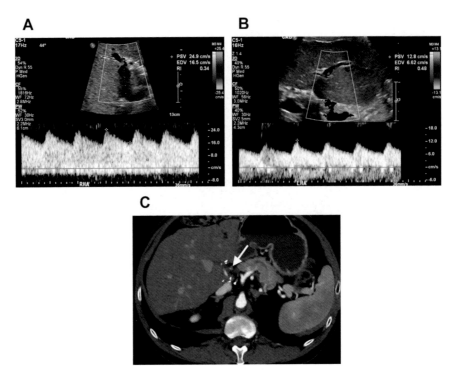

Fig. 13. A 53-year-old man status after liver transplant presented for surveillance ultrasound, which demonstrates low resistive indices and tardus-parvus waveforms in both the right (*A*) and left (*B*) hepatic arteries. CT angiography (*C*) confirmed focal stenosis of the hepatic arterial anastomosis (*arrow*).

anastomotic leak. Depending on the timing and level of concern, single-phase or multiphase CT can be performed, including arterial, and venous phases is particularly useful to demonstrate vascular complications and parenchymal necrosis. Understanding the indication and type of operation performed is crucial for identifying anastomotic leaks, particularly regarding the type and location of anastomoses. For example, a Whipple procedure results in the formation of 3 anastomoses (gastrojejunostomy, hepaticojejunostomy, and pancreaticojejunostomy), whereas a distal pancreatectomy has no anastomoses.

Pancreatic fistula occurs in 6% to 14% of patients and is the most important complication after a Whipple procedure because the mortality ranges from 1.4% to 3.7% but can be as high as 20% to 40% when also complicated by abscess or sepsis.[18] Pancreatic fistula is suspected clinically when surgical drain fluid contains amylase levels 3 times higher than serum amylase and refers to leaking pancreatic secretions from the pancreatic duct, usually resulting from pancreaticojejunal anastomotic breakdown.[18,20] The drain output is used for diagnosis, but suggestive CT findings include a focal collection or hemorrhage at the pancreaticojejunal anastomosis, sometimes with

visible communication with the pancreatic duct (Fig. 14).[18] Gastrojejunal leaks are rare after a Whipple procedure (0.4%) but are almost always associated with severe complications and reoperation.[21]

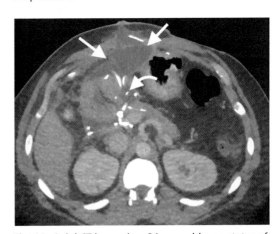

Fig. 14. Axial CT image in a 34-year-old man status after Whipple procedure for distal cholangiocarcinoma demonstrates a fluid collection anterior to the pancreaticojejunal anastomosis (*arrows*) as migration of the distal part of the pancreatic duct stent (*curved arrow*) outside of the jejunal limb (*asterisk*), indicating anastomotic dehiscence.

Hemorrhage after a Whipple procedure is infrequent (4%) but carries very high mortality (38%) and is most commonly from the gastroduodenal artery stump, either from inadequate ligation or pseudoaneurysm.[18] Hemorrhage can be into the bowel lumen or extraluminal, with corresponding active extravasation on CT seen in the bowel lumen, free fluid, or a fluid collection, often intermixed with or surrounded by a hematoma (**Fig. 15**).[3] Superior mesenteric vein (SMV) and portal vein thrombosis are most commonly seen when there has been venous reconstruction in the setting of a borderline resectable tumor.[18]

Pitfalls
- Nondistended bowel loops at pancreaticojejunostomy or hepaticojejunostomy
- Fluid and thickening along celiac axis or Superior mesenteric artery (SMA).

GASTROINTESTINAL
Bariatric Surgery

Between 2011 and 2017, the number of bariatric surgeries performed in the United States increased from 158,000 per year to 228,000 per year.[22] As such, the potential for postbariatric surgical complications may increase, and radiologists should be familiar with these complications. Commonly performed bariatric surgeries include sleeve gastrectomy, Roux-en-Y gastric bypass (RYGB), and gastric banding.

Leaks after sleeve gastrectomy and RYGB tend to occur in the early postoperative period so fluoroscopic upper gastrointestinal evaluation is often performed routinely after surgery. For RYGB, it is important to evaluate both the gastric pouch and the distal jejunojejunal anastomosis for leakage (**Fig. 16**).[23] At imaging, frank extravasation of enteric contrast can be seen on fluoroscopy, whereas pneumoperitoneum, features of peritonitis, or an intraabdominal abscess can be seen to better advantage on CT.[23]

Complications of RYGB can be grouped into those occurring proximally or distally. Examples of proximal RYGB complications include postsurgical leaks along the anastomosis, alimentary limb ulcerations, gastrogastric fistulas, and afferent loop syndrome. Gastrojejunal anastomosis marginal ulcers may occur due to the jejunal mucosa being exposed to the acidic gastric secretions.[24] The incidence of gastrojejunal anastomosis

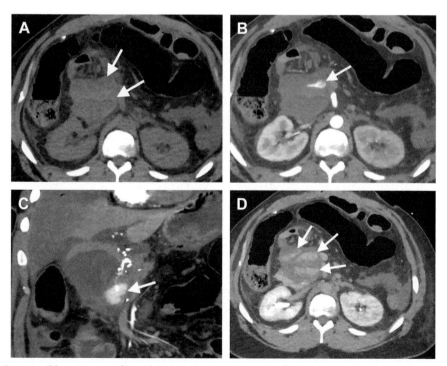

Fig. 15. A 34-year-old man status after Whipple procedure for distal cholangiocarcinoma (same patient as **Fig. 18**) underwent multiphase CT due to acute abdominal pain and hemodynamic instability. Precontrast axial CT image (*A*) demonstrates an intraperitoneal hematoma with layered blood products of different ages (*arrows*). On the axial (*B*) and coronal (*C*) arterial phase images, there is active contrast extravasation (*arrows*) from active bleeding arising from the gastroduodenal artery stump (*asterisk* in C). On the 5-minute delayed axial image (*D*), there is continued contrast accumulation within the hematoma (*arrows*).

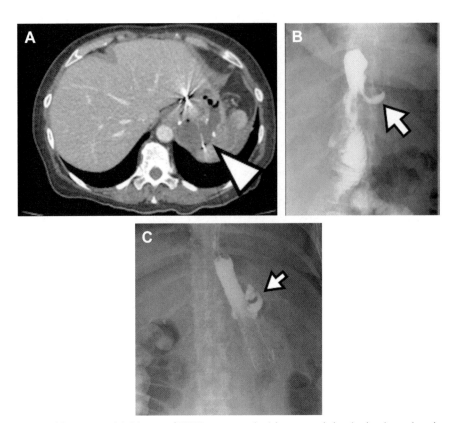

Fig. 16. A 59-year-old woman with history of RYGB presented with severe abdominal pain and underwent CT of the abdomen and pelvis. Axial CT image (*A*) demonstrates a 5 cm gas-containing fluid collection along the posterior margin of the gastric pouch (*arrowhead*). Upper gastrointestinal (*B*) showed that the fluid collection corresponded to a focal outpouching of contrast, suggesting a contained perforation (*arrow*). Subsequently, a covered stent was placed across the ulcer (*C*); however, the stent was unsuccessful in occluding the perforation (*arrow*).

marginal ulcers has been reported in up to 3% to 13% of patients, and patients may present with abdominal pain, hematemesis, and/or perforation.[23,25] Occasionally, the ulcers can be due to jejunal ischemia, which may require more aggressive management, including bowel resection.[23] With CT and fluoroscopy, the ulcers can be seen as outpouchings along or near the surgical anastomosis with adjacent bowel fold-thickening or edema (**Fig. 17**).

Internal hernias are the result of intraabdominal contents protruding into potential spaces of the peritoneum or mesentery, which can be via defects created intraoperatively (eg, transverse mesocolon, small bowel mesentery, posterior to the Roux limb). Internal hernias complicate an estimated 3% of RYGB cases and are the most common cause of small bowel obstruction after laparoscopic RYGB.[23,26,27] Most internal hernias present as a late complication but can occur as early as the first postoperative week.[28] When characterizing internal hernias, it is crucial to document presence of concurrent bowel obstruction because these are closed loop obstructions that will potentially need surgical management. On CT, a common and sensitive finding for internal hernia is the mesenteric swirl sign (whirl sign), but this is nonspecific and can also be seen in cases of adhesions and volvulus.[29,30] Other findings of internal hernias include abnormal clusters of dilated and/or fluid-filled small bowel loops in atypical locations, and the so-called mushroom sign with bowel loops draped over a central stalk created by the mesenteric vessels and bowel loops at the opening of the peritoneal defect (**Fig. 18**).[29,30] It is important to distinguish small bowel obstructions due to internal hernias from those caused by adhesions, anastomotic strictures, external hernias, or other etiologic factors.

Colectomy

Colonic resections can be performed for a variety of indications ranging from complicated infectious

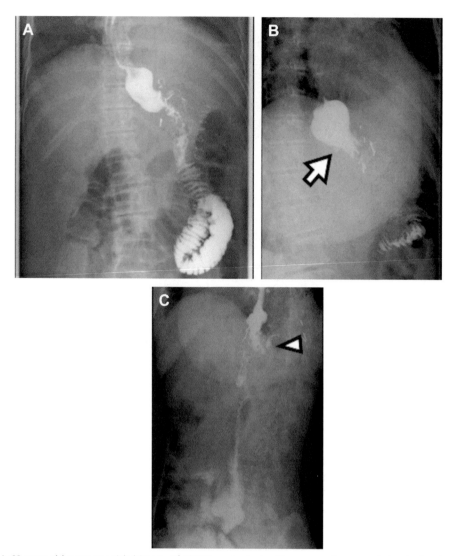

Fig. 17. A 62-year-old woman with history of RYGB presented with recurrent upper abdominal pain. An older comparison upper gastrointestinal fluoroscopic image (*A*) demonstrates normal postoperative anatomy. Subsequent anterior (*B*) and left anterior oblique (*C*) fluoroscopic images demonstrate focal outpouchings of contrast consistent with marginal ulcers (*arrow in B arrowhead in C*).

or inflammatory processes to tumor resection. Examples include total colectomy for ulcerative colitis, partial colectomy for colon cancer, sigmoid colectomy for complicated diverticulitis, or abdominoperineal resection for low rectal cancer. Anastomotic leak after primary anastomosis complicates 3% to 7% of colonic resections and 10% to 20% of rectal resections, which confers a higher morbidity, short-term mortality, likelihood of permanent ostomy, tumor recurrence, and a diminished overall long-term survival.[31] Most occur within the first few days after surgery and can be diagnosed by CT or water-soluble contrast enema, although existing literature is mixed

regarding which is more accurate.[32] Visualizing leaking intraluminal contrast is the most reliable finding on either modality, which requires the radiologist to ensure that contrast has reached the anastomosis.

Creation of a colonic pouch following colectomy allows for improved patient outcomes: reduced likelihood of tumor recurrence and improved continence.[7,33] The Hartmann procedure is a commonly used surgery for cases of complicated diverticulitis, sigmoid perforation, and colon carcinoma. It involves creation of a temporary diverting colostomy, as well as either a blind-ending colonic stump (Hartmann pouch)

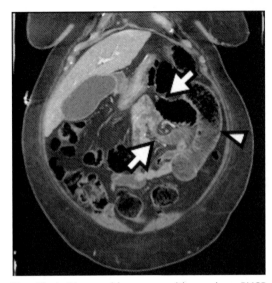

Fig. 18. A 61-year-old woman with previous RYGB presented with acute abdominal pain, vomiting, and leukocytosis. Coronal CT image demonstrates 2 loops of bowel that are focally indented at the same location (*arrows*), surrounding a central vascular stalk suggestive of a mushroom sign. Upstream small bowel is also dilated (*arrowhead*). Internal hernia with upstream mechanical obstruction was proven intraoperatively.

or a mucous fistula. The Hartmann procedure allows time for the surgical sites to heal and the patient to recover before restoring bowel continuity. Before restoring bowel continuity (takedown), fluoroscopic evaluation of a pouch may be performed, evaluating for leaks, fistulas, inflammation, and strictures. Whether evaluated

on fluoroscopy or CT, anastomotic leaks can be seen as perianastomotic loculated fluid, frank extravasation of intraluminal contrast, or stool adjacent to the anastomosis (**Fig. 19**).[7] Another commonly used pouch is the ileal pouch and ileal pouch-anal anastomosis (IPAA) after total proctocolectomy. For these patients, pouch-related inflammation (pouchitis) is very common, especially for patients with ulcerative colitis, occurring in up to 50% of cases.[7,34,35] Similar to other cases of bowel inflammation, pouchitis can manifest as bowel wall edema, mucosal hyperenhancement, adjacent fat stranding, vascular engorgement, and (occasionally) mucosal ulcerations (**Fig. 20**).[34,35]

Small bowel obstruction can occur after any type of bowel surgery and adhesions are the most common cause overall, some of which can develop as soon as 1 week after surgery, but high rates are reported after IPAA (15%–44%).[7] Imaging findings are similar to bowel obstruction of any kind with dilated proximal small bowel, decompressed distal small bowel, and a characteristic intervening transition point. The transition point should be specifically assessed for clues regarding the cause of the obstruction (eg, internal hernia, inflammation, anastomotic stricture) or findings of ischemia.[36] Obstruction must be distinguished from postoperative ileus (pseudoobstruction), which is also a common postoperative complication resulting in delayed return of bowel function. In contrast to obstruction, findings of ileus are characteristically diffusely dilated small and large bowel with no intervening transition point.[37]

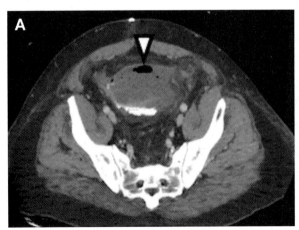
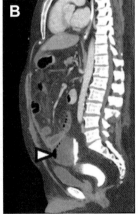

Fig. 19. A 56-year-old man with history of inflammatory bowel disease and cecal adenocarcinoma underwent total colectomy with ileostomy, then presented with acute lower abdominal pain and fever. CT was performed with rectal contrast and axial (*A*) and sagittal (*B*) images demonstrate a complex pelvic fluid collection containing fluid, gas, and layering rectal contrast (*arrowheads*), confirming communication with the rectal stump.

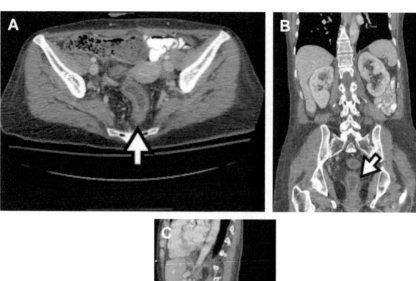

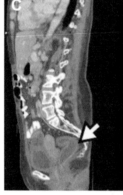

Fig. 20. A 49-year-old woman with Crohn disease status after segmental transverse colectomy and distal sigmoid Hartman pouch formation presented with lower abdominal and perianal pain. Axial (*A*), coronal (*B*), and sagittal (*C*) CT images demonstrate abnormal wall thickening and mucosal hyperenhancement of the pouch, consistent with pouchitis (*arrows*).

Pitfalls

- Temporary anastomotic edema
- Nondistended pouches or blind-ending bowel loops at anastomoses
- Intentional restriction of the gastric pouch
- Presacral posttreatment thickening.

GENITOURINARY

Surgery can be curative for patients with localized renal cell carcinoma and can consist of partial or radical nephrectomy, depending on the tumor size, number, location, and extent. Partial nephrectomy has a higher overall complication rate compared with radical nephrectomy, specifically bleeding and urinary fistula, but both have low overall rates of high-grade complications.[38]

After partial nephrectomy, displacement of the kidney, fat stranding, wedge-shaped postsurgical defect, and fluid collection are the most common imaging findings, most of which do not indicate a complication.[39] Potential pitfalls include perirenal fat used to pack the surgical defect that can be mistaken for an angiomyolipoma. Hemostatic material may also be present in and around the defect, which can contain foci of gas that could mimic an abscess.[40] Notably, fluid collections are a very common imaging finding, sometimes persisting up to 48 months postoperatively, and should not be assumed to represent abscesses even when there is rim enhancement or nonsimple fluid attenuation.[39] If there is a calyceal injury or incomplete calyceal repair for resection of a central tumor, nephrectomy may be complicated by urine leak. Imaging findings include perirenal fluid or fluid collection, which can be confirmed to be urine by using excretory imaging demonstrating excreted contrast from the collecting system into the fluid.[40] This generally requires stent placement or percutaneous drainage. Pseudoaneurysms and hematomas may occur when there is intraoperative injury and/or incomplete hemostasis, but these are uncommon. Lymphatic injury during partial nephrectomy can result in a fistulous communication with the collecting system, which

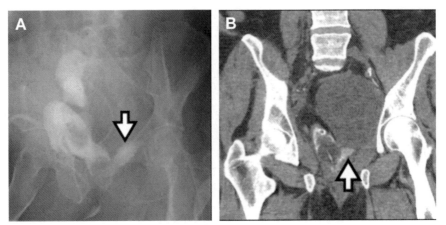

Fig. 21. A 56-year-old man 1 day status after robotic cystectomy with neobladder formation underwent fluoro-scopic cystogram. Left anterior oblique spot image (*A*) demonstrates a leak at the inferior aspect of the neoblad-der (*arrow*). Subsequent CT cystogram coronal image (*B*) demonstrates a similar finding with instilled neobladder contrast leaking into a large pelvic urinoma (*arrow*).

manifests as chyluria and can be seen as a fat-fluid level in the bladder on CT.[41]

Cystectomy can be performed for benign and malignant etiologic factors but is most common for bladder cancer. Bladder resection requires concurrent urinary diversion, which can be incontinent or continent. For both types of urinary diversion, most surgical procedures use a resected segment of bowel as a conduit or reser-voir.[42] Incontinent urinary diversion is the most common technique after cystectomy, most commonly using an ileal conduit. Continent urinary

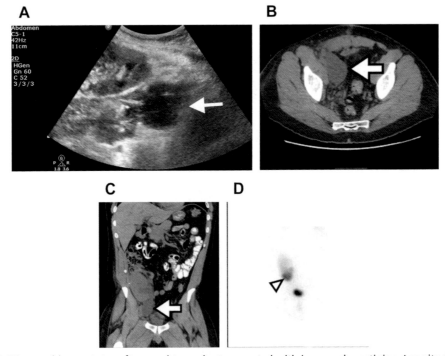

Fig. 22. A 37-year-old man status after renal transplant presented with increased creatinine. Longitudinal ultra-sound image (*A*) demonstrates a fluid collection inferior to the lower pole of the transplanted kidney (*arrow*). Follow-up axial (*B*) and coronal (*C*) CT images show the extent of the fluid collection (*arrows*), which appears to abut the ureter. A 99m-technetium mercaptoacetyltriglycine (MAG3) renal scan (*D*) was performed and dem-onstrates focal radiotracer accumulation within the collection (*arrowhead*), confirming it to be a urinoma.

diversion allows patients to control voiding by using their urethra (eg, neobladder) or a catheterizable stoma (eg, Indiana pouch) but is more technically challenging and requires more patient compliance.

Potential complications for all types of urinary diversion include leaks at either urinary or bowel anastomoses, pyelonephritis, abscess, lymphocele, seroma, hematoma, ileus, and small bowel obstruction.[43] Neobladder formation has the highest complication rate, with 22% of patients reported to have major complications within 90 days postoperatively.[44] Urine leak typically occurs at the urinary anastomosis, which can be diagnosed by demonstrating excreted contrast outside the collecting system on excretory imaging (CT or MR imaging). Retrograde injection under fluoroscopy can also be performed to evaluate a pouch, neobladder, or conduit for leak (Fig. 21). Excretory imaging, retrograde injection, and/or 99m-technetium MAG3 renal scan can also be useful for troubleshooting when there is uncertainty regarding the anatomy or etiologic factors of a fluid collection (Fig. 22). Lymphoceles characteristically are homogeneously simple fluid attention collections in areas of lymph node dissection and, if aspirated, the collection creatinine level will be similar to serum level, which helps differentiate from a urinoma.

Pitfalls
- Perirenal fat used in partial nephrectomy defect
- Ileal conduit or neobladder mistaken as fluid collection
- Fluid collection mistaken for bladder.

FOREIGN BODY

Retained surgical items (eg, cotton surgical sponge) can rarely complicate any surgery, but are more common after emergency surgery and most commonly found in the abdomen (56%) and pelvis (18%).[45,46] Surgical sponges are most common but can also include surgical instruments (eg, retractor), needles, or other items.[47] Some items may be seen by intraoperative radiographs if there is a discrepancy in the surgical count, whereas others may present much later. Imaging findings vary depending on the item, but cotton sponges all have distinctive radiopaque markers incorporated into the sponge itself (Fig. 23).[48] Needles may be difficult to distinguish from clips, fiducial markers, or other items that were intentionally left within the patient (Fig. 24). Similarly, a cotton sponge with foreign body reaction (so-called gossypiboma) can simulate an abscess

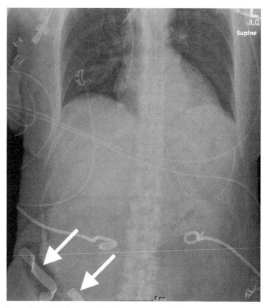

Fig. 23. A 60-year-old woman underwent emergent excision of infected aortoiliac stent. Immediate postoperative radiograph demonstrates 2 laparotomy sponges (*arrows*), which were intentionally left within the infected wound.

(or can become superinfected) (Fig. 25).[49] In these cases, reviewing the operative report and discussing directly with the surgeon may be the only way to determine whether the item is intentional or unintentional.

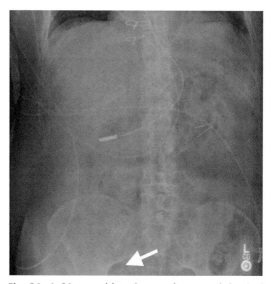

Fig. 24. A 64-year-old patient underwent abdominal radiograph for enteric tube placement and was found to have an unexpected curvilinear structure in the right lower quadrant (*arrow*). Further investigation revealed a remote history of abdominal surgery at an outside hospital several years prior.

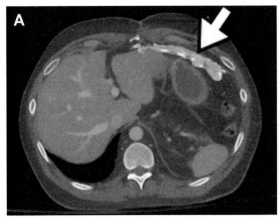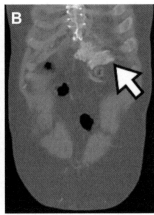

Fig. 25. A 37-year-old man with a remote history of heart transplantation at an outside institution underwent CT following abdominal trauma. Axial (*A*) and coronal (*B*) CT images demonstrate a heavily calcified sheet-like structure in the left upper abdomen or lower chest along the curvature of the diaphragm (*arrows*). On further questioning, the patient reported he had a known retained sponge from the heart transplant.

REFERENCES

1. Gore RM, Berlin JW, Yaghmai V, et al. CT diagnosis of postoperative abdominal complications. Semin Ultrasound CT MR 2004;25(3):207–21.
2. Parikh KR, Al-Hawary M, Millet JD, et al. Incisional hernia repair: what the radiologist needs to know. Am J Roentgenol 2017;209(6):1239–46.
3. Lubner M, Menias C, Rucker C, et al. Blood in the belly: CT findings of hemoperitoneum. Radiographics 2007;27(1):109–25.
4. Singh AK, Nachiappan AC, Verma HA, et al. Postoperative imaging in liver transplantation: what radiologists should know. Radiographics 2010;30(2):339–51.
5. Low G, Crockett AM, Leung K, et al. Imaging of vascular complications and their consequences following transplantation in the abdomen. Radiographics 2013;33(3):633–52.
6. Caiado AHM, Blasbalg R, Marcelino ASZ, et al. Complications of liver transplantation: multimodality imaging approach. Radiographics 2007;27(5):1401–17.
7. Weinstein S, Osei-Bonsu S, Aslam R, et al. Multidetector CT of the postoperative colon: review of normal appearances and common complications. Radiographics 2013;33(2):515–32.
8. Lacour M, Zins CR, Casa C, et al. CT findings of complications after abdominal wall repair with prosthetic mesh. Diagn Interv Imaging 2017;98(7–8):517–28.
9. Bueno-Lledó J, Torregrosa-Gallud A, Sala-Hernandez A, et al. Predictors of mesh infection and explantation after abdominal wall hernia repair. Am J Surg 2017;213(1):50–7.
10. Shubinets V, Carney M, Colen D, et al. Management of infected mesh after abdominal hernia repair. Ann Plast Surg 2018;80(2):145–53.
11. Cohen JT, Charpentier KP, Beard RE. An update on iatrogenic biliary injuries. Surg Clin North Am 2019;99(2):283–99.
12. Melamud K, LeBedis CA, Anderson SW, et al. Biliary imaging: multimodality approach to imaging of biliary injuries and their complications. Radiographics 2014;34(3):613–23.
13. Koch M, Garden OJ, Padbury R, et al. Bile leakage after hepatobiliary and pancreatic surgery: a definition and grading of severity by the International Study Group of Liver Surgery. Surgery 2011;149(5):680–8.
14. Halbert C, Altieri MS, Yang J, et al. Long-term outcomes of patients with common bile duct injury following laparoscopic cholecystectomy. Surg Endosc 2016;30(10):4294–9.
15. Kohn JF, Trenk A, Kuchta K, et al. Characterization of common bile duct injury after laparoscopic cholecystectomy in a high-volume hospital system. Surg Endosc 2018;32(3):1184–91.
16. Thompson CM, Saad NE, Quazi RR, et al. Management of iatrogenic bile duct injuries: role of the interventional radiologist. Radiographics 2013;33(1):117–34.
17. Thurley PD, Dhingsa R. Laparoscopic cholecystectomy: postoperative imaging. Am J Roentgenol 2008;191(3):794–801.
18. Raman SP, Horton KM, Cameron JL, et al. CT after pancreaticoduodenectomy: spectrum of normal findings and complications. Am J Roentgenol 2013;201(1):2–13.
19. Yamauchi FI, Ortega CD, Blasbalg R, et al. Multidetector CT evaluation of the postoperative pancreas. Radiographics 2012;32(3):743–64.
20. Butturini G, Daskalaki D, Molinari E, et al. Pancreatic fistula: definition and current problems. J Hepatobiliary Pancreat Surg 2008;15(3):247–51.

21. Winter JM, Cameron JL, Yeo CJ, et al. Duodenojejunostomy leaks after pancreaticoduodenectomy. J Gastrointest Surg 2008;12(2):263–9.

22. Estimate of bariatric surgery numbers, 2011-2017. American Society for Metabolic and Bariatric Surgery. Available at: https://asmbs.org/resources/estimate-of-bariatric-surgery-numbers. Accessed April 18, 2019.

23. Levine MS, Carucci LR. Imaging of bariatric surgery: normal anatomy and postoperative complications. Radiology 2014;270(2):327–41.

24. Rasmussen JJ, Fuller W, Ali MR. Marginal ulceration after laparoscopic gastric bypass: an analysis of predisposing factors in 260 patients. Surg Endosc 2007;21(7):1090–4.

25. Clayton RD, Carucci LR. Imaging following bariatric surgery: roux-en-Y gastric bypass, laparoscopic adjustable gastric banding and sleeve gastrectomy. Br J Radiol 2018;91(1089):20180031.

26. Takeyama N, Gokan T, Ohgiya Y, et al. CT of internal hernias. Radiographics 2005;25(4):997–1015.

27. Doishita S, Takeshita T, Uchima Y, et al. Internal hernias in the era of multidetector CT: correlation of imaging and surgical findings. Radiographics 2015;36(1):88–106.

28. Garza E, Kuhn J, Arnold D, et al. Internal hernias after laparoscopic Roux-en-Y gastric bypass. Am J Surg 2004;188(6):796–800.

29. Lockhart ME, Tessler FN, Canon CL, et al. Internal hernia after gastric bypass: sensitivity and specificity of seven CT signs with surgical correlation and controls. Am J Roentgenol 2007;188(3):745–50.

30. Duda JB, Bhatt S, Dogra VS. Utility of CT whirl sign in guiding management of small-bowel obstruction. Am J Roentgenol 2008;191(3):743–7.

31. Nerstrøm M, Krarup P-M, Jorgensen LN, et al. Therapeutic improvement of colonic anastomotic healing under complicated conditions: a systematic review. World J Gastrointest Surg 2016;8(5):389–401.

32. Samji KB, Kielar AZ, Connolly M, et al. Anastomotic leaks after small- and large-bowel surgery: diagnostic performance of CT and the importance of intraluminal contrast administration. Am J Roentgenol 2018;210(6):1259–65.

33. Cherukuri R, Levine MS, Maki DD, et al. Hartmann's pouch: radiographic evaluation of postoperative findings. AJR Am J Roentgenol 1998;171(6):1577–82.

34. Reber JD, Barlow JM, Lightner AL, et al. J Pouch: imaging findings, surgical variations, natural history, and common complications. Radiographics 2018;38(4):1073–88.

35. Hoeffel C, Arrivé L, Mourra N, et al. Anatomic and pathologic findings at external phased-array pelvic MR imaging after surgery for anorectal disease. Radiographics 2006;26(5):1391–407.

36. O'Malley RG, Al-Hawary MM, Kaza RK, et al. MDCT findings in small bowel obstruction: implications of the cause and presence of complications on treatment decisions. Abdom Imaging 2015;40(7):2248–62.

37. Gazelle GS, Goldberg MA, Wittenberg J, et al. Efficacy of CT in distinguishing small-bowel obstruction from other causes of small-bowel dilatation. Am J Roentgenol 1994;162(1):43–7.

38. Lowrance WT, Yee DS, Savage C, et al. Complications after radical and partial nephrectomy as a function of age. J Urol 2010;183(5):1725–30.

39. Hecht EM, Bennett GL, Brown KW, et al. Laparoscopic and open partial nephrectomy: frequency and long-term follow-up of postoperative collections. Radiology 2010;255(2):476–84.

40. Israel GM, Hecht E, Bosniak MA. CT and MR imaging of complications of partial nephrectomy. Radiographics 2006;26(5):1419–29.

41. Miller FH, Keppke AL, Yaghmai V, et al. CT diagnosis of chyluria after partial nephrectomy. Am J Roentgenol 2007;188(1):W25–8.

42. Catalá V, Solà M, Samaniego J, et al. CT findings in urinary diversion after radical cystectomy: postsurgical anatomy and complications. Radiographics 2009;29(2):461–76.

43. Moomjian LN, Carucci LR, Guruli G, et al. Follow the stream: imaging of urinary diversions. Radiographics 2016;36(3):688–709.

44. Hautmann RE, de Petriconi RC, Volkmer BG. Lessons learned from 1,000 neobladders: the 90-day complication rate. J Urol 2010;184(3):990–4 [quiz: 1235].

45. Wan W, Le T, Riskin L, et al. Improving safety in the operating room: a systematic literature review of retained surgical sponges. Curr Opin Anaesthesiol 2009;22(2):207–14.

46. Gawande AA, Studdert DM, Orav EJ, et al. Risk factors for retained instruments and sponges after surgery. N Engl J Med 2003;348(3):229–35.

47. Lincourt AE, Harrell A, Cristiano J, et al. Retained foreign bodies after surgery. J Surg Res 2007;138(2):170–4.

48. Wolfson KA, Seeger LL, Kadell BM, et al. Imaging of surgical paraphernalia: what belongs in the patient and what does not. Radiographics 2000;20(6):1665–73.

49. Manzella A, Filho PB, Albuquerque E, et al. Imaging of gossypibomas: pictorial review. Am J Roentgenol 2009;193(6_supplement):S94–101.

Approach to Abnormal Chest Computed Tomography Contrast Enhancement in the Hospitalized Patient

Kimberly G. Kallianos, MD[a], Michael D. Hope, MD[a,b], Travis S. Henry, MD[a,*]

KEYWORDS

- Pulmonary embolism • Flow • Artifact • Tamponade • Contrast • Thrombus • Shunt

KEY POINTS

- Abnormal distribution of intravenous contrast may be a clue to a compromised cardiovascular system in hospitalized patients.
- Inadequate transit of contrast or incomplete opacification of structures, such as the left ventricle or aorta, normally expected to be opacified, should prompt the imager to search for a potential cause, such as myocardial infarction or cardiac tamponade.
- Use of delayed venous-phase imaging is a strategy that can be used to reduce the occurrence of flow artifacts.

INTRODUCTION

Hospitalized patients frequently undergo contrast enhanced computed tomography (CT) examinations for a variety of clinical indications. This patient population is also uniquely predisposed to both important to recognize pathologies as a result of hemodynamic instability and vascular intervention as well as mimics of pathology resulting from their underlying disease state.

Often, hospitalized or ICU patients have impaired or altered cardiovascular function, and these findings often manifest on CT as alterations in blood flow—therefore, alterations in contrast distribution or flow. For example, decrease in myocardial contractility frequently manifests on contrast enhanced CT, because this imaging modality is dependent on adequate systolic function to homogeneously perfuse the imaged vessels and tissues. Abnormal contrast enhancement, however, not only is a symptom of the many pathologies that hospitalized patients may face but also can be useful diagnostically and prognostically to identify unsuspected disease or complications.

When abnormal contrast enhancement is present, knowledge of the underlying physiology can help the interpreting radiologist confidently distinguish artifacts from true pathology, improving the accuracy of interpretation of contrast enhanced chest CT in critically ill patients.

This article provides an approach to the assessment of contrast distribution on contrast-enhanced chest CT and then reviews several specific situations encountered when imaging hospitalized patients, including evaluation of patients with systolic dysfunction, interpretation

[a] Department of Radiology and Biomedical Imaging, University of California San Francisco, 505 Parnassus Avenue, M-396, San Francisco, CA 94143, USA; [b] Department of Radiology, San Francisco Veterans Affairs Medical Center, 4150 Clement Street, San Francisco, CA 94121, USA
* Corresponding author.
E-mail address: travis.henry@ucsf.edu

radiologic.theclinics.com

of heterogeneous flow, and mimics of enhancement, such as calcification and embolized materials.

SYSTOLIC DYSFUNCTION
Reflux of Contrast into the Inferior Vena Cava, Cardiogenic Shock, and Asystole

Reflux of contrast into the inferior vena cava (IVC) (assuming injection is performed via the upper extremities) is a common phenomenon on arterial-phase CT and does not necessarily indicate the presence of severe cardiac dysfunction when seen in isolation. In distinction, a true blood-contrast level in the IVC is a rare but often emergent imaging finding that signifies impending cardiovascular collapse. A discussion of each of these appearances follows.

The presence of intravenous (IV) contrast in the IVC is a potential imaging biomarker for right heart disease and should prompt the imager to look for further clues to the presence of pathology. Knowledge of the route and rate of injection of contrast is important in this evaluation because rate of injection can affect the degree of reflux[1] and injection from a lower extremity approach is going to make this assessment impossible.

Many early case reports or small series described the association of IVC reflux with various right-sided cardiac pathologies, including pulmonary hypertension, tricuspid regurgitation, atrial fibrillation, and right ventricular systolic failure. Yeh and colleagues[1] were the first group to perform a large retrospective review (127 patients) and found that reflux of contrast into the IVC or hepatic veins was significantly associated with right heart disease, including tricuspid regurgitation, pulmonary hypertension, or right ventricular

systolic dysfunction. The investigators reported, however, a sensitivity of only 31%.[1] Importantly, they found that at higher injection rates typical of CT angiography (CTA) studies (>3 mL/s), the specificity of IVC reflux for one of these pathologies was only 69%, whereas when the rate of injection was slower (less than <3 mL/s) the specificity was 98%.[1]

More recently, Aviram and colleagues[2] retrospectively reviewed 967 CT pulmonary angiogram (CTPA) studies and semiquantitatively graded the severity of reflux on a scale of 1 to 6 (1, no IVC reflux; 2, trace reflux only in the IVC; 3, reflux into the IVC but not the hepatic veins; 4, reflux into the IVC and proximal hepatic veins; 5, reflux into the IVC and midpart of the hepatic veins; and 6, reflux into the IVC and distal hepatic veins). They found that extensive reflux (grades 4–6) was significantly associated with pulmonary hypertension (odds ratio [OR] 5.4), congestive heart failure (OR 3.7), chronic atrial fibrillation (OR 2.3), and acute pulmonary embolism (OR 1.8).[2]

Although several studies have shown that reflux of contrast into the IVC can be seen in the setting of acute pulmonary embolism, the prognostic utility of this finding remains uncertain. Bach and colleagues[3] reviewed 365 CTPA studies of acute pulmonary embolism and found that reflux into the hepatic veins (grades 4–6, as described previously) was an independent predictor of 30-day mortality (OR 3.29). More recently, however, Beenen and colleagues[4] reviewed 1950 patients with acute pulmonary embolism (PE) and found no significant correlation between presence of IVC contrast reflux and either short-term (1-week) or long-term (1-year) mortality (Fig. 1).

Cardiogenic shock and, rarely, asystole/cardiac arrest represent the most severe forms of cardiac

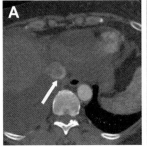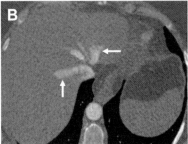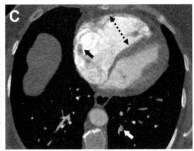

Fig. 1. (A) Mild reflux of contrast into the IVC in a 54-year-old woman (arrow). This is a common finding generally of no clinical consequence. Despite presence of moderate pericardial effusion there was no cardiac dysfunction. (B, C) Extensive reflux in a 58-year-old woman with acute pulmonary embolism. Contrast has refluxed into the hepatic veins (arrow [B]) consistent with extensive reflux, a finding often associated with right heart strain. (C) Acute PE is visible in the left lower lobe (white arrow), with thrombus in the right atrium (black arrow), dilation of the right ventricle (dotted black line), and leftward bowing of the interventricular septum. The patient was clinically diagnosed with massive PE due to systemic hypotension and tachycardia.

dysfunction in critically ill patients, and patients in these physiologic states occasionally may be imaged on CT. Cardiogenic shock is defined as a state of severely reduced cardiac output despite adequate intravascular volume whereas asystole represents the complete cessation of cardiac function.[5] There are numerous causes, including acute myocardial infarction (MI), acute decompensation of heart failure (eg, dilated cardiomyopathy and myocarditis), dynamic outflow tract obstruction, cardiac tamponade, pulmonary embolism, and sepsis.[5]

The main imaging finding in patients imaged with severely depressed cardiac output is pooling and dependent layering of contrast.[6] Many terms have been used to describe this phenomenon, including dependent pooling, blood-contrast level, and the IVC level sign, and all explain the concept that severely reduced (or, in the case of asystole, absent) cardiac output means that there is no force to combat gravity.[6–9] Hence, the contrast settles in the vena cava and other dependent structures like the right lobe of the liver, the kidneys, and the lumbar venous plexus, because it is heavier than blood. Furthermore, little contrast is propelled forward into the pulmonary arteries and may be entirely absent on the systemic side of the circulatory system. The authors have also observed contrast layering in the left atrium after passing through a patent foramen ovale (thus bypassing the pulmonary circulation) (Figs. 2 and 3).

A blood-contrast level is an emergent finding. Cardiogenic shock carries a short-term mortality

of up to 80%, if not recognized, and patients with asystole require immediate resuscitation.[9,10]

Less severe levels of systolic dysfunction can also lead to slow contrast transit through the heart, which may manifest as increased enhancement of the right-sided heart chambers with poor opacification of the left heart and aorta. Chaturvedi and colleagues[11] measured differential enhancement of the aorta and main pulmonary artery in 137 emergency department patients with suspected but absent pulmonary embolism and identified that those with poor left ventricular [LV] function (LV ejection fraction <40%) had several distinct features—aortic to pulmonary artery enhancement ratio of 0.2 to 1 had a sensitivity of 54% and specificity on 93% for LV systolic dysfunction. Not unexpectedly, those with poor LV function also had a more prolonged contrast transit time on bolus timing sequences. The investigators concluded that unsuspected LV systolic dysfunction can be identified on pulmonary embolism CT, and this realization may be important for the appropriate triage and management of patients presenting with otherwise uncharacterized cardiovascular complaints in the emergency department.

Cardiac Tamponade

Patients with cardiac tamponade also present with symptoms and imaging findings compatible with reduced cardiac output. Cardiac tamponade is the hemodynamic state of reduced cardiac filling that results from accumulation of any substance in the pericardial sac (usually fluid, such as blood)

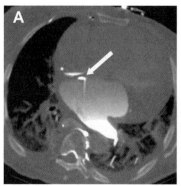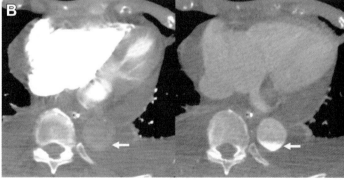

Fig. 2. (A) An 84-year-old woman who developed asystole during a CT scan. This axial image shows that most of the contrast is pooling in the most dependent portion of the patient—the left atrium and left pulmonary veins. The contrast bypassed the right ventricle via a patent foramen ovale (arrow). This pattern of pooling is a critical finding that requires immediate resuscitation. (B) A 95-year-old man who presented after a resuscitation for asystole. The arterial-phase imaging shows limited opacification of the descending aorta and subtle high attenuation from the leading edge of the contrast bolus (arrow [left image] not to be confused with intramural hematoma). On delayed imaging there is a contrast level in the aorta indicative of reduced cardiac output (arrow [right image]). On echocardiography patient was found to have diastolic dysfunction and early tamponade from the pericardial effusion.

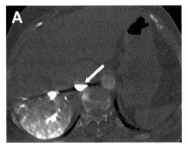
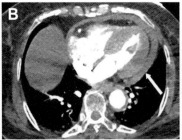
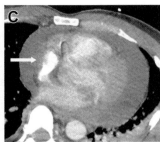

Fig. 3. (*A–C*) Dependent pooling of contrast in an 83-year-old woman with cardiac tamponade. (*A*) A blood-contrast level is visible in the IVC (*arrow*) with dependent pooling of contrast in the hepatic veins indicative of severely depressed cardiac function. (*B*) Hemopericardium (*arrow*) (from ruptured type A dissection) is present and is the cause of the reduced cardiac function. Tamponade was confirmed on echocardiogram and physical examination despite absence of other CT signs of tamponade, such as collapse of the right heart chambers. (*C*) Companion case of a middle-aged patient with large pericardial effusion resulting in tamponade, with compression and flattening of the right atrial wall (*arrow*).

that increases pericardial pressure and restricts cardiac chamber filling.[12] Because the fibrous pericardium is relatively noncompliant, even amounts as small as 100 mL to 200 mL can cause tamponade in the acute setting. Because tamponade is a potentially life-threatening condition, imagers need to be aware of the imaging appearance and search for any explainable cause.

When a pericardial effusion is present (especially if it is large), then the imager should look for signs of tamponade. Indirect CT findings that suggest elevated filling pressures include enlargement of the superior vena cava greater than the diameter of the thoracic aorta, distention of the IVC, reflux of contrast into the azygos vein or IVC, dependent pooling of contrast, and enlargement of the hepatic veins.[12] Flattening of the right heart chambers (the flattened heart sign), leftward bowing of the interventricular septum, and compression of intrapericardial structures like the pulmonary trunk or coronary sinus are more direct findings that can increase confidence in the diagnosis.[12,13] Causes of tamponade are numerous and include hemopericardium, other pericardial fluid such as malignant effusion or pericarditis, and rarely air resulting in tension pneumopericardium.[12]

Acute Myocardial Infarction on Computed Tomography

Finally, acute decline in cardiac function as the result of MI also may be identified with CT. Patients with a high suspicion of acute coronary syndrome should not undergo chest CT as a first-line diagnostic modality.[14] However, 20% to 60% of patients experiencing an acute MI may have atypical cardiopulmonary symptoms (eg, atypical chest pain and dyspnea) or abdominal symptoms

(eg, nausea and vomiting) that prompt CT evaluation.[15] Thus it is imperative that imagers recognize the findings of myocardial ischemia/MI on any contrast-enhanced CT that includes the heart, especially when no other readily identifiable causes for the symptoms are present on the CT.

Acute MI is recognizable as an area of decreased LV myocardial enhancement that corresponds to a vascular territory.[15] The decreased attenuation may involve just the subendocardial layer or may be transmural depending on the severity of the infarct. Even on older-generation CT scanners, the findings of acute MI may be apparent—Gosalia and colleagues[15] retrospectively reviewed 18 patients who underwent single-slice CT and found that a region of relative hypoattenuation of the LV in a vascular territory (decrease of more than 20 Hounsfield units [HU] relative to normal myocardium) was 83% sensitive and 95% specific, with positive predictive value of 94% and negative predictive value of 86% for diagnosis of acute MI. Other studies have shown similar results with specificities and sensitivities greater than 80% on newer generation CT scanners both for arterial-phase CT angiography[16,17] and for parenchymal-phase 100-second delay CT.[18] Depending on the amount of myocardium involved, patients experiencing an acute MI may have findings of pulmonary edema, reduced transit of contrast, and/or reflux of contrast into the IVC (as discussed previously) (**Fig. 4**).

Beam hardening, respiratory motion, and cardiac motion are common artifacts that may be mistaken for MI, especially in the posterobasal LV wall.[19] Especially when there is question of the reality of the finding, the imager should discuss with the clinician the possibility of MI and prompt further evaluation with electrocardiogram and or serum biomarkers.[20]

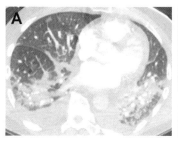
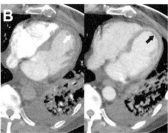

Fig. 4. An 83-year-old man with hypotension due to acute left anterior descending coronary artery-territory MI after hip surgery. (*A*) CTPA at lung windows shows dependent consolidation, smooth interlobular septal thickening, and small pleural effusions. (*B*) On the arterial-phase study (*left*), faint decrease in subendocardial enhancement (*white arrow*) is visible with mild dilation of the LV chamber. On the portal venous–phase image (*right*) the decreased enhancement is more pronounced (*black arrow*). A 100% left anterior descending coronary artery occlusion was subsequently confirmed during invasive catheter angiography.

HETEROGENEOUS FLOW

In general, the imager should not assume that contrast enhancement is uniform throughout a vessel. Nonuniform contrast enhancement of the thoracic vasculature on contrast-enhanced chest CT and CTA may result from a variety of physiologic and pathologic processes. Modern CT scanners have the benefits of better temporal resolution and shorter scan times; however, they are also more prone to flow-related artifacts. These artifacts can lead to misdiagnosis by mimicking pathology but, however, can also be illustrative of subtle cardiovascular abnormalities, such as shunts. The authors have recently described the principles of this phenomenon, termed *smoke*, in a recent publication.[21] In general, smoke is seen when there is fast temporal resolution and when there is inadequate time for contrast to mix (due to a combination of reduced cardiac output or other cause of reduced contrast transit, mixing of opacified and unopacified blood, and/or scanning at the leading edge of the bolus). Although detailed management strategies for these problems are beyond the scope of this article, scanning with a longer delay can allow more time for mixing to occur as described later.

Pulmonary Embolism

The basic principles needed to correctly distinguish flow artifact from intravascular filling defect due to thrombus include a firm grasp on the imaging appearance of thrombus. True thrombus appears as a discrete filling defect with defined margins and a density in the range of 30 HU to 60 HU. The mean attenuation of acute pulmonary embolism has been investigated and reported at 33 HU ± 15 HU, with greater than 99% of pulmonary embolism falling below 100 HU in density.[22] Contrast mixing, on the other hand, appears ill defined and has a wide range of attenuation based on the contrast density, however, often exceeding 100 HU. Contrast mixing mimicking pulmonary embolism (which may be termed smoke based on its wispy, ill-defined appearance) can be seen in a variety of clinical settings, including (1) scanning very early at the initial edge of the contrast bolus; (2) regional alterations in pulmonary arterial blood flow as a result of vascular stenosis, vasoconstriction, or down-regulated flow in areas of chronic parenchymal disease; and (3) venous or collateral inflow (**Fig. 5**).[21]

Transient interruption of contrast is a specific instance where unopacified venous inflow from the IVC mixes with opacified blood returning

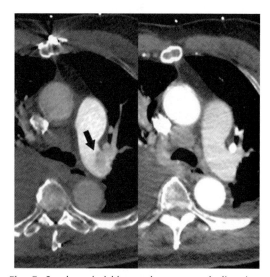

Fig. 5. Smoke mimicking pulmonary embolism in a 51-year-old man presenting with dyspnea. CTPA (*left*) shows a heterogeneous, amorphous filling defect initially interpreted as pulmonary embolism, but most consistent with a flow artifact (*black arrow*). Repeat study timed off of the descending aorta (*right*) shows homogeneous opacification of the left pulmonary artery confirming the diagnosis of smoke. Note the early acquisition (*left*) with little contrast reaching the aorta, another clue to the presence of heterogeneous flow.

from the superior vena cava and can result in poor opacification of the pulmonary arterial system. This venous inflow is exacerbated by maneuvers that increase systemic venous return, such as the Valsalva maneuver.

Chamber Thrombus

Similar to the presence of flow-related artifacts in the pulmonary arteries, slow flow in the cardiac chambers also may mimic the appearance of thrombus. This is particularly common in regions redisposed to stasis, including the atrial appendages and in LV apical aneurysms. Special caution needs to be paid to studies where little contrast has reached the left heart chambers because the cause of the slow transit (reduced LV systolic function) also may predispose to thrombus formation (Fig. 6A).

Contrast mixing or pseudothrombus in the left atrial appendage should be suspected when the filling defect is high in density (>100 HU) or has a smooth, graded transition on arterial-phase imaging.[23] Delayed-phase imaging performed 60 seconds after the injection of IV contrast resulted in resolution of 85% of the initially seen atrial appendage filling defects and had a sensitivity and specificity for the diagnosis of true left atrial appendage thrombus of 100% compared with transesophageal echocardiography (Fig. 6B).[24]

Shunts

Differential density of contrast within the cardiac chambers, in particular the atria, is most commonly explained by mixing, as discussed previously. There are specific instances, however, in which differential chamber enhancement is indicative of abnormal communication or shunt between the chambers. This may take the form of a directed contrast jet across the atrial or ventricular septum in the case of atrial or ventricular septal defect. The contrast timing bolus series, however, may be most helpful in identifying an unsuspected shunt by noting the order in which vessels and chambers are opacified. The appearance of contrast in the superior vena cava followed immediately by the left atrium, bypassing the pulmonary artery, is indicative of an intracardiac right-to left-shunt (Fig. 7A).[25]

A similar finding has been observed in other shunts, such as across a patent ductus arteriosus, if there is sufficient differential in contrast between the aorta and pulmonary artery, and should not be mistaken for thrombus (Fig. 7B).

Congenital Heart Disease

Patients with repaired congenital heart disease are particularly prone to flow-related artifacts as a result of novel flow patterns after surgical repair. One situation encountered fairly commonly is a patient with Glenn/Fontan repair physiology, where blood from the superior vena cava and IVC is passively directed into the pulmonary artery, bypassing the right heart. In this situation, a large volume of unopacified blood may enter the pulmonary arterial system, precluding accurate diagnosis of pulmonary embolism (and often mistaken for unilateral pulmonary embolism by inexperienced imagers). Because right-sided Glenn/Fontan connections are more common, there may be a distinct difference in density of the right and left pulmonary arteries depending on the phase of contrast (Fig. 8).

Other challenges in imaging patients with congenital heart disease include incorrect placement of the region of interest for bolus tracking. Variant vascular anatomy may be unfamiliar to the technologist, leading to suboptimal opacification of the vessels of interest.

Although strategies to mitigate these challenges have included complex protocols with simultaneous injection of contrast in both upper and lower extremities, a single extremity injection with 60-second to 90-second delayed-phase imaging is usually adequate to opacity the major intrathoracic vasculature.[26]

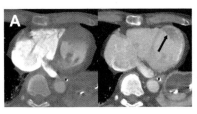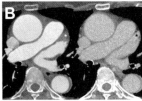

Fig. 6. (A) LV thrombus in a 49-year-old man with nonischemic dilated cardiomyopathy. A CTPA (left) and portal venous phase of abdomen/pelvis (right) was performed for hypotension and generalized symptoms. On the CTPA there is slow flow and incomplete opacification of the LV chamber, which renders evaluation of apical thrombus difficult. On the portal venous phase, however, a large mural thrombus is clearly visible in the LV apex (black arrow). (B) An 85-year-old woman undergoing left atrial mapping for atrial fibrillation ablation. Slow flow in the left atrial appendage could be mistaken for a thrombus (white asterisk [left]), but resolves on delayed imaging (black asterisk [right]). This is a frequent finding in patients with atrial fibrillation due to slow flow, particularly in the atrial appendage.

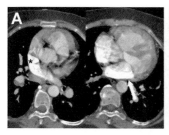 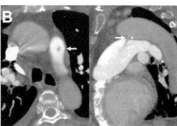

Fig. 7. (*A*) A 65-year-old woman with pulmonary arterial hypertension from a previously undetected sinus venosus atrial septal defect (ASD). Axial images from a CTPA show dense contrast in the left atrium (*arrow*) that is much denser than the right ventricle, suggesting a shunt. Close inspection shows a direct communication (*asterisk*) consistent with a sinus venosus ASD that had been previously missed on echocardiography. Right superior partial anomalous pulmonary venous return to the superior vena cava (SVC) was also present (not shown). (*B*) A 79 year old with incidentally discovered patent ductus arteriosus. Axial (*left*) and sagittal (*right*) images from a CTPA performed for dyspnea. On the axial image, a discrete filling defect is present in the main pulmonary artery (*arrow [left]*). Sagittal image shows that this represents a jet of relatively unopacified blood from the aorta (*arrow [right]*) and should be recognized as a patent ductus arteriosus (and not mistaken for pulmonary embolism).

MIMICS OF ENHANCEMENT
Myocardial Calcification

High density within the heart and thoracic vasculature is most likely due to the administration of contrast; however, there are several situations when intrathoracic high density is due to the presence of other materials, such as calcium, hematoma, and embolized materials.

Myocardial calcification can be subdivided into dystrophic calcification or metastatic calcification. Dystrophic calcification is the deposition of calcium in nonviable myocardium that has undergone necrosis and cell death and is usually seen after MI, cardiac surgery, or myocarditis.[27] Dystrophic calcification is relatively common on CT especially in post-MI patients, where the calcification should be focal/multifocal and confined to the involved vascular territory.[28]

Metastatic calcification, on the other hand, represents the deposition of calcium in viable myocardium due to systemic disorders, such as abnormal calcium homeostasis, most commonly in patients with end-stage renal disease on dialysis.[27]

Diffuse myocardial calcification is occasionally encountered on CT in critically ill patients and has been called heart of stone and petrified myocardium.[29–32] The mechanism for this entity is poorly understood and likely multifactorial, but sepsis resulting in microvascular disease and myocardial injury is thought to play a role in many cases.[27,33] The outcomes in patients with heart of stone is variable. Some patients may have preserved myocardial function, but many cases have been associated with restrictive cardiomyopathy, heart failure, arrhythmia, and sudden cardiac death (**Fig. 9**).[27,30,32]

Diffuse myocardial calcification may be detected on echocardiography as increased echogenicity and/or acoustic shadowing produced by the myocardial calcification but is a less sensitive modality than CT.[32] CT is considered the gold standard for diagnosis of diffuse myocardial calcification. The distribution of calcification is variable but often multifocal or diffuse, transmural or subepicardial, and occurring even in the absence of calcification of other organs.[31,33] Importantly, the calcification often develops rapidly over the course of days to weeks during the hospitalization of a critically ill patient.[33] It is important for the imager to differentiate diffuse myocardial

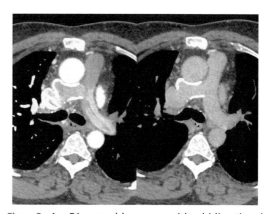

Fig. 8. A 51-year-old man with bidirectional Glenn and Fontan shunts for treatment of congenital heart disease who presented with dyspnea. Arterial-phase image through SVC injection (*left*) shows heterogeneous enhancement of the pulmonary arterial tree with reduced filling of left-sided pulmonary veins and heterogeneous flow that could be mistaken for PE. A 90-second delay (*right*) allows time for contrast to fully opacify the pulmonary circulation and confirm absence of PE. The preferential filling of the right-sided arteries on the arterial-phase imaging is easily explained by the continuity of the Glenn shunt with the right pulmonary artery.

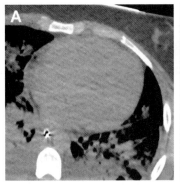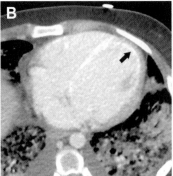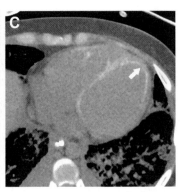

Fig. 9. Progressive myocardial calcification (heart of stone) in a 22-year-old woman initially admitted with sepsis and acute kidney injury. Noncontrast CT at time of admission (*A*) shows normal appearance of the heart. Contrast-enhanced CT on hospital day 17 (*B*) shows high attenuation in the heart that was initially thought to be hyper-enhancement (*black arrow*). A repeat noncontrast CT on hospital day 30 (*C*) shows that this is myocardial calcification rather than enhancement (*white arrow*).

calcification from myocardial enhancement on contrast-enhanced CT because the 2 entities can occasionally be confused. Although many patients with diffuse myocardial calcification have poor outcomes, there are no long-term outcomes or guidelines for follow-up in patients who survive their acute hospitalization.[33]

Pericardial Collections

Critically ill patients may develop pericardial collections for a variety of reasons, ranging from sequela of fluid overload to direct cardiac or vascular injury. Increased density of pericardial fluid greater than water is indicative exudative pericardial effusion or hemopericardium, with higher densities ranging from 40 HU to 60 HU suggestive of blood products.[34] Hemopericardium may develop spontaneously in patients with coagulopathy or may be the result of ruptured MI or aortic dissection. Iatrogenic causes, such as line malplacement, also should be considered in hospitalized patients (**Fig. 10**).

The presence of very high attenuation material in the pericardial space (150+ HU) is indicative of contrast excretion or extravasation. After iatrogenic vascular perforation, such as may occur during cardiac catheterization or transcatheter aortic valve replacement, iodinated contrast opacification of the pericardium is not unexpected. In patients without hemodynamic compromise, limited or contained rupture may be managed conservatively.[35] Unstable patients or those with growing hemopericardium may necessitate percutaneous pericardial drainage or emergent exploration.

Investigators have also noted the presence of intermediate and high-attenuation pericardial fluid on CT after cardiac catheterization in cases of perforation not clinically suspected.[36] High-attenuation pericardial fluid was most strongly associated with a shorter time gap between cardiac catheterization and chest CT in this study. These patients followed a benign clinical course, and the investigators proposed vicarious excretion of contrast as a potential mechanism of this finding in asymptomatic patients after cardiac catheterization (**Fig. 11**).

Embolized Materials

Pulmonary thrombotic emboli may occur in hospitalized patients due to prolonged immobility in addition to other clinical risk factors, such as recent surgery or malignancy. Other materials may embolize, however, into the pulmonary arterial system and mimic thrombotic emboli. Identification of these materials is important in order to avoid inappropriate anticoagulation as well as to direct appropriate therapeutic interventions.

Iatrogenic microembolism during injection of radiotracer for fluorodeoxyglucose (FDG)-positron emission tomography has been well described as an etiology of localized FDG uptake in the lung parenchyma without corresponding CT pathology.[37]

Fig. 10. Noncontrast CT (*A*) in a 65-year-old man after left subclavian line placement. Subsequent CTA (*B*) shows large volume of contrast extravasation into the mediastinum, confirming extravascular line location.

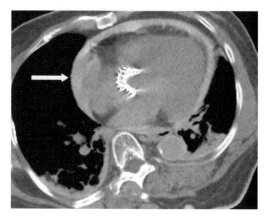

Fig. 11. Noncontrast chest CT performed immediately after transcatheter aortic valve replacement with clinical concern for intraprocedureal myocardial perforation. High-attenuation (150 HU) pericardial effusion (*arrow*) is compatible with the extravasation of iodinated contrast into the pericardial space.

A similar phenomenon can rarely occur with contrast material itself, presumably due to small aggregates of contrast particles that become clumped prior to injection. These contrast emboli cause transient high-density pulmonary arterial filling defects, which subsequently resolve as the contrast material becomes diluted by the flow of blood. It is important to recognize this phenomenon so as to avoid misinterpretation of the findings as an embolized catheter fragment or other device. Multiphase CT or follow-up imaging may be helpful in correctly recognizing the transient nature of contrast embolism and its direct relation to the time of contrast injection (**Fig. 12**).

Implanted lines and devices can indeed embolize to the pulmonary arterial system in hospitalized patients, with CT findings corresponding to the shape and density of the embolized material. Polymethylmethacrylate cement used in vertebral body augmentation procedures is a not uncommon cause of nonthrombotic pulmonary embolism.[38,39] Extravasation of contrast into the paravertebral venous plexus at the time of cement injection leads to cement transit into the azygos system, right heart, and ultimately the lung parenchyma. CT findings include tubular, high-density filling defects in the pulmonary artery branches. Cement emboli are readily identified on noncontrast CT. Utilization of window and level settings closer to a traditional bone window aids identification of cement emboli on contrast-enhanced chest CT, where these filling defects may be obscured by dense contrast. Treatment of cement embolism is an area of uncertainty in the literature and may vary from no treatment to surgical embolectomy, depending on burden of emboli and patient symptoms. Because thrombus has been reported to form adjacent to the cement deposits, anticoagulation has also been proposed as a treatment in some patients, particularly in symptomatic patients or those with central cement emboli (**Fig. 13**).[40]

Finally, hospitalized patients are at risk for air embolism as a result of indwelling vascular lines and vascular interventions. Small-volume air embolism in the pulmonary arterial systems is common, seen in 23% of patients undergoing contrast-enhanced chest CT and is most often s asymptomatic. Instillation of larger volumes of gas into the pulmonary arterial system (usually 300–500 mL) may be fatal by resulting in obstruction of the right ventricular outflow tract or small pulmonary vessels leading to right heart failure.[41]

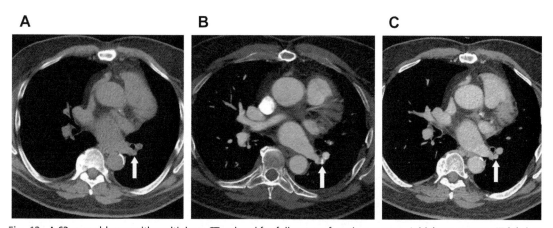

A   **B**   **C**

Fig. 12. A 63-year-old man with multiphase CT ordered for follow-up of aortic aneurysm. Initial noncontrast CT (*A*) demonstrates no radio-opaque intravascular filling defects. Note the normal appearance of the left lower lobe pulmonary artery branches (*arrow*). CTA-phase (*B*) image shows new hyperdense pulmonary arterial filling defect in the left lower lobe (*arrow*), however, which resolved on the subsequently performed 90-second delayed-phase (*arrow*) (*C*) as a result of contrast dilution. No distal emboli were present on the delayed phase, confirming dissolution of contrast emboli.

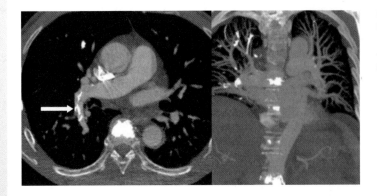

Fig. 13. Axial (*left*) and coronal (*right*) contrast enhanced CT images in a middle-aged after spine cement augmentation procedure demonstrates multifocal cement embolism, preferentially involving the right pulmonary artery (*arrow*).

Air entrained into the pulmonary veins, left heart, or aorta can lead to fatal embolic complications, including stroke, MI, or bowel ischemia. The treatment of air embolism varies based on the location of the intravascular gas but consists of strategies promoting reabsorption of the air, such as supplemental oxygen and positional changes to ensure adequate pulmonary and systemic blood flow while avoiding systemic embolization.[42]

SUMMARY

Alterations in IV contrast distribution are common on cardiothoracic CT, especially in critically ill patients. Abnormal transit or distribution of contrast should prompt the imager to look for an explanation—either to recognize a potentially life-threatening disease or to distinguish the appearance from flow artifact.

REFERENCES

1. Yeh BM, Kurzman P, Foster E, et al. Clinical relevance of retrograde inferior vena cava or hepatic vein opacification during contrast-enhanced CT. AJR Am J Roentgenol 2004;183(5):1227–32.
2. Aviram G, Cohen D, Steinvil A, et al. Significance of reflux of contrast medium into the inferior vena cava on computerized tomographic pulmonary angiogram. Am J Cardiol 2012;109(3):432–7.
3. Bach AG, Nansalmaa B, Kranz J, et al. CT pulmonary angiography findings that predict 30-day mortality in patients with acute pulmonary embolism. Eur J Radiol 2015;84(2):332–7.
4. Beenen LFM, Bossuyt PMM, Stoker J, et al. Prognostic value of cardiovascular parameters in computed tomography pulmonary angiography in patients with acute pulmonary embolism. Eur Respir J 2018;52(1):1702611.
5. van Diepen S, Katz JN, Albert NM, et al. Contemporary management of cardiogenic shock: a scientific statement from the American Heart Association. Circulation 2017;136(16):e232–68.
6. Roth C, Sneider M, Bogot N, et al. Dependent venous contrast pooling and layering: a sign of imminent cardiogenic shock. AJR Am J Roentgenol 2006;186(4):1116–9.
7. Tsai P-P, Chen J-H, Huang J-L, et al. Dependent pooling: a contrast-enhanced sign of cardiac arrest during CT. AJR Am J Roentgenol 2002;178(5):1095–9.
8. Wu C, Lee RC, Wu M, et al. A blood-contrast level: a sign of cardiac arrest. J Radiol Sci 2015;40:133–5.
9. Bagheri SM, Taheri MS, Pourghorban R, et al. Computed tomographic imaging features of sudden cardiac arrest and impending cardiogenic shock. J Comput Assist Tomogr 2012;36(3):291–4.
10. Sullivan IW, Hota P, Dako F, et al. Dependent layering of venous refluxed contrast: a sign of critically low cardiac output. Radiol Case Rep 2019;14(2):230–4.
11. Chaturvedi A, Thompson JP, Kaproth-Joslin K, et al. Identification of left ventricle failure on pulmonary artery CTA: diagnostic significance of decreased aortic & left ventricle enhancement. Emerg Radiol 2017;24(5):487–96.
12. Restrepo CS, Lemos DF, Lemos JA, et al. Imaging findings in cardiac tamponade with emphasis on CT. Radiographics 2007;27(6):1595–610.
13. Hernández-Luyando L, Calvo J, González de las Heras E, et al. Tension pericardial collections: sign of "flattened heart" in CT. Eur J Radiol 1996;23(3):250–2.
14. Mammen L, White RD, Woodard PK, et al. ACR Appropriateness Criteria® on chest pain, suggestive of acute coronary syndrome. J Am Coll Radiol 2011;8(1):12–8.
15. Gosalia A, Haramati LB, Sheth MP, et al. CT detection of acute myocardial infarction. AJR Am J Roentgenol 2004;182(6):1563–6.
16. Watanabe T, Furuse Y, Ohta Y, et al. The effectiveness of non-ECG-gated contrast-enhanced computed tomography for the diagnosis of non-ST segment elevation acute coronary syndrome. Int Heart J 2016;57(5):558–64.
17. Mano Y, Anzai T, Yoshizawa A, et al. Role of non-electrocardiogram-gated contrast-enhanced computed tomography in the diagnosis of acute coronary syndrome. Heart Vessels 2015;30(1):1–8.

18. Yamazaki M, Higuchi T, Shimokoshi T, et al. Acute coronary syndrome: evaluation of detection capability using non-electrocardiogram-gated parenchymal phase CT imaging. Jpn J Radiol 2016; 34(5):331–8.

19. Shriki JE, Shinbane J, Lee C, et al. Incidental myocardial infarct on conventional nongated CT: a review of the spectrum of findings with gated CT and cardiac MRI correlation. AJR Am J Roentgenol 2012;198(3):496–504.

20. Moore A, Goerne H, Rajiah P, et al. Acute myocardial infarct. Radiol Clin North Am 2019;57(1):45–55.

21. Henry TS, Hammer MM, Little BP, et al. Smoke: how to differentiate flow-related artifacts from pathology on thoracic computed tomographic angiography. J Thorac Imaging 2019;34(5):W109–20.

22. Wittram C, Maher MM, Halpern EF, et al. Attenuation of acute and chronic pulmonary emboli. Radiology 2005;235(3):1050–4.

23. Teunissen C, Habets J, Velthuis BK, et al. Double-contrast, single-phase computed tomography angiography for ruling out left atrial appendage thrombus prior to atrial fibrillation ablation. Int J Cardiovasc Imaging 2017;33(1):121–8.

24. Lazoura O, Ismail TF, Pavitt C, et al. A low-dose, dual-phase cardiovascular CT protocol to assess left atrial appendage anatomy and exclude thrombus prior to left atrial intervention. Int J Cardiovasc Imaging 2016;32(2):347–54.

25. Chaturvedi A, Oppenheimer D, Rajiah P, et al. Contrast opacification on thoracic CT angiography: challenges and solutions. Insights Imaging 2017;8: 1–14.

26. Ghadimi Mahani M, Agarwal PP, Rigsby CK, et al. CT for assessment of thrombosis and pulmonary embolism in multiple stages of single-ventricle palliation: challenges and suggested protocols. Radiographics 2016;36(5):1273–84.

27. Bower G, Ashrafian H, Cappelletti S, et al. A proposed role for sepsis in the pathogenesis of myocardial calcification. Acta Cardiol 2017;72(3): 249–55.

28. Nance JW, Crane GM, Halushka MK, et al. Myocardial calcifications: pathophysiology, etiologies, differential diagnoses, and imaging findings. J Cardiovasc Comput Tomogr 2015;9(1): 58–67.

29. Austin CO, Kramer D, Canabal J, et al. A heart of stone: a case of acute development of cardiac calcification and hemodynamic collapse. J Cardiovasc Comput Tomogr 2013;7(1):66–8.

30. Na J-Y. A heart of stone: an autopsy case of massive myocardial calcification. Forensic Sci Med Pathol 2018;14(1):102–5.

31. Furman MS, Healey TT, Agarwal S, et al. "Heavy hearted havoc" – A case series of petrified myocardium. J Cardiovasc Comput Tomogr 2018;12(6): e21–3.

32. Mana M, Sanguineti F, Unterseeh T, et al. Petrified myocardium: the age of stone? Circulation 2012; 126(9):1139–42.

33. Ahmed T, Inayat F, Haq M, et al. Myocardial calcification secondary to toxic shock syndrome: a comparative review of 17 cases. BMJ Case Rep 2019;12(1) [pii:bcr-2018-228054].

34. Wang ZJ, Reddy GP, Gotway MB, et al. CT and MR imaging of pericardial disease. Radiographics 2003; 23:S167–80.

35. Coughlan JJ, Kiernan T, Mylotte D, et al. Annular rupture during transcatheter aortic valve implantation: predictors, management and outcomes. Interv Cardiol 2018;13(3):140–4.

36. Avery LL, Jain VR, Cohen HW, et al. High attenuation pericardial fluid on CT following cardiac catheterization. Emerg Radiol 2014;21(4):381–6.

37. Ozdemir E, Poyraz NY, Keskin M, et al. Hot-clot artifacts in the lung parenchyma on F-18 fluorodeoxyglucose positron emission tomography/CT due to faulty injection techniques: two case reports. Korean J Radiol 2014;15(4):530–3.

38. Khashper A, Discepola F, Kosiuk J, et al. Nonthrombotic pulmonary embolism. AJR Am J Roentgenol 2012;198(2):W152–9.

39. Pelton WM, Kirsch J, Candocia FJ, et al. Methylmethacrylate pulmonary emboli: radiographic and computed tomographic findings. J Thorac Imaging 2009;24(3):241–7.

40. Krueger A, Bliemel C, Zettl R, et al. Management of pulmonary cement embolism after percutaneous vertebroplasty and kyphoplasty: a systematic review of the literature. Eur Spine J 2009;18(9):1257–65.

41. Rossi SE, Goodman PC, Franquet T. Nonthrombotic pulmonary emboli. AJR Am J Roentgenol 2000; 174(6):1499–508.

42. McCarthy CJ, Behravesh S, Naidu SG, et al. Air embolism: practical tips for prevention and treatment. J Clin Med 2016;5(11) [pii:E93].

Imaging Approach to Misplaced Central Venous Catheters

Demetrios A. Raptis, MD*, Kevin Neal, MD, Sanjeev Bhalla, MD

KEYWORDS

- Central venous catheters • Malpositioned catheters • Cavoatrial junction • Extravascular catheters
- Right-sided venous catheters • Left-sided venous catheters • Intra-arterial catheters

KEY POINTS

- The radiologist is frequently requested to evaluate the location of central venous catheter (CVC) tips and deem them suitable for use. An approach to CVC placement based on tip location (right of midline, left of midline, or midline) can be helpful in localization and guiding management.
- The ideal anatomic location for a CVC tip is in the lower superior vena cava or upper right atrium, also known as the superior right cavoatrial junction.
- When encountered with a catheter tip located to the left of the midline, the following locations should be considered: left-sided superior vena cava, left superior intercostal vein, left pericardiophrenic vein, left superior anomalous pulmonary vein, and left internal mammary vein.
- CVCs with the tips located to the right of the midline have several potential locations in addition to the desired location of the superior vena cava, including the right internal mammary, right pericardiophrenic, azygous vein, and, rarely, an anomalous right superior pulmonary vein.
- In the setting of arterial placement of a CVC, CT can be used to illustrate the site of arterial access and in turn direct further management.

INTRODUCTION

Central venous catheters (CVCs) are commonly used in patients in a variety of clinical settings, including the intensive care unit (ICU), general ward, and outpatient settings. CVC, also known as a central line or central venous line, is defined as a catheter placed into a large vein, with the tip typically terminating within the superior vena cava (SVC) or inferior vena cava (IVC). CVCs enable continuous access to the venous system and are a mainstay for treatment in the ICU setting. CVCs are typically placed for administration of fluids, medication delivery, repeated blood draws, hemodynamic monitoring, total parenteral nutrition, and dialysis access.

The type of CVC placed is typically dependent on the expected duration of the catheter use. Short-term CVCs are deployed with the expectation to remain in place for use for days to weeks. As a result, they are not tunneled under the skin. The tunneling may decrease the risk of infection but adds to the complexity of the procedure. Long-term CVCs are tunneled lines typically placed for intravenous (IV) therapy or multiple repeated intermittent treatments, with the expectation of use lasting longer than 4 weeks. Regardless of the expected duration of use, CVCs are available in a variety of lengths, gauges, and lumens. Multiple lumen catheters allow for simultaneous functions, such as drug infusions, blood draws, and hemodynamic monitoring. The

Disclosure statement: None of the authors have any disclosures.
Mallinckrodt Institute of Radiology, 216 South Kingshighway Boulevard, St Louis, MO 63110, USA
* Corresponding author. Mallinckrodt Institute of Radiology, 510 S. Kingshighway Boulevard, St Louis, MO 63110.
E-mail address: d.raptis@wustl.edu

Radiol Clin N Am 58 (2020) 105–117
https://doi.org/10.1016/j.rcl.2019.08.011

radiologic.theclinics.com

multiple lumens may have different lengths, with a staggered termination of the tips, or all tips may terminate at the same length.

Short-term catheters can be inserted, exchanged, and removed at the bedside and frequently are used in the ICU setting. Reported rates of CVC usage range from 13% to 91% in the ICU setting.[1–4] In the authors' experience, it is rare for an ICU patient to have no central catheter. CVC placement may result in a multitude of complications, including infection, hemorrhage, and thrombosis. Not infrequently, complications may result from catheter insertion or malpositioning. Multiple studies have demonstrated that a malpositioned CVC occurs approximately 10% of the time.[5–12] Frequent sites of misplaced catheters include the internal jugular vein, azygous vein, superior intercostal vein, contralateral subclavian vein, and axillary vein.[13] A majority of the complications are minor with vessel wall perforation the most common severe complication. Vessel wall perforation may result in pneumothorax, hemothorax, mediastinal/soft tissue hematoma, and cardiac perforation. Pneumothorax is the result of wall perforation, occurring in approximately 2% of cases[5,7,14] Complications are more common with subclavian vein placement compared with jugular placement.[8]

The American College of Radiology Appropriateness Criteria on the radiological management of central venous access recommends a chest radiograph after insertion of a CVC and/or Swan-Ganz catheter to demonstrate proper placement and possible complications.[5] Rarely, computed tomography (CT) may be used as a problem-solving technique when the radiograph is ambiguous. After initial insertion, follow-up chest radiographs demonstrate little benefit in revealing complications and are suggested only when there is a clinical suspicion of a catheter-related complication.[5] The radiologist, then, has the potential to play a key role after CVC placement in the recognition of correct positioning of the CVC as well as catheter-related complications in order to prevent adverse outcomes and prompt potentially life-saving intervention in cases of a rare life-threatening complication.

NORMAL CATHETER PLACEMENT

The tip of the CVC should be distal to the last venous valve, which is located at the confluence of the internal jugular and subclavian veins.[15] On the chest radiograph, this location typically is seen at the first intercostal space. The ideal anatomic location for a CVC tip is in the lower SVC or upper right atrium, also known as the superior right cavoatrial junction. The location of the CVC tip typically is verified by obtaining a portable chest radiograph after CVC placement, prior to the first use of the catheter. Although other methods, such as ultrasound, electrocardiography, and impedence technology, have been explored for catheter verification, the chest radiograph remains the standard of care at most institutions. A portable chest radiograph is easily obtained and imparts a very low effective radiation dose; approximately 0.02 mSv, or the equivalent of 3 days of background radiation at sea level.[16] The lower SVC is located below the right mainstem bronchus, above the superior cavoatrial junction (**Fig. 1**A). The superior cavoatrial junction is approximately 2 vertebral bodies below the carina[17] (see **Fig. 1**A). In certain scenarios it may be difficult to accurately localize the tip of the catheter secondary to overlying structures or patient body habitus. An additional lateral or oblique view can be obtained to demonstrate proper location of the catheter (**Fig. 1**B). In the current era of digital radiography, adjusting contrast and brightness with narrow window widths can be utilized to help locate catheter tips in suboptimal exposures.

MALPOSITIONED CATHETERS

The authors propose a simplified approach to evaluation of malpositioned catheters, with an emphasis placed on the location of the catheter relative to the midline. Close attention should be paid to possible intra-arterial course of the catheter. Furthermore, the chest radiograph should be used to evaluate for secondary complications of catheter placement, including pneumothorax and vascular perforation. When there is concern for malposition of a CVC, orthogonal images and injection of contrast material can be used to verify the precise location. Increasingly, CT is used as a problem-solving technique.

RIGHT-SIDED VENOUS CATHETERS

CVCs with the tips located to the right of the midline have several potential locations in addition to the desired location of the SVC. These potential venous locations include normal structures, most commonly, the right internal mammary, right pericardiophrenic, and azygous vein. Rarely, a CVC may find its way into an anomalous right superior pulmonary vein.

The right anterior aspect of the chest is drained by the right internal mammary vein, also referred to as the right internal thoracic vein. The right internal mammary vein drains the anterior intercostal veins

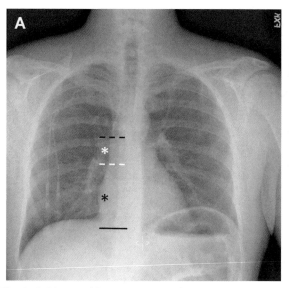

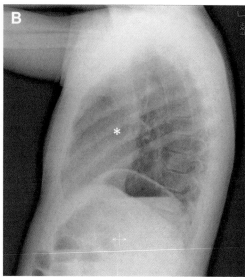

Fig. 1. A 44-year-old man post–CVC placement with a 2-view chest radiograph to confirm catheter placement. (*A*) The posterior-anterior chest radiograph demonstrates the CVC tip located within the lower SVC (*white asterisk*). The lower SVC is defined by the space located below the right mainstem bronchus (*black dashed line*) and the superior cavoatrial junction (*white dashed line*). The space between the superior cavoatrial junction and superior aspect of the IVC (*solid black line*) represents the right atrium (*black asterisk*). (*B*) Lateral chest radiograph with the catheter tip (*asterisk*) positioned within the lower SVC (note the course in the middle mediastinum).

and anastomoses with abdominal wall vessels. The right internal mammary vein courses superiorly and drains cranially into the innominate vein. The orifice of the right internal mammary vein is located close to the origin of the SVC and can be entered during catheter placement from both right-sided and left-sided approaches. CVCs located within the right internal mammary vein may be slightly lateral to the SVC, just to the right of the sternal boarder, on the frontal view with a distinct anterior course seen on the lateral view. The frontal radiograph often demonstrates a distinctive curve or notching of the catheter as it enters the internal mammary vein (**Fig. 2**).

The right pericardiophrenic vein is a small vein responsible for drainage of the pericardium, pleura, and diaphragm. The vein courses lateral to the right heart boarder traveling adjacent to the phrenic nerve. The right pericardiophrenic vein drains directly into the right internal mammary

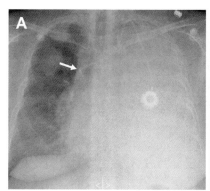

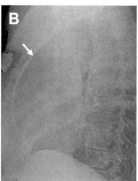

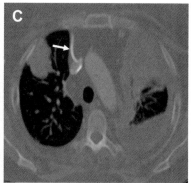

Fig. 2. A 58-year-old woman post–placement of a left ventral venous port catheter. (*A*) The posterior-anterior chest radiograph demonstrates a distinctive curve of the catheter (*arrow*), which is located lateral to the expected location of the SVC. These findings are suspicious for catheter placement into the right internal mammary vein. (*B*) The lateral chest radiograph demonstrates the catheter (*arrow*) located anteriorly coursing along the chest wall, within the right internal mammary vein. (*C*) Transaxial CT image confirms the location of the catheter (*arrow*) within the right internal mammary vein.

vein. In patients with venous obstruction, it may serve as a collateral pathway for venous drainage. It often anastomoses with the inferior phrenic vein. Although not frequently entered during CVC placement, given its diminutive size, placement may result in thrombosis or perforation.

The azygous vein is located to the right of the vertebral bodies and enters the thorax through the aortic hiatus and courses superiorly within the thorax carrying deoxygenated blood from the posterior chest and abdominal walls. Although the term, *azygous*, translates to *without a pair*, the azygous vein often communicates with the left-sided equivalent—the hemiazygous vein. The azygous vein forms around the level of T12-L2 from the confluence of ascending lumbar veins and right subcostal veins. Differing from other right-sided venous structures, the azygous vein courses through the posterior or middle mediastinum before arching over the right mainstem bronchus, at which point it joins the SVC (**Fig. 3**). This course posterior to the trachea is best appreciated on the lateral projection.

A right superior anomalous pulmonary vein is equally as common as a left superior anomalous pulmonary vein. It represents a congenital malformation in which the blood supply from the right upper lobe drains directly to the systemic venous system or right atrium. The most common site of drainage is the SVC, although drainage into the right atrium, right brachiocephalic vein, coronary

sinus, and azygous system have all been reported. Even more rarely, the anomalous vein may drain into the portal vein, ductus venosus, or inferior vena cava. This lesion results in a left to right shunt. Typically, these patients have an associated sinus venosus type atrial septal defect. A catheter within an anomalous right upper lobe pulmonary vein has the tip located to the right of the expected location of the SVC extending toward the right upper lobe. It often appears as if the tip is freely floating in the lung itself. The lateral view shows a midline location (**Fig. 4**). A catheter in a pulmonary vein can be confusing if an arterial blood gas is used to confirm venous placement because the blood is richly oxygenated.

LEFT-SIDED VENOUS CATHETERS

CVC tips located to the left of the midline have a distinctively abnormal appearance relative to right-sided catheters because this is opposite the expected location of the SVC. When encountered with a catheter tip located to the left of the midline, the following locations should be considered: left-sided SVC (LSVC), left superior intercostal vein, left pericardiophrenic vein, left superior anomalous pulmonary vein, and left internal mammary vein.

The LSVC is one of the more common variants of systemic venous drainage. LSVC has a reported incidence of 0.21% with a greater than

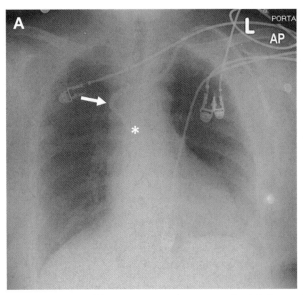
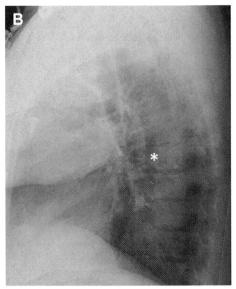

Fig. 3. A 61-year-old woman post–placement of a left internal jugular CVC. (*A*) Posterior-anterior chest radiograph demonstrates curving (*arrow*) of the CVC with the tip (*asterisk*) located in a location medial to the expected location of the SVC. (*B*) Lateral chest radiograph shows the catheter tip (*asterisk*) within the middle mediastinum, located posteriorly to the expected location of the SVC. These findings are in keeping with placement of the catheter within the azygous vein.

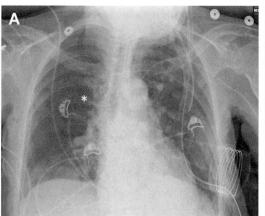
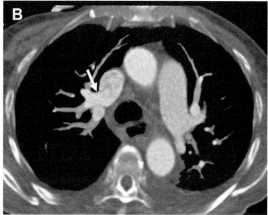

Fig. 4. A 66-year-old man post–placement of a left subclavian CVC. (A) Anterior-posterior chest radiograph demonstrates the catheter tip (*asterisk*) located lateral to the expected location of the SVC overlapping the lung. Note the catheter tip is directed superiorly toward the right upper lobe. The findings were suggestive of a malpositioned catheter, possibly within an anomalous pulmonary vein. (B) A prior CT examination confirms the presence of an anomalous right upper lobe pulmonary vein (*arrow*).

7-fold increase seen in patients with congenital heart disease (3.1%).[18] The presence of an isolated LSVC has a higher association with congenital heart disease in contrast to the presence of the bilateral SVCs. Bilateral SVCs may have a bridging brachiocephalic vein. The LSVC drains the left subclavian and left jugular veins to the right atrium via the coronary sinus. Catheters placed in the LSVC, which drain into the right atrium, are suitable for use. In rare cases, the LSVC may drain into the left atrium. Catheters placed within an LSVC course leftward of the sternal boarder and on a lateral projection follow the expected course of a right-sided SVC, ultimately extending toward the right atrium via the coronary sinus (Fig. 5).

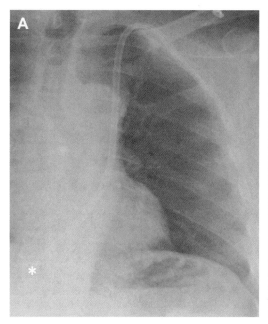
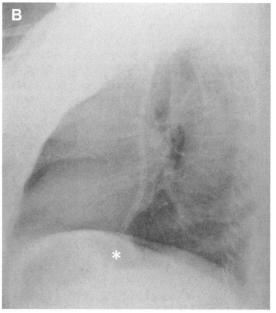

Fig. 5. A 49-year-old man status post–placement of a left internal jugular catheter. (A) Coned down view from a posterior-anterior chest radiograph shows the catheter coursing to the left of the sternal boarder with the tip extending toward the right atrium (*asterisk*). (B) The lateral radiograph shows the catheter tip within a posterior location in the expected location of the right atrium. The findings are in keeping with placement into an LSVC.

Occasionally, a catheter may be malpositioned within the left superior intercostal vein. The left superior intercostal vein forms an arch on the left side of the mediastinum, similar to the azygous arch on the right. The second through fourth intercostal veins are drained by the left superior intercostal vein. The vein then ascends upward along the aortic arch to drain into the left brachiocephalic vein. The left superior intercostal vein connects to the accessory hemiazygous vein. Frontal radiographs may demonstrate a catheter coursing along a bulge alongside the aortic knob, known as the aortic nipple (**Fig. 6**). The catheter tip may be present above or below the level of the aorta depending on its location within the vein. The lateral radiograph shows the catheter in a posterior location coursing over the vertebral bodies quite similar to the course of the azygous vein.

Although uncommon, the left pericardiophrenic vein can be inadvertently entered on catheter placement. Similar to the right side, the left pericardiophrenic vein is responsible for draining the pericardium, pleura, and diaphragm. Malpositioning into the left pericardiophrenic vein is more common with a jugular approach and similar to the right side. Because of risk of thrombosis from the small vessel size, the left pericardiophrenic vein is not a suitable position for a CVC. Frontal and lateral radiographs shows the catheter coursing along the left heart boarder (**Fig. 7**A). CT imaging can be used to confirm placement (**Fig. 7**B).

Similar to the right internal mammary vein, the left internal mammary vein (also known as the left internal thoracic vein) can be entered on attempted catheter placement. The left internal mammary vein drains the anterior intercostal veins and abdominal wall veins (including the inferior epigastric vein). The left internal mammary vein is located just to the left of the sternal boarder and drains into the left brachiocephalic vein (**Fig. 8**). Given that the orifice for the left internal thoracic vein is located quite remotely from the right-sided venous structures, the vein typically is entered only from a left brachiocephalic approach.[19] Catheter placement into the left internal thoracic vein has a characteristic approach on the lateral chest radiograph, with the catheter located anteriorly coursing along the chest wall (**Fig. 9**). As with the right side, a catheter in the left internal mammary vein often has a characteristic curve or notch.

A left superior pulmonary vein is an anomalous vein, which drains the left upper lobe and may be undetected in the adult patient because these patients may be asymptomatic. Although it is as common as an anomalous right upper lobe vein, it often is not associated with other anomalies. The anomalous vein most commonly drains into the left brachiocephalic vein, although anomalous drainage to the left subclavian or left superior intercostal vein has been reported. The frontal radiograph shows the course of the catheter within the anomalous vein extending into the lung (**Fig. 10**). The catheter may appear to be within the lung; however, there are no secondary findings of vascular perforation (eg, pneumothorax, hemothorax, and consolidation). Similar to a catheter in a right superior pulmonary vein, there may be clinical confusion because blood return is richly oxygenated.

INTRA-ARTERIAL CATHETERS

Rarely, CVCs may be inadvertently placed into the arterial system. Arterial perforation/cannulation is believed to be more common (14.28%) when attempting to place a CVC into the jugular vein.[20–22] It has been proposed that the close proximity of the carotid artery in relation to the jugular vein places it at risk for inadvertent cannulation.

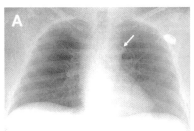
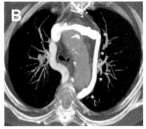
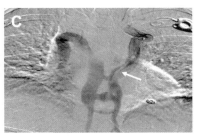

Fig. 6. A 38-year-old man status post–placement of a left port catheter in a patient with end stage renal disease. (*A*) Anterior-posterior chest radiograph demonstrates the catheter coursing along an excrescence from aortic knob (aortic nipple) (*arrow*). (*B*) Maximum intensity projection image from a contrast-enhanced CT examination shows the presence of a large left superior intercostal vein which extends posteriorly (*asterisks*). (*C*) Image from venogram demonstrates the catheter (*arrow*) located within the left superior intercostal vein.

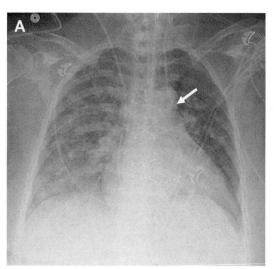
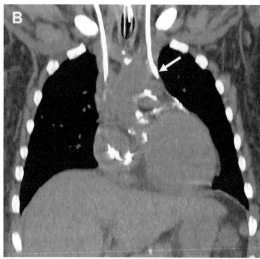

Fig. 7. A 52-year-old woman post–placement of a left internal jugular catheter. (*A*) Anterior-posterior chest radiograph demonstrates the catheter tip (*arrow*) coursing along the lateral most aspect of the left heart boarder. The catheter was believed to be within a pericardiophrenic vein. (*B*) Maximal intensity projection coronal images from a contrast-enhanced CT demonstrate the catheter (*arrow*) located along the lateral aspect of the mediastinum in the pericardiophrenic location. Note the absence of adjacent hematoma to suggest soft tissue perforation. The findings were consistent with a malpositioned catheter in the left pericardiophrenic vein.

Radiographs are helpful when evaluating a potentially arterially placed CVC. Catheters flush with the left heart boarder (left ventricular apex) are highly suspicious for arterial placement, with retrograde extension down the ascending aorta into the left ventricle (**Fig. 11**A–D). When placed from a subclavian approach, arterially placed catheters usually course above the scalene tubercle (**Fig. 12**). A catheter placed from the right subclavian approach may course above the scalene tubercle extending inferiorly into the aorta (see

Fig. 12). As a general rule, catheters within the subclavian artery have a more curvilinear course along the lung apex than catheters within the subclavian vein, which tend to be more inferior and horizontal.

Often, arterial catheter placement is recognized by the return of bright red pulsatile blood. In patients with low blood pressure or ICU patients, these features may not be clinically apparent. Confirmation of arterial CVC placement can be made with a transducer,

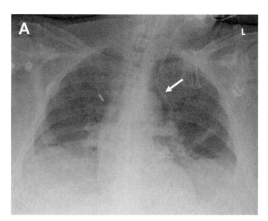
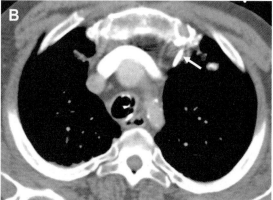

Fig. 8. A 46-year-old woman post–catheter left internal jugular catheter placement. (*A*) Anterior-posterior chest radiograph demonstrates the catheter tip (*arrow*) located to the left of the mediastinum. The differential diagnosis for this placement includes a pericardiophrenic vein, extravascular mediastinal soft tissue location, or internal mammary vein. (*B*) Axial images from a CT examination confirm the tip of the catheter (*arrow*) is located within the left internal mammary vein.

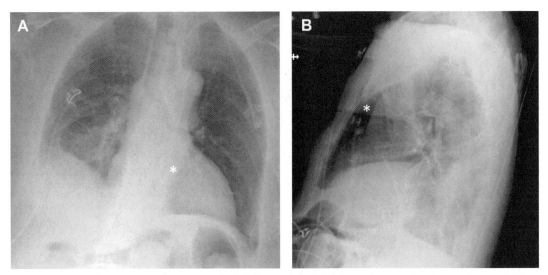

Fig. 9. A 72-year-old man post–placement of a left internal CVC. (*A*) Posterior-anterior chest radiograph shows the catheter tip (*asterisk*) located to the left of the sternal boarder. (*B*) The lateral view shows the catheter tip (*asterisk*) located along the anterior chest wall consistent with malpositioning of catheter within the left internal mammary vein.

manometer, or blood gas analysis. On recognition of arterial placement, the catheter should be left in place and a vascular surgery consult may be necessary. Typically, with carotid placement, the catheter should be removed as soon as possible with manual pressure after removal. Subclavian arterial catheters are at greater risk of hemorrhage and pseudoaneurysm formation and have a more complex treatment strategy, which may include collagen plugs, embolization, and surgical closure. More often, the catheters may enter the artery through an oblique course (either through an initial venous puncture or through a mediastinal course). CT often is helpful in understanding the site of arterial access. The site of injury directs management and may determine which surgical team is consulted. In the authors' center, for example, a catheter entering an artery medial to the manubrium results in a cardiothoracic surgery evaluation.

CROSSING CATHETERS

The normal path of a CVC from a left-sided approach (left internal jugular vein or left subclavian vein) results in the catheter coursing from the left side of the chest across the midline into the SVC in an oblique course near the

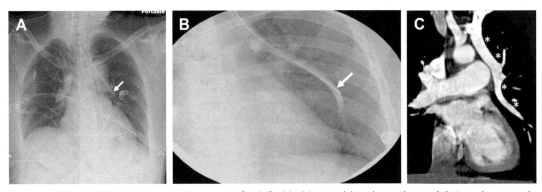

Fig. 10. A 45-year-old woman post–placement of a left-sided internal jugular catheter. (*A*) Anterior-posterior chest radiograph demonstrates the catheter tip (*arrow*) located to the left of the midline extending toward the lung. (*B*) Angiographic images confirm the catheter (*arrow*) located within an anomalous pulmonary vein. (*C*) Contrast-enhanced CT images prior to catheter placement show the presence of a large anomalous vein (*asterisks*) draining the left upper lobe to the brachiocephalic vein.

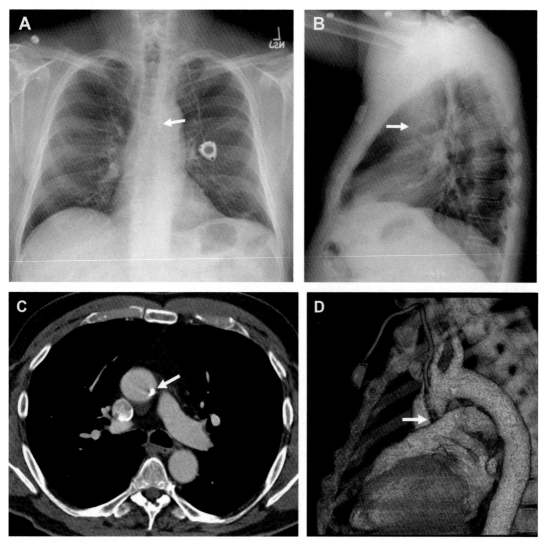

Fig. 11. A 55-year-old man post–placement of a left internal jugular port catheter placement with blood return suspicious for arterial placement. (*A*) Posterior-anterior and (*B*) lateral chest radiograph shows the catheter tip (*arrow*) overlying the expected location of the ascending aorta. (*C*) Axial image from a contrast-enhanced CT shows the catheter tip (*arrow*) located within the ascending aorta. (*D*) 3-Dimensional reconstructed images from the CT examination show the catheter (*red*) with the tip (*arrow*) located within the ascending aorta.

sternomanubrial junction. Occasionally, malpositioned CVCs may course across the midline in an atypical course.

Intra-arterial catheters placed into the left common carotid artery or left subclavian artery may cross the midline and terminate in the ascending aorta, more medial to the expected location of the SVC. These courses have a distinctive appearance on the frontal radiograph in which they follow the aortic arch and extend retrograde along the expected course of the ascending aorta (**Fig. 13**) to the expected location of the SVC. In rare cases, a catheter may cross from right to left and into the aorta and terminate within the transverse or descending aorta (**Fig. 14**). Secondary findings may include mediastinal widening as a result of hematoma formation.

Catheters crossing from left to right with a shallower or more horizontal course than expected (usually higher than the sternomanubrial joint) may enter the jugular arch. This occurs more commonly in patients with central venous stenosis (eg, chronic renal failure patients). Although there are many variants of venous anatomy, a transverse trunk communicates between the left external jugular vein and anterior jugular veins, ultimately draining to the right subclavian vein or right external jugular vein. Catheters placed into the

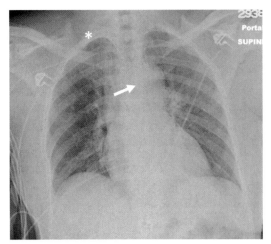

Fig. 12. A 61-year-old woman post–placement of a right subclavian CVC with blood return suspicious for arterial placement. Anterior-posterior chest radiograph shows the catheter tip (*arrow*) overlying the expected location of the descending aorta. Note the catheter (*asterisk*) extends above the scalene tubercle and follows a curvilinear course at the lung apex. These findings are consistent with intra-arterial catheter placement with the tip located within the descending aorta.

left external jugular vein may cross from left to right and ultimately terminate within the jugular vein arch. Given the diminutive size of these vessels, there is increased risk for thrombosis, perforation, and extravasation. Findings can be confirmed on

imaging and via monitoring of the central venous wave form (**Fig. 15**). Rarely, a catheter may begin to cross the mediastinum and take an oblique course to end vertically in the midline. This course is typical of a thymic vein. A CVC in this location should be removed because it is more prone to thrombosis and potential perforation.

EXTRAVASCULAR PLACEMENT

Rarely, CVCs may be malpositioned within a site external to the vasculature. Such sites include the mediastinum, pericardium, pleural space, thoracic duct, and extrapleural space. An abnormal appearance of a course of the catheter or clinical suspicion may raise suspicion for an extravascular catheter. Catheters placed in the soft tissues can be confirmed with contrast injection but more often are confirmed by CT.

Mediastinal placement is unusual; however, it can occur when a CVC is placed with excessive force or entry into a fragile collateral with resultant perforation of a vascular wall. Infusion of a catheter within the soft tissue may result in swelling, compression of adjacent structures, and/or tissue necrosis.

Placement into the pericardium is a rare complication of CVC placement with grave consequences. Pericardial placement occurs when the right atrium or lower SVC is perforated and can occur immediately after placement or after a long duration of time secondary to erosion. Filling

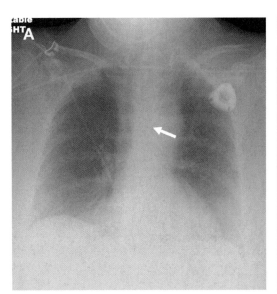

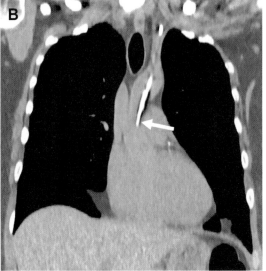

Fig. 13. A 49-year-old woman status post–placement of a left internal jugular port catheter with blood return concerning for intra-arterial placement. (*A*) Anterior-posterior chest radiograph demonstrates the catheter coursing across the midline with the tip (*arrow*) overlying the expected location of the ascending aorta. (*B*) Coronal images from a CT examination confirm the catheter tip (*arrow*) is located within the ascending aorta.

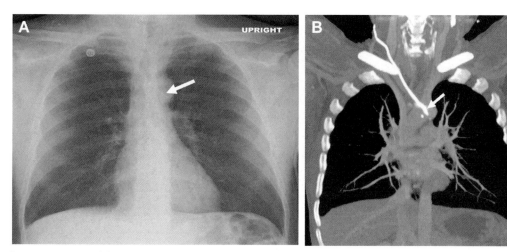

Fig. 14. A 52-year-old man status post–placement of a right internal jugular catheter with blood return concerning for intra-arterial placement. (*A*) Anterior-posterior chest radiograph demonstrates the catheter coursing across the midline with the tip (*arrow*) located over the expected location of the aortic arch. (*B*) Maximum intensity projection coronal images from a CT examination confirm the intra-arterial location of the catheter with the tip (*arrow*) located within the aortic arch.

of the pericardial space with infused material can result in cardiac tamponade. Patients may require lifesaving intervention, including aspiration of fluid, perciardiocentesis, and/or surgical repair.

The pleural space can be entered given its close proximity to the SVC, azygous, hemiazygous, and internal mammary veins. Perforation of these adjacent vascular structures can result in pneumothorax and/or hemothorax (**Fig. 16**). If unrecognized, infusion of fluids can result in filling of the pleural space. This has been referred to as a glucothorax, owing to the frequent use of glucose supplemented IV fluids.

Rarely, needle punctures into the left brachiocephalic vein in the location of the orifice of the thoracic duct can result in cannulation of the thoracic duct. The CVC follows the course inferiorly to the level of the cisterna chyli. Infusion of a catheter within the duct may result in mediastinal fluid accumulation. Laceration of the thoracic duct can result in chylothorax and subsequent surgical intervention.

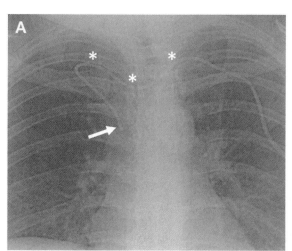
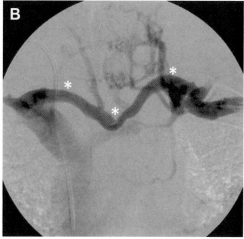

Fig. 15. A 77-year-old woman status post–placement of a left subclavian CVC with wave form consistent with venous placement. (*A*) Anterior-posterior chest radiograph demonstrates the catheter (*asterisks*) crossing from left to right in a shallow fashion with the tip (*arrow*) overlying the SVC. The findings were suspicious for a catheter traversing the jugular arch. (*B*) Angiographic images demonstrate the catheter (*asterisks*) located within the jugular arch.

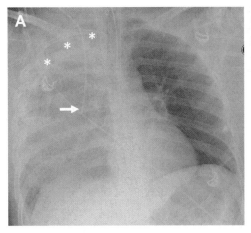
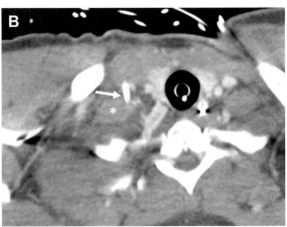

Fig. 16. A 49-year-old woman status post–attempted placement of a left internal jugular catheter. (*A*) Anterior-posterior chest radiograph demonstrates the catheter tip (*arrow*) located to the right of the expected location of the SVC. Note the extensive apical pleural fluid collection (*asterisks*) suggestive of associated hematoma/hemothorax. The findings were suspicious for soft tissue perforation and placement of the catheter into the lung with a resultant hemothorax. (*B*) Axial images from a contrast enhanced CT confirm the findings with hematoma (*asterisk*) located adjacent to the catheter tip (*arrow*).

CVC placement in to the extradural space is exceedingly rare complication as a result of perforation of the internal jugular vein.[22] Patients experience neck swelling and an epidural hematoma. If suspected, cross-sectional imaging and surgical consultation are recommended prior to CVC removal.

SUMMARY

CVCs are commonly used in both the general ward and ICU settings. After placement, a radiologist is frequently requested to evaluate the location of CVC tips and deem them suitable for use. An understanding of the ideal location of catheter tips as well as approach to identifying malpositioned catheter tips is essential to prevent improper use, recognize and/or prevent further injury, and direct potential lifesaving care. An approach to CVC placement based on tip location (right of midline, left of midline, or midline) can be helpful in localization and guiding management.

REFERENCES

1. Gershengorn HB, Garland A, Kramer A, et al. Variation of arterial and central venous catheter use in United States intensive care units. Anesthesiology 2014;120(3):650–64.
2. Traoré O, Liotier J, Souweine B. Prospective study of arterial and central venous catheter colonization and of arterial- and central venous catheter-related bacteremia in intensive care units. Crit Care Med 2005;33(6):1276–80.
3. Burgmann H, Hiesmayr JM, Savey A, et al. Impact of nosocomial infections on clinical outcome and resource consumption in critically ill patients. Intensive Care Med 2010;36(9):1597–601.
4. Vincent JL, Bihari DJ, Suter PM, et al. The prevalence of nosocomial infection in intensive care units in Europe. Results of the European Prevalence of Infection in Intensive Care (EPIC) Study. EPIC International Advisory Committee. JAMA 1995;274(8):639–44.
5. Suh RD, Genshaft SJ, Kirsch J, et al. ACR appropriateness criteria® intensive care unit patients. J Thorac Imaging 2015;30(6):W63–5.
6. Strain DS, Kinasewitz GT, Vereen LE, et al. Value of routine daily chest x-rays in the medical intensive care unit. Crit Care Med 1985;13(7):534–6.
7. Silverstein DS, Livingston DH, Elcavage J, et al. The utility of routine daily chest radiography in the surgical intensive care unit. J Trauma 1993;35(4):643–6.
8. Gray P, Sullivan G, Ostryzniuk P, et al. Value of postprocedural chest radiographs in the adult intensive care unit. Crit Care Med 1992;20(11):1513–8.
9. Henschke CI, Pasternack GS, Schroeder S, et al. Bedside chest radiography: diagnostic efficacy. Radiology 1983;149(1):23–6.
10. Horst HM, Fagan B, Beute GH. Chest radiographs in surgical intensive care patients: a valuable "routine." Henry Ford Hosp Med J 1986;34(2):84–6.
11. Brunel W, Coleman DL, Schwartz DE, et al. Assessment of routine chest roentgenograms and the physical examination to confirm endotracheal tube position. Chest 1989;96(5):1043–5.
12. Bekemeyer WB, Crapo RO, Calhoon S, et al. Efficacy of chest radiography in a respiratory intensive

care unit. A prospective study. Chest 1985;88(5): 691–6.

13. Fisher KL, Leung AN. Radiographic appearance of central venous catheters. AJR Am J Roentgenol 1996;166(2):329–37.

14. Sise MJ, Hollingsworth P, Brimm JE, et al. Complications of the flow-directed pulmonary artery catheter: a prospective analysis in 219 patients. Crit Care Med 1981;9(4):315–8.

15. Jain SN. A pictorial essay: radiology of lines and tubes in the intensive care unit. Indian J Radiol Imaging 2011;21(3):182–90.

16. Wall BF, Hart D. Revised radiation doses for typical X-ray examinations. Report on a recent review of doses to patients from medical X-ray examinations in the UK by NRPB. National Radiological Protection Board. Br J Radiol 1997;70(833):437–9.

17. Johnston AJ, Bishop SM, Martin L, et al. Defining peripherally inserted central catheter tip position

and an evaluation of insertions in one unit. Anaesthesia 2013;68(5):484–91.

18. Nagasawa H, Kuwabara N, Goto H, et al. Incidence of persistent left superior vena cava in the normal population and in patients with congenital heart diseases detected using echocardiography. Pediatr Cardiol 2018;39(3):484–90.

19. Godwin JD, Chen JT. Thoracic venous anatomy. AJR Am J Roentgenol 1986;147(4):674–84.

20. Hodzic S, Golic D, Smajic J, et al. Complications related to insertion and use of central venous catheters (CVC). Med Arch 2014;68(5):300–3.

21. Powers CJ, Zomorodi AR, Britz GW, et al. Endovascular management of inadvertent brachiocephalic arterial catheterization. J Neurosurg 2011;114(1): 146–52.

22. Wang L, Liu Z-S, Wang C-A. Malposition of central venous catheter: presentation and management. Chin Med J (Engl) 2016;129(2):227–34.

Imaging of Diffuse Lung Disease in the Intensive Care Unit Patient

Konstantinos Stefanidis, MD, MSc, PhD[a],*, Joanna Moser, MBChB, FRCR[b], Ioannis Vlahos, MBBS, BSc, MRCP, FRCR[b]

KEYWORDS

- Diffuse lung disease (DLD) • Intensive care unit (ICU) • Acute respiratory distress syndrome (ARDS)
- Ventilatory-associated pneumonia (VAP) • Idiopathic pulmonary fibrosis (IPF)

KEY POINTS

- There is a wide variety of causes of diffuse lung disease in the intensive care unit patient, of which adult respiratory distress syndrome is the commonest clinical consideration.
- Plain radiography, computed tomography, and ultrasound can be used synergistically to evaluate patients with diffuse lung disease and respiratory impairment.
- Imaging is not limited to characterization of the cause of diffuse lung disease but also aids in monitoring its evolution and in ventilator setting management.

INTRODUCTION

Clinical evaluation of the intensive care patient is multifactorial but relies to a great extent on pulmonary imaging. Numerous primary pulmonary diseases or systemic disorders may affect the lung independently or may superimpose on a preexisting lung disorder. Clinical assessment can be complex in the intensive care unit (ICU) setting, making the interpretation of lung disease contribution challenging. However, determining the cause of the diffuse lung disease (DLD) is crucial because characterizing the mechanisms can optimize both the etiologic and the symptomatic treatment. The principal cause of DLD is the clinical syndrome of adult respiratory distress syndrome (ARDS), which often constitutes a common challenging radiological pattern in the ICU population; however, DLD is not limited to ARDS. The main causes of DLD and diffuse lung injury are pneumonia, aspiration, nonpulmonary sepsis, major trauma, pulmonary contusion, acute exacerbation of idiopathic pulmonary fibrosis (AE-IPF), inhalational injury, severe burns, noncardiogenic shock, pancreatitis, drug overdose, multiple transfusions, or transfusion-associated acute lung injury (TRALI), pulmonary vasculitis, and near drowning.

Imaging plays a significant role in the detection and characterization of DLD. However, the role of modern radiology is not limited to this remit. Applications of multimodality imaging also include respiratory management and monitoring during lung recruitment and lung protection strategies. Current and novel imaging modalities aim to evaluate the effectiveness of the therapeutic interventions by providing functional information optimizing lung assessment during ventilator management.

This article focuses on the clinicoradiological aspects of the detection, characterization, and radiologically assisted management of the principal

Disclosures: The authors have no relevant disclosures.
a Radiology Department, King's College Hospital, NHS Foundation Trust, Denmark Hill, London SE5 9RS, UK;
b Radiology Department, St. George's University Hospitals, NHS Foundation Trust and School of Medicine, Blackshaw Road Tooting, London SW17 0QT, UK
* Corresponding author.
E-mail address: kstefanidis@nhs.net

Radiol Clin N Am 58 (2020) 119–131
https://doi.org/10.1016/j.rcl.2019.08.005
0033-8389/20/Crown Copyright © 2019 Published by Elsevier Inc. All rights reserved.

radiologic.theclinics.com

causes of diffuse interstitial lung disease (ILD) presenting as clinical management issues in the adult ICU patient, with a particular focus on ARDS and its differentiation from other common similarly presenting causes of DLD.

ADULT RESPIRATORY DISTRESS SYNDROME: DIRECT AND INDIRECT LUNG INJURY

ARDS is the most frequently associated clinical entity to DLD in the ICU patient. It is characterized by an acute inflammatory lung injury in a heterogeneous group of patients with respiratory insufficiency hours to days after a severe local or systemic insult.[1] Three overlapping pathologic phases have been described following direct insult to the alveolar epithelium (eg, pneumonia or gastric acid) or indirect to the pulmonary capillary endothelium (eg, pancreatitis, extrapulmonary sepsis).[2] The exudative or early phase, which lasts for the first week after the onset of symptoms, is histologically characterized by diffuse alveolar damage (DAD). The proliferative or intermediate phase occurs from day 5 to 7 onwards and can last for a further week, characterized by organization of the exudates. In patients who do not recover, a final fibrotic or late phase can begin as early as day 10 after the initiating injury and is histologically characterized by fibroplasia.

Following the first description of ARDS by Ashbaugh and colleagues,[3] there have been several attempts to describe and clarify the syndrome with a reliable definition. The 1994 American-European Consensus Conference definition of ARDS was the first to become globally accepted.[4] However, there were several concerns regarding the timing, origin of edema, oxygenation, severity, and imaging description criteria of the syndrome. The most recent 2012 "Berlin" international expert consensus panel addressed these limitations.[5] Specifically, the acute timeframe was specified; 3 subgroups of ARDS by severity were created (mild, moderate, and severe); the acute lung injury (ALI) term and pulmonary artery wedge pressure requirement were removed; a ventilation minimal positive end-expiratory pressure (PEEP) level was incorporated; and imaging criteria were clarified (**Table 1**).

ARDS reflects a clinicoradiologically diverse spectrum of disease, course, and prognosis, influenced by the etiologic mechanism. ARDS cause is generally classified as due to direct causes of lung injury, such as pneumonia or aspiration, and indirect causes of lung injury, such as nonpulmonary sepsis or transfusion. Accordingly, these pulmonary and extrapulmonary causes result in different pathophysiology, with resultant varying

Table 1 "Berlin" definition of adult respiratory distress syndrome	
Timing	Onset of ARDS must be acute, defined as within 7 d
Imaging	Bilateral opacities, not fully explained by effusions, lobar/lung collapse, detected on chest radiograph or CT
PAWP: origin of edema	There is no need to exclude heart failure in the new ARDS definition
Oxygenation Pao_2/Fio_2	3 subgroups by severity/degree of hypoxemia Mild (<300 mm Hg), moderate (<200 mm Hg), severe (<100 mm Hg)

Abbreviation: PAPW, pulmonary artery wedge pressure.

radiological patterns and consequent effects on respiratory mechanics and responses to ventilator settings.[6]

The radiological description of ARDS in daily practice remains often confusing regarding the appropriate terminology. Although ARDS is a clinical diagnosis, it is often used in the radiology reports interchangeably with ALI and with the histopathologic and pathophysiology terms of DAD and increased permeability edema. Because the diagnosis remains a clinical determination, and radiology has a supportive role, the radiology report should be descriptive and indicate appearances suggestive of ARDS and, if appropriate, the cause, infective or extrapulmonary, to direct clinical corroboration and appropriate treatment and management.

Despite optimized therapy, ARDS is associated with appreciable morbidity and mortality. In a large observational study, based on the 2012 Berlin criteria, a 28-day mortality of 30%, 35%, and 43% was observed for mild, moderate, and severe ARDS, respectively.[7]

ACUTE INTERSTITIAL PNEUMONIA

Acute interstitial pneumonia (AIP), previously known as Hamman-Rich syndrome, is reserved for ARDS of unknown cause. It is a rapidly progressive idiopathic clinical disorder associated with DAD. AIP radiologically resembles ARDS with similar clinical presentation. However, the different clinical management and the poor prognosis with greater than 70% mortality at 3 months despite mechanical ventilation[8] make the determination of AIP versus other causes of ARDS of paramount importance. Open lung biopsy is, therefore, frequently indicated to confidently confirm AIP and exclude other causes.

VENTILATOR-ASSOCIATED PNEUMONIA

Ventilator-associated pneumonia (VAP) is defined as pneumonia that occurs more than 48 hours following endotracheal intubation. It is the most common nosocomial infection in mechanically ventilated patients in the ICU.[9,10] A combination of clinical criteria, the Clinical Pulmonary Infection Score (CPIS), has been proposed for VAP diagnosis.[11] These clinical criteria include radiological evaluation on a chest radiograph (CXR). New findings of pulmonary infiltrates in a patient with fever or hypothermia, leukocytosis or leukopenia, purulent tracheal secretions, and impaired oxygenation are highly indicative of VAP (**Table 2**). To detect these pulmonary infiltrates, current American Thoracic Society guidelines recommend CXR and computed tomography (CT) for VAP diagnosis.[12] However, in mechanically ventilated patients, such pulmonary infiltrates are frequent and may be associated with multiple causes. Therefore, imaging determination of VAP in the critical care setting remains problematic.

ACUTE EXACERBATION OF INTERSTITIAL LUNG DISEASE

Patients with fibrotic lung disease can develop acute respiratory failure because of an exacerbation of their underlying disease. Identifying and managing this type of respiratory failure remains clinically challenging. The diagnostic workup includes imaging with high-resolution computed tomography (HRCT) as part of an initial assessment identifying signs of fibrosis and most typically a background pattern consistent with usual interstitial pneumonia pattern. According to an international multidisciplinary working group consensus, the recently updated diagnostic criteria of acute exacerbation of IPF have been defined as an acute (<1 month in duration) and clinically significant respiratory deterioration in a previously diagnosed IPF patient, associated with the presence of new widespread alveolar abnormality on HRCT and exclusion of alternative causes.[13] Because respiratory failure in IPF has a poor prognosis, imaging plays a significant role in the distinction of acute exacerbation of IPF from infection to guide appropriate management demanding increased immunosuppression rather than antimicrobial treatment.

Table 2
The Clinical Pulmonary Infection Score, a diagnostic algorithm on easily available clinical, radiographic, and microbiological criteria

Criteria	CPIS Points
Temperature	$\geq$36.5 or $\leq$38.4 = 0 point $\geq$38.5 or $\leq$38.9 = 1 point $\geq$39 or <36.5 = 2 point
Leukocyte count	$\geq$4000 or $\leq$11.000 = 0 point <4000 or >11.000 = 1 point Band forms $\geq$50% = add 1 point
Tracheal secretions	Absent = 0 point Tracheal secretion with less purulence = 1 point Abundant purulent secretion = 2 points
Oxygenation	Pao_2/Fio_2 <200 = 0 point Pao_2/Fio_2, mm Hg $\leq$240 or ARDS = 2 points
Chest radiograph	No infiltrate = 0 point Diffuse infiltrates = 1 point Local infiltrates = 2 points
Chest radiograph progression (day 2–3)	No progression (−) = 0 point Progression (+) (after the exclusion of heart failure and ARDS) = 2 points
Microbiological culture (day 2–3)	No growth or few pathogenic bacteria = 0 point Moderate or high levels of pathogenic bacteria = 1 point Pathogenic bacteria seen on Gram staining = add 1 point

Diagnosis of VAP is made when the CPIS score >6.

IMAGING
Chest Radiography

For several decades, CXR evaluation was the only imaging modality in the assessment of DLD in critically ill patients to assess progression, stability, or regression in concordance with direct or indirect pulmonary insults. However, the radiographic appearance is recognized to be frequently nonspecific, including bilateral, symmetric, or asymmetric airspace consolidative opacification with air bronchograms that may reflect infection, or ARDS. The coexistence of septal lines and pleural effusions makes interpretation more challenging, favoring the coexistence of cardiogenic pulmonary edema, a common confounder in the ICU setting. Volume loss may be appreciated in the later phases of interstitial pulmonary fibrosis, indicating a background of ILD in a patient with potential acute exacerbation. However, the volume loss of IPF is frequently basilar and, therefore, may overlap in appearance with the basilar volume loss of hypoinflation atelectasis, which is common in ventilated patients.

ARDS is the commonest consideration for DLD on ICU chest radiographs. The radiographic findings vary depending on the phase of the disease mirroring the histopathologic phase. The CXR may be normal in the first hours of the syndrome. The progression of the disease during the early exudative phase (1–2 days) is typically of bilateral patchy alveolar airspace opacities with progression to confluent consolidation in the late exudative phase (3–7 days) (Fig. 1A). Thereafter, in the proliferative phase (day 5–7 onwards), the consolidation becomes progressively extensive and dense (Fig. 1B). If the syndrome persists for at least 7 to 10 days, early fibrotic changes with a coarse reticular pattern begin to evolve (Fig. 1C–E). An exception to the generally bilateral progressive appearance is if ARDS is triggered by a direct lung injury (eg, pneumonia), in which case early asymmetric focal or multifocal consolidation may be observed.

Undoubtedly, chest radiographs are of assistance in determining the presence, and monitoring the evolution, of cardiogenic edema and fluid overload, differentiating these common causes for diffuse parenchymal abnormality in the ICU patient from ARDS. The typical features of cardiogenic edema are well recognized: progressing from septal lines and central peribronchovascular interstitial edematous changes to alveolar edema with diffuse airspace abnormalities that may resemble infection or ARDS. Typically, effusions may be present, although these are a nonspecific feature also seen in infection and other conditions. Similarly, the heart is usually enlarged, although this feature may be absent in patients with acute cardiogenic shock, acute renal impairment, or acute fluid overload. Asymmetry of appearances may be postural or indicate noncardiogenic edema, particularly in

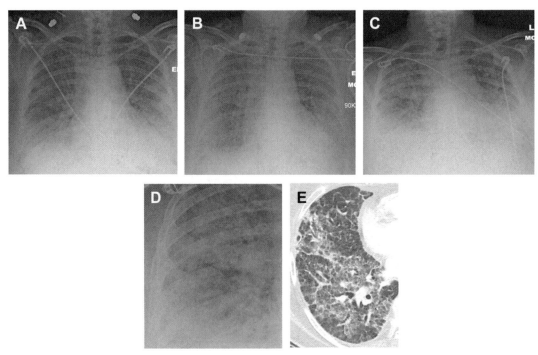

Fig. 1. Radiological evolution of extrapulmonary ARDS in a series of chest radiographs showing progression of symmetric bilateral airspace opacification (*A*: exudative phase, day 5) into diffuse alveolar involvement (*B*: proliferative phase, day 9). There is further progression of the lung abnormalities with combination of consolidation and reticulation in the fibrotic phase (*C*: day 13). Close-up view of the chest radiograph and of the axial CT image (*D*, *E*) confirms the presence of 2 different patterns: reticulation and airspace opacities.

cases of opiate overdose. The role of chest radiography has also been investigated as a possible guide for fluid management, measuring the changes of a simple anatomic landmark, such as the vascular pedicle width. According to a study by Rice and colleagues,[14] the vascular pedicle width measurement on a CXR appears to correlate highly with pulmonary artery occlusion pressure distinguishing cardiogenic from noncardiogenic edema and suggesting a fluid management protocol. In a recent study, a radiographic severity score of lung edema (RALE score) has been developed quantifying the severity of pulmonary edema in ARDS.[15] The study showed that the RALE score is associated with ARDS severity, response to conservative fluid management, and clinical outcomes.

Daily routine CXR for DLD, and more specifically ARDS, remains a common practice in most ICU departments. Indeed, the American College of Radiology's Appropriateness Criteria[16] recommend daily routine CXRs for patients with mechanical ventilation. CXRs are also recommended immediately following the placement of tubes, catheters, and other monitoring devices to check their position and detect procedure-related complications. In a study by Henschke and colleagues,[17] the routine use of daily CXR detected malposition of tubes and lines in 12% and 1%, respectively, and provided useful information affecting patient management in 65% of studies. However, more recent metaanalysis data suggest that daily routine CXRs can possibly be eliminated because the observed daily variations are minor and are unlikely to alter clinical management and decision making.[18,19]

The use of daily chest radiographs is supported by the new definition of ARDS, whereby radiographic criteria are more explicitly stated, defining the syndrome by the presence of bilateral opacities consistent with pulmonary edema not fully explained by effusions, lobar collapse, or nodules. However, specificity, even in the context of ARDS, remains low.[20] The Berlin definition statement also underscores the limits of CXRs, recommending that CXR criteria should be clarified by creating a set of example radiographs.[20] The limitations of chest radiography in ARDS include not only a lower accuracy compared with other image modalities[21–24] but also a high interobserver variability in the radiographic definition of ARDS.[25] Figueroa-Casas and colleagues[26] demonstrated that the accuracy of anteroposterior chest radiograph in the diagnosis of ARDS is limited, resulting generally in underrecognition of ARDS, particularly when nondiffusely distributed, but also in other circumstances, overdiagnosis of the syndrome.

Indeed, in daily practice, it remains difficult to differentiate ARDS from infection and cardiogenic and noncardiogenic pulmonary edema because they frequently coexist. Although this limitation has been partially addressed with the new definition, ICU CXR interpretation remains a consistent challenge for radiologists attempting to appropriately guide ICU clinicians. Compared with other modalities, several studies have demonstrated the lower-diagnostic accuracy of chest radiography for alveolar consolidation, pleural effusions, and alveolar or interstitial pathology compared with CT and ultrasound (US).[21–24] In practice, CXR, CT, and lung US should be used in a complementary fashion rather than used interchangeably.[27]

Computed Tomography

CT is perhaps the most consistently useful imaging tool in the evaluation of DLD and ARDS in the ICU patient. A progressive understanding of CT imaging patterns has offered insights into both clinical aspects and the pathophysiology of acute lung illness in critical patients. Several studies have illustrated the superiority of CT in the imaging and follow-up of DLD in the ICU context. In 1 study, the imaging findings provided by CT compared with CXR frequently yielded additional information (66%), with direct influence on patient treatment in 22% of cases.[28] CT is also important in providing further information regarding complications, such as iatrogenic line or tube insertions and ventilation-associated complications (barotrauma) (Fig. 2). The improved imaging characterization by CT, and in particular

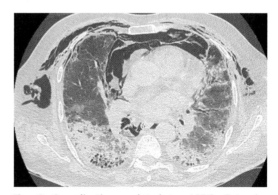

Fig. 2. Complications related to ARDS. Extensive pneumomediastinum, subcutaneous emphysema, and a small-volume right-sided pneumothorax secondary to barotrauma from positive pressure ventilation in reduced lung compliance. The background lung demonstrates basal consolidation, ground-glass opacification, and traction bronchiectasis in a patient with acute exacerbation of interstitial fibrosis.

HRCT reconstructions, can assist in the differentiation of ARDS from pulmonary edema and other clinical causes of DLD.

Unlike chest radiographs, which can be performed repeatedly at the bedside, the principal limitation of CT in the ICU is that it requires movement of the patient to the CT scanner, an undertaking that may be difficult or prohibited by the physiologic state of the patient. Because this movement may cause disruption to the care of the patient, it is important both that the environment of the CT scanner is optimized for ventilator support and also that the examination itself is performed to the highest standard. In conscious self-breathing patients with noninvasive (eg, continuous positive airway pressure) or invasive airway support (eg, tracheostomy or endotracheal tube), high respiratory rates frequently adversely affect image quality. In order to minimize respiratory motion on HRCT imaging, volumetric acquisition with subsequent reconstruction of HRCT images should be acquired rather than repeated noncontiguous HRCT acquisitions during repeated breath-holds.[29] Care should be expended to coach conscious patients for the breath-hold required for volumetric acquisition. The breath-hold duration can be reduced by high-pitch acquisitions,[30] particularly with dual source systems whereby pitch values of greater than 3.0 can enable subsecond whole thorax acquisitions (**Fig.** 3A, B). In paralyzed patients on invasive positive pressure support, coordination with the anesthesiologist can allow for a period of hyperventilation before suspended respiration for the examination. For a subset of patients, repeated low-dose CT acquisitions with varying positive end-expiratory pressures (PEEP) can be used to optimize ventilator settings to enable greater lung recruitment.

In ARDS, CT provides detailed information regarding the complex histopathologic phases of DAD. As per chest radiography, the morphologic changes are also dependent on whether the clinical ARDS is due to a direct or indirect insult. During the acute exudative phase, capillary congestion with interstitial and intraalveolar edema is present, corresponding radiologically to diffuse ground-glass opacification with a posterior and basal predominance. Dense posterior-dependent consolidation can be seen as the syndrome progresses beyond the first week. This pattern is gravity dependent and reverses when the patient is positioned prone, if this is clinically possible. Bronchial dilatation may also be present; however, this is reversible.[31,32] In the late phase (>2 weeks), CT signs of parenchymal architectural distortion appear with reticulation and bronchiectasis. Ground-glass opacity and dense basal consolidation may also coexist if the precipitating insult persists.[32] Limited studies have shown the potential role of CT imaging in grading and prognostication.[33,34] Ichikado and colleagues[33] showed that in early ARDS, CT signs of fibrosis with traction bronchiectasis or bronchiolectasis are predictive of poor prognosis. Similarly, in another study, from Chung and colleagues,[34] the CT extension of lung involvement with bronchiectasis is predictive of increased mortality in patients with ARDS.

CT can aid in the differentiation of pulmonary versus extrapulmonary ARDS and assist in guiding the appropriate management.[35,36] Asymmetric consolidation in a nondependent pattern is present in pulmonary causes of ARDS, such as pneumonia, and even in aspiration (**Fig.** 4A). ARDS from

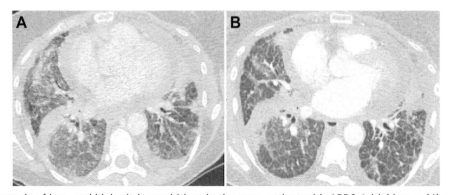

Fig. 3. Example of low- and high-pitch acquisitions in the same patient with ARDS. Initial image (*A*) performed with single source acquisition at pitch of 1.0 demonstrates significant respiratory motion degradation. Follow-up study (*B*) performed 24 hours later to exclude pulmonary embolism with dual-source acquisition at pitch of 2.3 demonstrates reduced artifacts with better visualization of ground-glass, intralobar reticulation, and interlobular septal thickening.

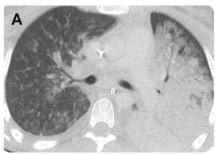
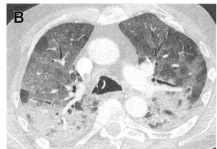

Fig. 4. Examples of pulmonary and extrapulmonary ARDS. (*A*) Pulmonary ARDS secondary to aspiration pneumonia: asymmetric changes with dense consolidation in the left lung and multiple small patchy ground-glass opacities on the right. (*B*) Extrapulmonary ARDS in a patient with background of pancreatitis and sepsis: symmetric, bilateral diffuse areas of mixed dense consolidation and ground-glass opacification with an anteroposterior gradient, characterized by worse disease in the posterior lung.

extrapulmonary causes is more typically symmetric with both a ventral-posterior and a cephalocaudal gradient of the parenchymal airspace disease, worst posteriorly and at the lung bases (**Fig. 4**B). This discrimination is of critical importance to clinically guide ICU physicians. For example, in setting the appropriate level of PEEP, high values are selected for the low pulmonary compliance of pulmonary ARDS and low values in the higher pulmonary compliance present in extrapulmonary ARDS.[36]

In ARDS clinical management, patient lung recruitment maneuvers and the application of PEEP are essential components of mechanical ventilation, increasing the proportion of aerated lung. ICU ventilatory support often necessitates a so-called lung protection strategy characterized by the application of low tidal volumes and high levels of PEEP. However, the selection of an optimal PEEP level remains a common problem in the management of ARDS patients compromising between beneficial and negative effects. Indeed, 2 metaanalyses suggested outcome benefit of higher PEEP in more severe ARDS and possible harm in patients with mild ARDS.[37,38] Because CT can demonstrate lung morphology

changes related to attempted lung recruitment maneuvers, CT can have an integral role in the management of ARDS patients (**Fig. 5**). Gattinoni and colleagues[39] have suggested performing limited CT of the lungs, with just 2 or 3 image sections in inspiration, expiration, and with different PEEP levels, as a guide in the selection of the optimal PEEP level to establish the potential for further lung ventilator recruitment. As ARDS patients may differ substantially in terms of response to recruitment maneuvers, the key to success is the identification of patients with potentially recruitable lung, which will benefit from these maneuvers.[39] In identifying responders and nonresponders to recruitment maneuvers, CT can prevent the application of high PEEP levels in patients with low lung recruitability and the associated barotrauma complications.

Other Diseases

The principal common differential considerations for ARDS in the ICU patient are the diagnosis of infection, edema, and the acute exacerbation of fibrotic ILD. The diagnosis of pneumonia remains challenging in ICU patients. The role of early CT

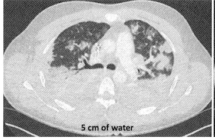
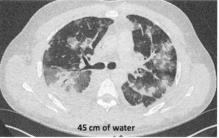

Fig. 5. Lung recruitment in ARDS. Images at airway PEEPs of 5 and 45 cm of water pressure demonstrate the increased aeration at higher pressure and, therefore, high potential for ventilatory lung recruitment.

imaging complementing chest radiography has been shown to be useful in establishing the diagnosis of infection and affecting therapeutic decision and management in up to 70% of critically ill patients.[40,41,42] CT allows accurate assessment of airspace inflammation, including nodules, ground-glass opacities, tree-in-bud pattern, lobar-segmental consolidation, and lobular consolidation.

In critically ill patients, cardiogenic pulmonary edema and fluid overload are common. The CT findings usually include septal thickening in interstitial pulmonary edema and bilateral ground-glass opacification with perihilar and gravitational distribution, bilateral relatively symmetric pleural effusions, and cardiomegaly in cardiogenic alveolar pulmonary edema. Enlargement of the antidependent upper-lobe pulmonary veins may also be appreciated. TRALI is another less common entity secondary to transfusion therapy with CT findings that are usually indistinguishable from cardiogenic pulmonary edema. However, septal lines and pleural effusions are uncommon in TRALI and may help differentiate this entity from cardiogenic pulmonary edema.[43]

Patients with chronic known or unknown ILD may present with severe respiratory failure that necessitates ICU management. AE-ILD is a relatively common complication. In a retrospective study of 147 patients with biopsy-proven ILD, 9.6% developed an acute exacerbation during the 2-year period.[44] AE-ILD is most common in the background of IPF; however, it can also be seen in usual interstitial pneumonia associated with connective tissue disorders, idiopathic nonspecific interstitial pneumonia, and nonspecific interstitial pneumonia associated with connective tissue disorders (Fig. 6A, B).[45] CT is potentially helpful in predicting patient prognosis in acute exacerbation of IPF.[46,47] The use of an HRCT classification

score demonstrated that CT features of ground-glass attenuation associated with bronchiectasis or bronchiolectasis is the most important pattern related to prognosis.[33,47] Hence, CT is a valuable imaging tool in early diagnosis of background of AE-ILD to improve outcome prediction, choose optimal ventilator settings, and assess the appropriateness of specific treatments, such as corticosteroids or immunosuppressants.

Ultrasound

US has in recent years emerged as an adjunct bedside tool in imaging and clinical management of DLD, overcoming some of the limitations of CT, in particular, the use of ionizing radiation and the difficulty of transporting critically ill patients to the radiology department. Although there is a learning curve to the use of pulmonary ultrasound, the application of this relatively available tool thereafter is relatively simple.

Multiple studies have demonstrated the bedside utility of US in detecting consolidation, pleural effusions, pulmonary embolism, and pneumothorax.[21–23,48–52] Its safety and portability allow for its use at the bedside to provide rapid and detailed information regarding the lung morphologic changes during the evolution of DLD.

The most important finding in the diagnosis of DLD is the "B" line or "comet tail artifacts," which are an US correlate of the CT findings of ground-glass opacity, consolidation, or septal thickening. "B" lines are perpendicular to the pleural line and move synchronously with lung sliding. The presence of 3 or more "B" lines in 1 intercostal space is considered abnormal and referred to as a "B" pattern.[53–55] By contrast, "A" lines constitute a basic artifact of normally aerated lung described as horizontal repetitive hyperechoic artifacts arising from, and appearing parallel to, the pleural

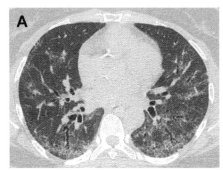 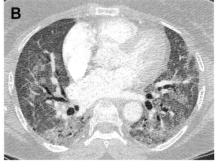

Fig. 6. AE-ILD. (*A*) Fibrotic changes with subpleural and peribronchovascular reticulation with superimposed ground-glass opacification in a female patient with rheumatoid arthritis. (*B*) Clinical and radiologic deterioration with respiratory failure. Superimposed infection was excluded clinically, including by bronchiolar lavage. The CT axial image shows progression of the fibrotic changes and ground-glass component.

line.[54,55] US features in DLD can be classified as focal or diffuse based on the sonographic distribution of aeration loss. Specifically, a focal pattern is characterized by focal loss of aeration with multiple "B" lines or focal consolidation posterolaterally with a predominantly normal sonographic aeration pattern (anterior "A" lines and normal lung sliding) seen anteriorly. In diffuse disease, there is diffuse loss of aeration with multiple B lines and/or areas of consolidation in all lung fields.

Lung US is also a useful tool in the follow-up of ARDS patients. An aeration score has been suggested related to the different degrees of aeration with 4 different sonographic patterns.[56] Specifically, a normal aeration pattern is characterized by horizontal "A" lines (Fig. 7A); a pattern of multiple and well-separated "B" lines is in keeping with moderate loss of aeration (Fig. 7B) and a pattern with multiple diffuse coalescent "B" lines is reflective of severe loss of aeration (Fig. 7C). The fourth pattern is the sonographic appearance of consolidation with complete aeration loss (Fig. 7D). This tool is a useful monitoring tool in the US assessment of ARDS, its evolution, and response to treatment. The same aeration score has been validated as a reliable tool in the assessment of patients with VAP following appropriate antimicrobial therapy.[57]

In daily practice, a frequent question that the ICU clinician seeks to address in a patient with DLD is the differentiation of cardiogenic pulmonary edema and ARDS. According to Coppetti and colleagues,[58] US is a useful tool in the differentiation of these 2 entities, although frequent appearance overlap can render interpretation difficult. US signs, such as small subpleural foci of consolidation, irregularity of the pleural line, absence or reduction of lung sliding, and spared normal aerated areas surrounded by abnormal areas with aeration loss are strongly predictive of the early phase of ARDS.

CT and clinically determined ventilator pressure-volume (P-V) curves are considered the gold-standard methods to assess recruitment effectiveness. In view of the associated disadvantages of CT utilization in the ICU environment, including availability and increased radiation exposure, several studies have evaluated the reliability of US as an alternative method in assessing lung recruitment (Fig. 8).

The aforementioned US-determined aeration score has been used during PEEP-induced lung recruitment in a study by Bouhemad and colleagues.[56] The investigators found a significant correlation between the US reaeration score and the patient P-V curves. In a limited study, lung US estimating the dependent atelectatic areas

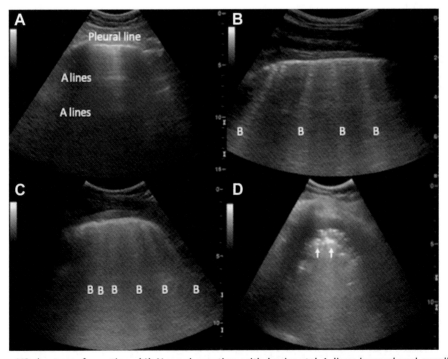

Fig. 7. Four US degrees of aeration. (A) Normal aeration with horizontal A lines beyond and parallel to the pleural line. (B) Moderate decrease with well-separated B lines. (C) Severe decrease of lung aeration with coalescent B lines less than 3 mm. (D) Complete loss with sonographic consolidation and air bronchograms (arrows).

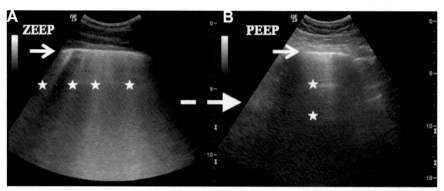

Fig. 8. Example of PEEP-induced lung recruitment detected with US. (*A*) Severe decrease of lung aeration with coalescent B lines (*stars*) arising from the pleural line (*arrow*). ZEEP, zero end-expiratory pressure. (*B*) In the same patient, after PEEP 15 cmH2O, the same lung region appears normally aerated in a normal aeration pattern with horizontal A lines (*stars*) parallel to the pleural line (*arrow*).

during a trial of PEEP effectively tracked lung aeration changes during recruitment maneuvers in patients with early ARDS and differentiated ARDS responders and nonresponders to PEEP.[59] However, in a recent study, Chiumello and colleagues[60] showed that although US can assess regional and global lung aeration, it is not as reliable an imaging tool for assessing PEEP-induced recruitment when compared with the gold-standard CT.

Although US has significant advantages as a radiation-free bedside tool, with high sensitivity, specificity, and reproducibility, it also has its own inherent limitations. Subcutaneous emphysema and large overlying dressings do not allow US assessment. Lung overinflation secondary to high PEEP levels is associated with potential barotrauma complications but is not detectable by US. Another limitation is that US can only visualize parenchymal abnormalities adjacent to and extending to the pleura. Despite these limitations, US is increasingly considered an essential imaging tool, playing a significant role in clinical decision making and management.[61] Therefore, in resource-constrained settings, the use of US is recognized as a valid alternative to CXR and CT and can be used with a modified Berlin definition (Kigali modification) in the diagnosis of ARDS.[62] According to this modified definition, the radiological requirement of bilateral infiltrates can be met with the use of ultrasound replacing CXR and CT.

Fluorodeoxyglucose F18 PET-Computed Tomography

Fluorodeoxyglucose F18 PET-CT is a functional imaging tool predominantly associated with the staging imaging of malignancy. In recent years,

experimental use of PET-CT has provided additive information contributing to the better understanding of the pathophysiology of ARDS and more generally in DLD in select populations. Although normal CT density may be demonstrated in the anterior lung segments, different PET-CT studies have demonstrated that metabolically there is more diffuse lung involvement. Specifically, the metabolic activity is markedly increased across the entire lung and no lung region is spared by the inflammatory process. Indeed, Bellani and colleagues[63] demonstrated in the largest study cohort of 10 mechanically ventilated patients with ARDS that inflammation also involved normally aerated regions. Overall, PET-CT shows promise of possibly providing a future clinical guide to monitor cellular metabolic activity, inflammation, and the severity of lung injury. However, the use of PET-CT remains severely constrained in clinical practice because of its complexity, time-consuming nature, radiation exposure, and difficulty of transferring and monitoring critically ill patients.

SUMMARY

Optimizing the use of imaging has significantly changed the understanding of the natural history of DLD and ARDS and helped refine the definition of this complex entity. The role of multimodality imaging, both current and novel, is not only limited to the nonspecific description of DLD. It is essential in the understanding of individual entities within this disease spectrum, most notably ARDS, and guiding their clinical management. Although plain radiography and CT imaging remain the principal reference for imaging, management, and research, US imaging and imaging during ventilator setting variation can dynamically assist in determining optimum ventilatory settings and predict the capacity for recovery, bridging anatomic depiction and physiologic understanding.

REFERENCES

1. Shaver CM, Bastarache JA. Clinical and biological heterogeneity in ARDS: direct versus indirect lung injury. Clin Chest Med 2014;35(4):639–53.
2. Castro CY. ARDS and diffuse alveolar damage: a pathologist's perspective. Semin Thorac Cardiovasc Surg 2006;18:13–9.
3. Ashbaugh DG, Bigelow DB, Petty TL, et al. Acute respiratory distress in adults. Lancet 1967;2(7511): 319–23.
4. Bernard GR, Artigas A, Brigham KL, et al. Report of the American- European consensus conference on ARDS: definitions, mechanisms, relevant outcomes and clinical trial coordination. The Consensus Committee. Intensive Care Med 1994;20:225–32.
5. ARDS Definition Task Force, Ranieri VM, Rubenfeld GD, Thompson BT, et al. Acute respiratory distress syndrome: the Berlin definition. JAMA 2012;307:2526–33.
6. Fan E, Brodie D, Slutsky AS. Acute respiratory distress syndrome advances in diagnosis and treatment. JAMA 2018;319(7):698–710.
7. Bellani G, Laffey JG, Pham T, et al. Epidemiology, patterns of care, and mortality for patients with acute respiratory distress syndrome in intensive care units in 50 countries. JAMA 2016;315:788–800.
8. Bouros D, Nicholson AC, Polychronopoulos V, et al. Acute interstitial pneumonia. Eur Respir J 2000;15: 412–8.
9. Hunter JD. Ventilator associated pneumonia. BMJ 2012;344:e3325.
10. Afshari A, Pagani L, Harbarth S. Year in review 2011: critical care–infection. Crit Care 2012;16:242–7.
11. Pugin J, Auckenthaler R, Mili N, et al. Diagnosis of ventilator-associated pneumonia by bacteriologic analysis of bronchoscopic and nonbronchoscopic "blind" bronchoalveolar lavage fluid. Am Rev Respir Dis 1991;143:1121–9.
12. American Thoracic S, Infectious Diseases Society of America. Guidelines for the management of adults with hospital-acquired, ventilator-associated, and healthcare-associated pneumonia. Am J Respir Crit Care Med 2005;171:388–416.
13. Collard HR, Ryerson CJ, Corte TJ, et al. Acute exacerbation of idiopathic pulmonary fibrosis. An international working group report. Am J Respir Crit Care Med 2016;194:265–75.
14. Rice TW, Ware LB, Haponik EF, et al. Vascular pedicle width in acute lung injury: correlation with intravascular pressures and ability to discriminate fluid status. Crit Care 2011;15:R86.
15. Warren MA, Zhao Z, Koyama T, et al. Severity scoring of lung oedema on the chest radiograph is associated with clinical outcomes in ARDS. Thorax 2018;73(9):840–6.
16. Aquino SL, Khan A, Batra PV, et al. American College of Radiology. ACR Appropriateness Criteria: Routine Chest Radiograph. Available at: http://www.dcamedical.com/pdf/appropriateness-criteria-routine-chest-xray.pdf. Accessed April 18, 2019.
17. Henschke C, Pasternack G, Schroeder S, et al. Bedside chest radiography: diagnostic efficacy. Radiology 1983;149:23–6.
18. Oba Y, Zaza T. Abandoning daily routine chest radiography in the intensive care unit: meta-analysis. Radiology 2010;255(2):386–95.
19. Hejblum G, Chalumeau-Lemoine L, Ioos V, et al. Comparison of routine and on-demand prescription of chest radiographs in mechanically ventilated adults: a multicentre, cluster-randomised, two-period crossover study. Lancet 2009;374:1687–93.
20. Ferguson ND, Fan E, Camporota L, et al. The Berlin definition of ARDS: an expanded rationale, justification, and supplementary material. Intensive Care Med 2012;38:1573–82.
21. Lichtenstein D, Goldstein I, Mourgeon E, et al. Comparative diagnostic performances of auscultation, chest X-ray, and lung ultrasonography in acute respiratory distress syndrome. Anesthesiology 2004;100:9–15.
22. Stefanidis K, Dimopoulos S, Kolofousi C, et al. Sonographic lobe localization of alveolar-interstitial syndrome in the critically ill. Crit Care Res Pract 2012; 2012:179719.
23. Xirouchaki N, Magkanas E, Vaporidi K, et al. Lung ultrasound in critically ill patients: comparison with bedside chest radiography. Intensive Care Med 2011;37:1488–93.
24. Karhu JM, Ala-Kokko TI, Ahvenjärvi LK, et al. Early chest computed tomography in adult acute severe community-acquired pneumonia patients treated in the intensive care unit. Acta Anaesthesiol Scand 2016;60(8):1102–10.
25. Rubenfeld GD, Caldwell E, Granton J, et al. Interobserver variability in applying a radiographic definition of ARDS. Chest 1999;116:1347–53.
26. Figueroa-Casas JB, Brunner N, Dwivedi AK, et al. Accuracy of chest radiograph to identify bilateral pulmonary infiltrates consistent with the diagnosis of acute respiratory distress syndrome using computed tomography as reference standard. J Crit Care 2013;28:352–7.
27. See KC, Ong V, Tan YL, et al. Chest radiography versus lung ultrasound for identification of acute respiratory distress syndrome: a retrospective observational study. Crit Care 2018;22:203.
28. Tagliabue M, Casella MC, Zincone GE, et al. CT and chest radiography in the evaluation of adult

respiratory distress syndrome. Acta Radiologica 1994;35:230–4.

29. Sundaram B, Chughtai AR, Kazerooni E. Multidetector high-resolution computed tomography of the lungs: protocols and applications. J Thorac Imaging 2010;25(2):125–41.

30. Farshad-Amacker NA, Alkadhi H, Leschka S, et al. Effect of high-pitch dual-source CT to compensate motion artifacts: a phantom study. Acad Radiol 2013;20(10):1234–9.

31. Gattinoni L, Pesenti A. The concept of "baby lung". Intensive Care Med 2005;31:776–84.

32. Zompatori M, Ciccarese F, Fasano L. Overview of current lung imaging in acute respiratory distress syndrome. Eur Respir Rev 2014; 23(134):519–30.

33. Ichikado K, Suga M, Muranaka H, et al. Prediction of prognosis for acute respiratory distress syndrome with thin-section CT: validation in 44 cases. Radiology 2006;238(1):321–9.

34. Chung JH, Kradin RL, Greene RE, et al. CT predictors of mortality in pathology confirmed ARDS. Eur Radiol 2011;21(4):730–7.

35. Desai SR, Wells AU, Suntharalingam G, et al. Acute respiratory distress syndrome caused by pulmonary and extrapulmonary injury: a comparative CT study. Radiology 2001;218(3):689–93.

36. Pelosi P, D'Onofrio D, Chiumello D, et al. Pulmonary and extrapulmonary acute respiratory distress syndrome are different. Eur Respir J Suppl 2003;42: 48s–56s.

37. Briel M, Meade M, Mercat A, et al. Higher vs lower positive end-expiratory pressure in patients with acute lung injury and acute respiratory distress syndrome: systematic review and meta-analysis. JAMA 2010;303(9):865–73.

38. Phoenix SI, Paravastu S, Columb M, et al. Does a higher positive end expiratory pressure decrease mortality in acute respiratory distress syndrome? A systematic review and meta-analysis. Anesthesiology 2009;110(5):1098–105.

39. Gattinoni L, Caironi P, Cressoni M, et al. Lung recruitment in patients with the acute respiratory distress syndrome. N Engl J Med 2006;354: 1775–86.

40. Claessens YA, Debray MP, Tubach F. Early chest computed tomography scan to assist diagnosis and guide treatment decision for suspected community-acquired pneumonia. Am J Respir Crit Care Med 2015;192(8):974–82.

41. Heussel CP, Kauczor HU, Heussel G, et al. Early detection of pneumonia in febrile neutropenic patients: use of thin-section CT. Am J Roentgenol 1997;169:1347–53.

42. Mirvis SE, Tobin KD, Kostrublak I, et al. Thoracic CT in detecting occult disease in critically ill patients. AJR Am J Roentgenol 1987;148:685–9.

43. Carcano C, Okafor N, Martinez F, et al. Radiographic manifestations of transfusion-related acute lung injury. Clin Imaging 2013;37(6):1020–3.

44. Kim DS, Park JH, Park BK, et al. Acute exacerbation of idiopathic pulmonary fibrosis: frequency and clinical features. Eur Respir J 2006;27:143–50.

45. Silva CIS, Muller NL, Fujimoto K, et al. Acute exacerbation of chronic interstitial pneumonia: high-resolution computed tomography and pathologic findings. J Thorac Imaging 2007;22:221–9.

46. Akira M, Kozuka T, Yamamoto S, et al. Computed tomography findings in acute exacerbation of idiopathic pulmonary fibrosis. Am J Respir Crit Care Med 2008;178(4):372–8.

47. Fujimoto K, Taniguchi H, Johkoh T. Acute exacerbation of idiopathic pulmonary fibrosis: high-resolution CT scores predict mortality. Eur Radiol 2012;22: 83–92.

48. Lichtenstein D, Meziere G, Seitz J. The dynamic air bronchogram. a lung ultrasound sign of alveolar consolidation ruling out atelectasis. Chest 2009; 135:1421–5.

49. Roch A, Bojan M, Michelet P, et al. Usefulness of ultrasonography in predicting pleural effusions > 500 mL in patients receiving mechanical ventilation. Chest 2005;127:224–32.

50. Reissig A, Heyne J, Kroegel C. Sonography of lung and pleura in pulmonary embolism: sonomorphologic characterization and comparison with spiral CT scanning. Chest 2001;120:1977–83.

51. Lichtenstein DA, Mezière G, Lascols N, et al. Ultrasound diagnosis of occult pneumothorax. Crit Care Med 2005;33:1231–8.

52. Lichtenstein D, Meziere G, Biderman P, et al. The 'lung point': an ultrasound sign specific to pneumothorax. Intensive Care Med 2000;26: 1434–40.

53. Volpicelli G, Elbarbary M, Blaivas M, et al. International Liaison Committee on Lung Ultrasound for International Consensus Conference on Lung Ultrasound (ICC-LUS). International evidence-based recommendations for point-of-care lung ultrasound. Intensive Care Med 2012;38:577–91.

54. Lichtenstein DA, Meziere GA. Relevance of lung ultrasound in the diagnosis of acute respiratory failure: the BLUE protocol. Chest 2008;134: 117–25.

55. Stefanidis K, Dimopoulos S, Nanas S. Basic principles and current applications of lung ultrasonography in the intensive care unit. Respirology 2011; 16(2):249–56.

56. Bouhemad B, Brisson H, Le-Guen M, et al. Bedside ultrasound assessment of positive end-expiratory pressure-induced lung recruitment. Am J Resp Crit Care Med 2010;83:341–7.

57. Bouhemad B, Liu ZH, Arbelot C, et al. Ultrasound assessment of antibiotic-induced pulmonary

reaeration in ventilator-associated pneumonia. Crit Care Med 2010;38:84–92.

58. Coppetti R, Soldati G, Copetti P. Chest sonography: a useful tool to differentiate acute cardiogenic pulmonary edema from acute respiratory distress syndrome. Cardiovasc Ultrasound 2008;296:16.

59. Stefanidis K, Dimopoulos S, Tripodaki ES, et al. Lung sonography and recruitment in patients with early acute respiratory distress syndrome: a pilot study. Crit Care 2011;15:R185.

60. Chiumello D, Mongodi S, Algieri I, et al. Assessment of lung aeration and recruitment by CT scan and ultrasound in acute respiratory distress syndrome patients. Crit Care Med 2018;46(11):1761–8.

61. Xirouchaki N, Kondili E, Prinianakis G, et al. Impact of lung ultrasound on clinical decision making in critically ill patients. Intensive Care Med 2014;40: 57–65.

62. Riviello ED, Buregeya E, Twagirumugabe T. Diagnosing acute respiratory distress syndrome in resource limited settings: the Kigali modification of the Berlin definition. Curr Opin Crit Care 2017; 23(1):18–23.

63. Bellani G, Messa C, Guerra L, et al. Lungs of patients with acute respiratory distress syndrome show diffuse inflammation in normally aerated regions: a [18F]-fluoro-2-deoxy-D-glucose PET/CT study. Crit Care Med 2009;37(7):2216–22.

Imaging Early Postoperative Complications of Cardiothoracic Surgery

Alberto Cossu, MD[a], Maria Daniela Martin Rother, MD[b],
Joanna Eva Kusmirek, MD[b], Cristopher A. Meyer, MD[b],
Jeffrey P. Kanne, MD[b],*

KEYWORDS

- Thoracotomy • Esophagectomy • Pneumonectomy • Postoperative complications
- Bronchopleural fistula • Empyema

KEY POINTS

- The radiologist is an important contributor to the postoperative care of patients undergoing cardiothoracic surgery.
- Early identification of postoperative complications has the potential to reduce morbidity and mortality.
- Chest imaging can identify postsurgical complications of cardiothoracic surgery before they are clinically apparent and confirm their presence and further characterize them when they are suspected.
- Knowledge of the spectrum of complications following cardiothoracic surgery and of their respective imaging manifestations is essential for the radiologist to make a meaningful impact on patient care.

INTRODUCTION

Imaging plays a central role in the evaluation of patients following cardiothoracic surgery, both for monitoring in the early postoperative period and for assessing for suspected complications. Patients with postsurgical complications can develop a range of signs and symptoms, from hypotension and tachycardia as the result of severe bleeding to fever and leukocytosis because of infection. The radiologist is an important member of the care team in the postoperative period, helping identify and manage complications of cardiothoracic surgery. This article reviews the common complications of cardiothoracic surgery focusing on the role of imaging and clues to diagnosis.

PULMONARY EDEMA

Postoperative pulmonary edema is a noncardiogenic form of edema primarily associated with increased capillary permeability and transient pulmonary microvascular hypertension.[1] The cumulative incidence of postoperative pulmonary edema has been estimated at up to 7% in cohorts of patients undergoing surgery, with a relative mortality of approximately 11%,[2] although with modern postoperative care the mortality rates are likely much lower.

Anesthesia, volume overload from excessive intraoperative and postoperative fluid administration, and mechanical ventilation with high peak end expiratory pressure (PEEP) and tidal volumes

[a] Scuola di Specializzazione di Radiodiagnostica, Università degli Studi di Ferrara, Azienda Ospedaliera Universitaria S. Anna di Ferrara, Arcispedale Sant'Anna, Via Aldo Moro, 8, Cona, Ferrara Centralino 44124, Italy;
[b] Department of Radiology, University of Wisconsin School of Medicine and Public Health, 600 Highland Avenue, Madison, WI 53792, USA
* Corresponding author.
E-mail address: JKanne@uwhealth.org

Radiol Clin N Am 58 (2020) 133–150
https://doi.org/10.1016/j.rcl.2019.08.009

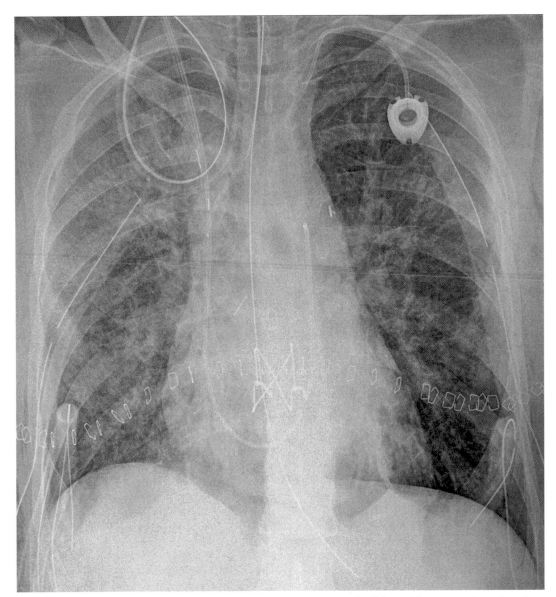

Fig. 1. A 28-year-old man with asymmetric postoperative lung edema after bilateral lung transplantation. Anteroposterior (AP) radiograph shows bilateral hazy opacities with poorly defined pulmonary vessels, worse on the right. The gastric tube is malpositioned with the tip at the esophagogastric junction and the side port in the lower esophagus.

can all contribute to microvascular injury.[3,4] The acute development of negative intrathoracic pressure from laryngospasm after extubation also can increase total pulmonary vascular resistance, promoting pulmonary edema.[1,5] Barotrauma, ischemia, and reperfusion damage produced by single lung ventilation with double-lumen endotracheal tubes during lung surgery are the most significant risk factors for postoperative edema.[3] Extracorporeal cardiopulmonary bypass used during cardiac surgery is invariably associated with hemodilution and systemic inflammatory responses, which may trigger pulmonary edema.[6] Pulmonary edema is reported to occur more commonly after right pneumonectomy because the left lung, which normally receives 45% of cardiac output, subsequently receives the entire cardiac output but lacks adequate lymphatic drainage to handle the volume.[7,8]

Distinguishing cardiogenic from noncardiogenic edema following cardiothoracic surgery can be challenging because many patients who

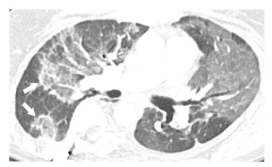

Fig. 2. A 42-year-old woman with postoperative ARDS. CT image shows extensive ground-glass opacity in the left lung and patchy ground-glass opacity in the right lung with higher attenuation periphery (*arrows*), the latter creating a "reversed halo" sign.

undergo such procedures usually have underlying cardiopulmonary comorbidities. Radiographic manifestations of pulmonary edema typically begin with peribronchial cuffing, Kerley B lines, and apparent thickening of the fissures from subpleural edema while more confluent lung opacity develops with more extensive edema, although overlap of findings is very common. Asymmetric distribution may occur following smaller resections and single lung ventilation or with prolonged lateral decubitus positioning (**Fig. 1**). Widening of the vascular pedicle is an indirect sign of volume overload, reflecting distended mediastinal veins. Common computed tomography (CT) findings of edema include septal thickening and diffuse ground-glass opacities.[9]

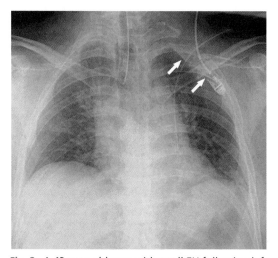

Fig. 3. A 43-year-old man with small EH following left first rib resection. AP portable radiograph obtained in the operating room shows a small extrapleural collection near the resection site forming a smooth interface with the adjacent lung (*arrows*).

ACUTE LUNG INJURY

In the past, acute lung injury (ALI) was often used to describe either the radiological pattern or the clinical manifestations of patients with acute respiratory distress from immunologic-mediated injury to the lung. Particularly, ALI was used for patients with mild gas-exchange impairment (Pao_2/Fio_2 ratio >200 mm Hg) who did not meet full criteria for acute respiratory distress syndrome (ARDS).[10] The 2012 Berlin criteria revised the definition of ARDS and omitted ALI.[11] ARDS now refers to rapidly progressive respiratory failure occurring within 7 days of an insult with Pao_2/Fio_2 less than 300 mm Hg with minimum PEEP of 5 mm Hg and bilateral lung opacities consistent with edema present on radiographs or CT. Furthermore, the criteria state that the clinical presentation cannot be "fully explained by cardiac failure or fluid overload." Although the Berlin criteria have improved the diagnosis of ARDS, interobserver agreement for some factors including radiographic findings is only moderate.[11]

Pathologically, ARDS in its most severe form is characterized by diffuse alveolar damage, which is caused by a sudden alteration of the permeability of the alveolar-capillary membrane induced by an acute insult. Other histopathologic patterns that occur include organizing pneumonia and acute fibrinous and organizing pneumonia.[12] Postoperative risk factors for ARDS include mechanical ventilation, lung infection, sepsis, transfusion-associated ALI, and aspiration.[1,4,13] In one large series, patients undergoing pneumonectomy were more likely to develop ALI compared with those undergoing less extensive lung resection.[14]

Patients presenting with clinical manifestations of ARDS often have radiographic findings, such as dependent atelectasis and patchy areas of lung consolidation, similar to those of infection and hemorrhage. The opacities become denser and more confluent over a period of just days with air bronchograms becoming apparent.[15] CT findings include diffuse or patchy ground-glass opacities, which can have a geographic distribution with normal lobules located adjacent to abnormal lobules, and the subpleural regions of the lungs can be spared (**Fig. 2**). For most patients, CT is not necessary, as it uncommonly provides additional useful information.[12,15] Despite much improvement and recent success in therapy, ARDS is still associated with high in-hospital mortality rates of up to 40%.[14]

POSTOPERATIVE HEMORRHAGE

All major surgical procedures include a risk of bleeding, and cardiothoracic surgical procedures

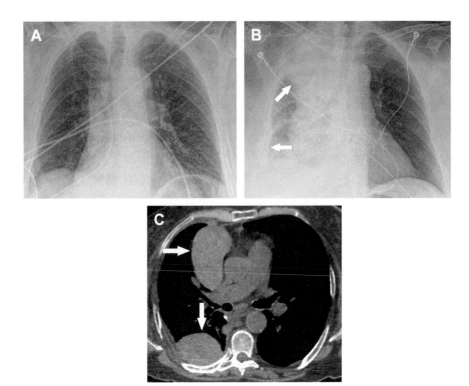

Fig. 4. A 76-year-old woman with large hemothorax following right lower lobectomy for lung cancer. (*A*) AP portable radiograph shortly after surgery shows a clear right pleural space. (*B*) AP radiograph 3 days later shows a new, complex right pleural collection (*arrows*). (*C*) Unenhanced CT image shows loculated high-attenuation material (*arrows*) in the right pleural space consistent with hemothorax.

are often associated with significant but expected intraoperative blood loss.[16] Postoperative evidence of significant blood loss includes blood in a surgical drain, hemoptysis, tamponade, or hypovolemia. Most postoperative bleeding is self-limited, but severe or persistent hemorrhage may require surgical exploration and repair or endovascular embolization. Reactive bleeding develops within the first 24 hours after surgery and is usually related to vascular ligature slipping, dislodgment of an electrocautery clot, or, as in cardiovascular procedures and lung transplantation, dehiscence of a vascular anastomosis. Delayed postsurgical bleeding, with onset within the first

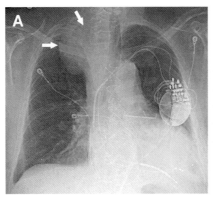
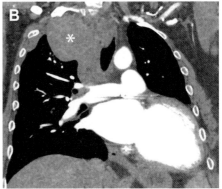

Fig. 5. A 67-year-old man with mediastinal hematoma approximately 1 week after heart surgery. (*A*) Posteroanterior (PA) radiograph shows a convex mass in the right upper mediastinum (*arrows*) displacing the trachea to the left and extending in the superior extrapleural space. (*B*) Coronal reformatted, contrast-enhanced CT image shows a high-attenuation mass (*asterisk*) typical of hematoma.

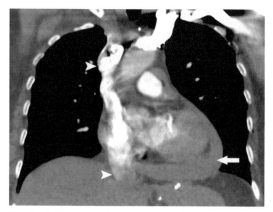

Fig. 6. A 73-year-old woman with hemopericardium and developing cardiac tamponade after hiatal hernia repair. Coronal reformatted, contrast-enhanced CT image shows a high-attenuation pericardial collection (*arrow*) and dilation of the venae cavae (*arrowheads*).

10 days, has numerous causes with surgical injury to vessels and inflammatory or infectious erosion being the 2 most important causes. Risk factors for postoperative hemorrhage include the type of surgery performed, vascular anatomic variants, and altered or weakened vessels from atherosclerosis, neoplasia, previous infection, chemotherapy, or radiation therapy. Compounding risk for hemorrhage are preexisting coagulopathy or concomitant antiplatelet or anticoagulation therapy.[16] Postoperative chest radiography can detect the presence of subclinical bleeding or correctly localize the site of hemorrhage. CT can be used to confirm bleeding or to potentially identify sites of active bleeding.

Extrapleural Hematoma

Clinically significant isolated extrapleural hematoma (EH) resulting from injury to an intercostal vessel is a rare consequence of rib resection and potentially can complicate thoracotomy or thoracoscopy. On chest radiographs, rapidly growing EH from arterial bleeding may appear as an expanding biconvex extrapulmonary opacity, whereas low-pressure venous injuries may be occult or present as small extrapleural collections (**Fig. 3**). On chest CT and MR imaging, inward displacement of the extrapleural fat layer (extrapleural fat sign) by a blood collection is characteristic.[17] Contrast-enhanced imaging can show active bleeding in some cases.

Hemothorax

Postoperative hemothorax is reported to develop in fewer than 1% of patients after lung resection and up to 18% of lung transplant recipients.[18,19]

Pulmonary, bronchial, and intercostal vessels are all potential sites of bleeding. Patients may become hypotensive or have increased bloody output from a pleural drain. In the immediate postoperative period, chest radiography can be used to evaluate for developing pleural collections. Early onset, rapid expansion, and loculation suggest bleeding (**Fig. 4**). However, radiographic detection of slow bleeding in the early postoperative period can be challenging, as the slow accumulation of pleural blood can be mistaken for the normal accumulation of serous fluid that follows pneumonectomy. CT typically shows a high-attenuation pleural collection and sometimes can reveal a site of active contrast extravasation.

Mediastinal Hematoma

Mediastinal hematoma is another frequent presentation of postoperative bleeding and can be life threatening. Bleeding can result from manipulation of or injury to the pulmonary arteries and veins, azygos vein and its tributaries, and intercostal and internal thoracic arteries.[20] Numerous radiographic findings suggest mediastinal bleeding, including increasing attenuation and increasing fullness of the mediastinum. Effacement of normal interfaces, such as the right paratracheal stripe and aortic arch along with displacement of the trachea and main bronchi, also suggest mediastinal hemorrhage (**Fig. 5**).

Hemopericardium

Hemopericardium can accompany mediastinal hematoma or occur in isolation. Slow accumulation of fluid, even large amounts (1000–1500 mL) can be tolerated well. However, rapidly developing small pericardial effusion (100–200 mL) can lead to tamponade.[21] Rapid enlargement of the cardiac silhouette and progressive flattening of the left mediastinal and cardiac contours are highly suggestive radiographic findings of hemopericardium.[22] On CT, high-attenuation blood products can be readily identified in the mediastinum, pericardium, or both (**Fig. 6**). Contrast-enhanced CT sometimes can show the site(s) of active bleeding. Findings suggesting cardiac tamponade in addition to hemopericardium include dilation of the venae cavae and underfilling of the ventricles. The "flattened heart sign" is characterized by flattening of the anterior surface of the heart with decreased anteroposterior diameter. With severe tamponade, the cardiac chambers may have a concave morphology. Straightening of the right contour also can develop because of the relatively higher compliance of the right cardiac chambers.[21,23] Bedside echocardiography provides rapid assessment of unstable patients.[21]

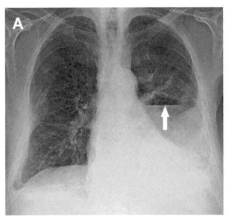
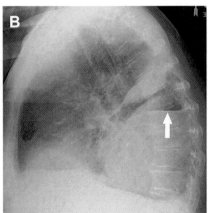
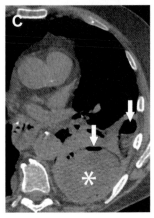

Fig. 7. A 69-year-old man with left pleural empyema after esophagectomy. PA (*A*) and lateral (*B*) radiographs show a complex left pleural collection with fluid levels (*arrows*). (*C*) Unenhanced chest CT image shows complex, expansile left pleural collection (*asterisk*) with multiple gas pockets (*arrows*).

Diffuse Alveolar Hemorrhage

Diffuse alveolar hemorrhage, although extremely rare, may develop shortly after surgery, as a result of damage to the pulmonary microcirculation. Risk factors include preexisting pulmonary hypertension, mechanical ventilation, cytotoxic therapy, and inhaled halogenated anesthetics.[24] Patients typically develop acute-onset dyspnea and hypoxia. Hemoptysis occurs in only approximately 60%. Hemoglobin levels can precipitously drop.[25]

Chest radiographs typically show patchy or confluent bilateral lung opacities indistinguishable from edema or massive aspiration in most cases. CT findings are similar and include consolidation, ground-glass opacity, and centrilobular nodules. Superimposed septal thickening and intralobular lines are sometimes present, often more than 24 hours after the initial event. The abrupt onset of signs and symptoms and development of radiographic abnormalities is most of the clue to the diagnosis. Bronchoalveolar lavage is confirmatory.[25]

Infectious Pneumonia

The incidence of postoperative infectious pneumonia after lung resection has been reported as high as 25% but is likely closer to 3% to 4% with routine use of preoperative antibiotics and aggressive postoperative pulmonary toilet.[26–28] Prolonged atelectasis with bacterial colonization and aspiration are major contributors. Mortality rates have reported as high as 30%.[28]

The diagnosis of postoperative pneumonia is often challenging, as the radiographic findings of lung consolidation and nodules may be delayed or obscured by underlying atelectasis and pleural effusion. Furthermore, fever and leukocytosis have a variety of potential sources in the postoperative period.[9] CT can be helpful in selected cases in which the diagnosis is unclear because of its increased sensitivity for lung opacities as compared with portable chest radiographs.[29] CT also can be helpful in cases in which there is little or no improvement despite appropriate therapy to assess for underlying abscess or empyema or

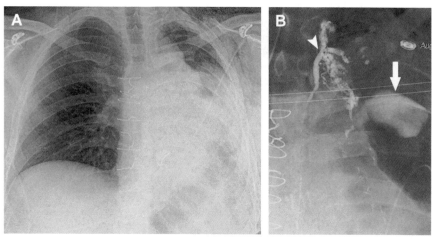

Fig. 8. A 58-year-old woman with chylothorax after left pneumonectomy. (*A*) AP radiograph shows left pleural collection 3 days after pneumonectomy, indistinguishable from pleural effusion. (*B*) Image from lymphangiogram shows disruption of the thoracic duct near its insertion with the left subclavian vein (*arrowhead*) and accumulation of contrast in the left pneumonectomy space (*arrow*).

to detect radiographic mimics of infection, such as venous infarct or lobar torsion.

Aspiration

Aspiration is a common complication among hospitalized patients, including those recovering from surgery. Aspiration can occur during anesthesia induction or with instrumentation, including endotracheal tube placement or removal or upper endoscopy. In addition, patients can aspirate from altered mentation, sedative effects from medication, or impaired aerodigestive function.[30] Aspiration is of particular concern for patients undergoing esophagectomy because of altered anatomy and intraoperative injury to the recurrent laryngeal nerve, which can lead to impaired cough reflex.[31] The injury to the airway and lungs depends on the volume and types of material

aspirated. Aspiration can lead to acute respiratory failure, ARDS, and infection including empyema or abscess.[29]

The typical radiographic findings of aspiration include gravitationally dependent, peribronchial consolidation, nodules, and bronchial wall thickening. Associated atelectasis can occur. CT imaging findings are similar to radiographs, but debris or secretions in the associated airways and nearby centrilobular nodules are readily apparent. Sometimes liquid or debris is retained in the esophagus.[29]

PLEURAL COMPLICATIONS
Empyema

Empyema is frank infection of the pleural space with an incidence after lung resection of 2% to 16% and occurring up to several weeks after resection,

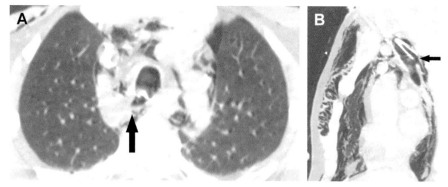

Fig. 9. A 67-year-old man with tracheal laceration from endotracheal intubation. Axial (*A*) and coronal reformatted (*B*) images show extension to the endotracheal tube tip posteriorly (*arrows*) because of a disruption in the posterior tracheal membrane.

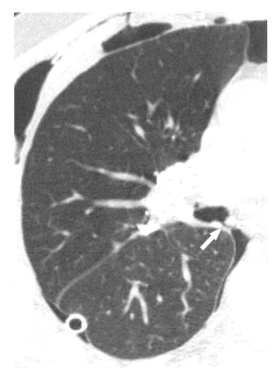

Fig. 10. A 45-year-old man double lung transplant recipient with bronchial anastomotic dehiscence. CT image shows a communication (*arrow*) between the right main bronchus and the pleural space. Pneumothorax and chest wall gas are present.

although rates have declined with improved surgical techniques and routine use of preoperative antibiotics.[9] Early postoperative empyema typically results from residual infection in the pleural space, whereas later empyema often results from bronchopleural or esophagopleural fistulas.

Chest radiographic findings of postpneumonectomy empyema include expansion of the pneumonectomy space with straightening or convexity of the normally concave mediastinal margin of the pneumonectomy space, contralateral mediastinal shift, and thickening of the ipsilateral parietal pleura. Fluid levels also can develop in the pneumonectomy space, or the fluid level can drop as more gas enters.[32] CT better delineates fluid loculations and underlying lung infection. Causative fistulas also can be apparent (Fig. 7).

Management of empyema is with percutaneous drainage. Video-assisted thoracic surgery (VATS) drainage may be required for patients who fail more conservative therapy or in whom fistula treatment is also required, often with a muscle flap.

Chylothorax

Chylothorax refers to the persistent collection of lymphatic fluid within the pleural space. It usually results from obstruction or transection of the thoracic duct. Surgical procedures are the most common causes of traumatic thoracic duct injury.[33] Chylothorax may occur following several cardiothoracic surgical procedures. Fewer than 1% of patients undergoing pneumonectomy develop chylothorax,[34] whereas the incidence is up to 4% for patients undergoing esophagectomy.[35] Chylothorax is usually indistinguishable from other causes of pleural effusion, and the diagnosis is confirmed by fluid analysis (Fig. 8).

AIRWAY COMPLICATIONS
Tracheal Injuries

Intraoperative tracheal laceration is primarily related to airway management. Several factors contribute to tracheal injuries. Traumatic intubation and prolonged balloon cuff overinflation are mechanical factors, whereas underlying tracheal pathology can predispose patients to injury.[36] Lacerations usually occur in the posterior membranous wall of the trachea due to lack of cartilage protection. A higher incidence of tracheal injury has been reported in women, thought to be related to a weaker membranous posterior membrane. The trachea also can be injured during esophageal surgery, such as esophagectomy.[37] Tracheal laceration usually presents intraoperatively or in the immediate postoperative period with acute respiratory distress and hemoptysis.[38,39]

Chest radiographs and CT typically show extensive pneumomediastinum, often with gas extending into the chest wall soft tissues. CT also can show mediastinal hematoma adjacent to the trachea as well as the defect in the tracheal wall (Fig. 9).[40]

Postoperative Persistent Air Leak

Postoperative air leaks are defined as a continuous air inflow into the pleural space because of an abnormal communication with the airways. An abnormal communication between the lung distal to a segmental bronchus is referred as an alveolar-pleural fistula (APF) and is the most common post-resection air leak. These typically result from direct injury to the visceral pleura and underlying lung during surgery. Incomplete or absent fissures together with diseased lung are major risk factors for APF in addition to impaired visibility in the operative field. APF is reported to be more common after upper lobe surgery (more on the right) or more extensive anatomic resection, such as lobectomy or bilobectomy.[41]

Small postoperative air leaks are expected, with an incidence of 25% to 60%. However, in approximately 5% to 10% of patients, they may last more

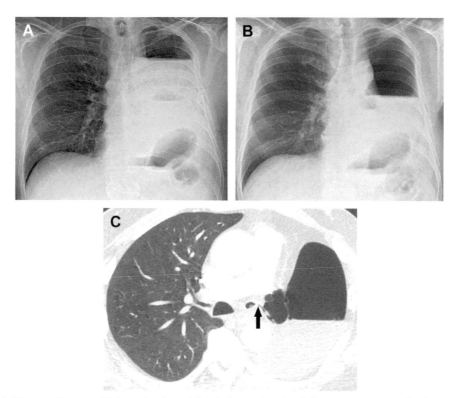

Fig. 11. A 62-year-old man with bronchopleural fistula 2 months after left pneumonectomy for lung cancer. (*A*) PA radiograph performed shortly before discharge shows fluid levels in the left pneumonectomy space with small volume gas remaining, leftward mediastinal shift, and elevation of the left hemidiaphragm. (*B*) PA radiograph obtained 2 months later shows a precipitous drop in the fluid level, indicating gas entering the pneumonectomy cavity. (*C*) Unenhanced CT image shows small communication (*arrow*) between the left bronchial stump and the pneumonectomy cavity.

than 5 to 7 days and are considered persistent.[41,42] In the normal postoperative course, small volume serosanguinous liquid accumulates in the pleural space with concurrent gas resorption, evident on serial chest radiographs and by decreasing pleural drain output. Stable or increasing gas in the post-resection space and failed reexpansion of the residual lung beyond the first postoperative week is suggestive of persistent air leak. Because most APFs are managed conservatively, chest CT is usually reserved for conservative treatment failures or when pleurodesis, endobronchial valve placement, or additional surgery is planned.

Bronchial Anastomotic Dehiscence

Bronchial anastomotic dehiscence can occur after sleeve lobectomy or lung transplant. The incidence after sleeve lobectomy has been reported to occur in up to 6% of patients.[43] Extended lymph node dissection has been reported to increase the risk of bronchial anastomotic dehiscence because of excessive tension on the bronchial anastomosis

site and subsequent bronchial wall ischemia. Bronchial anastomotic dehiscence is reported to occur in up to 10% of lung transplant recipients and develops between 1 and 4 weeks after transplantation. A variety of factors contribute to dehiscence and include surgical technique, donor-recipient size discrepancies, infection, and, most important, disruption of the bronchial arterial supply.

Radiographic findings suggesting dehiscence include new or worsening pneumomediastinum, pneumothorax, or both. CT is more sensitive and can show the defect or a collection of extraluminal gas adjacent to the anastomosis (**Fig. 10**). Most bronchial anastomotic dehiscence is usually treated with an endobronchial stent. Surgical revision, often with muscle flap, is reserved for refractory cases.

Bronchopleural Fistula

Bronchopleural fistula (BPF) is a rare cause of persistent air leak and is an abnormal communication between a proximal bronchus (up to the first segmental generation) and the pleural space. Postoperative BPFs are usually the result of bronchial stump leak. The incidence varies from only 1% for segmentectomy up to 10% for right pneumonectomy. Right pneumonectomy is thought to have a higher rate of BPF because of the shorter stump length and greater risk for ischemic injury.[44] Bronchial stumps longer than 25 mm have a higher frequency of dehiscence.[45,46] Infection at the staple line also can lead to breakdown of and subsequent leak at the bronchial stump. Other risk factors include compromised bronchial arterial supply from neoadjuvant radiotherapy, chemotherapy, or both. Furthermore, the bronchial arteries can be injured during mediastinal lymphadenectomy. Rarely, BPF can result from trauma from instrumentation, such as endotracheal tube or unintended surgical injury. BPF may complicate both the early and late postoperative periods and lead to recurrent lung infection or empyema.[9,47]

Chest radiographs show persistent air leak characterized by ongoing or enlarging pneumothorax and failure of the remaining lung to expand (**Fig. 11**). CT sometimes can show direct communication between the affected airway and the pleural space, helping facilitate treatment in cases that do not respond to prolonged pleural catheter drainage. Sometimes the direct communication is not apparent, but bubbles of gas can accumulate adjacent to the bronchial stump.[48]

Postpneumonectomy Syndrome

Postpneumonectomy syndrome is a late complication of pneumonectomy, usually developing within 1 year after surgery. Children, young adults, and female patients are more commonly affected,[49,50] and postpneumonectomy syndrome occurs more commonly after right pneumonectomy.[51,52] Following pneumonectomy, gas and liquid are reabsorbed from the pneumonectomy space with subsequent ipsilateral mediastinal shift and cardiac rotation. With this alteration in anatomy, the trachea and remaining main bronchus can become compressed between the spine, aorta, and pulmonary artery resulting in narrowing or malacia. Patients can be dyspneic because of impaired ventilation in the remaining lung and are predisposed to recurrent lung infection.

Chest radiographic findings in patients with postpneumonectomy syndrome include marked displacement and rotation of the heart, mediastinum, and trachea into the pneumonectomy space. The cardiac apex usually orients toward the posterolateral hemithorax. As the remaining lung hyperexpands and crosses midline, aerated lung can be visible on the pneumonectomy side. CT is confirmatory, showing compression of the distal trachea and main bronchus (**Fig. 12**).[9] Treatment consists of reorienting the mediastinal structures and placing saline or silicone implants into the pneumonectomy space to prevent recurrence. Some surgeons might elect to prophylactically fill the pneumonectomy space at the time of resection to prevent postpneumonectomy syndrome.[53]

VASCULAR COMPLICATIONS
Pulmonary Vein Thrombosis

Pulmonary vein thrombosis is a rare complication following lung transplantation, lung resection, or cardiac surgery. It can occur from sluggish flow from altered anatomy or inadvertent injury or ligation because of complex anatomy or difficult dissection. Complications include pulmonary venous infarct and systemic embolism with stroke or other end-organ injury.[54] One study showed an incidence of 3.3% after lobectomy with up to nearly 18% in patients undergoing left upper lobectomy.[55] Radiographic findings of pulmonary vein thrombosis include progressively increasing density in and size of the affected lobe. Contrast-enhanced CT or MR imaging shows a filling defect in the vein with occasional left atrial extension in addition to septal thickening and ground-glass opacity in the affected lobe from edema, infarcts, or both (**Fig. 13**).[54,56]

Postoperative Lobar Torsion

Postoperative lobar torsion results from the rotation of the residual lung parenchyma on its own

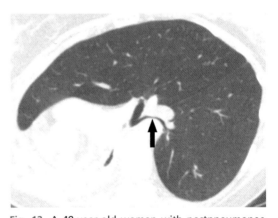

Fig. 12. A 48-year-old woman with postpneumonectomy syndrome after left pneumonectomy for carcinoid tumor. CT image shows marked rotation and displacement of the heart and mediastinum to the right with stretching and narrowing of the left lower lobe bronchus (*arrow*).

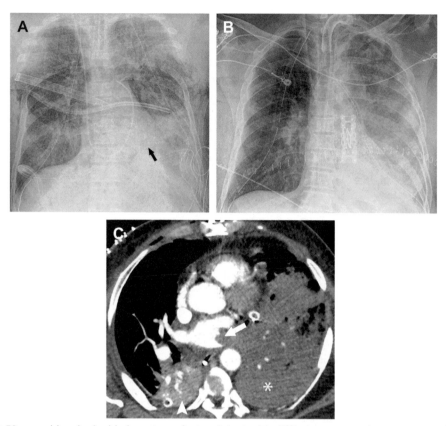

Fig. 13. A 58-year-old male double lung transplant recipient with difficult postoperative course complicated by left inferior pulmonary vein thrombosis. (*A*) AP radiograph after surgery shows an open chest with reperfusion edema and mid left basal atelectasis. The left hemidiaphragm (*arrow*) remains visible. (*B*) AP radiograph 9 days later, after chest closure, shows a well-aerated right lung allograft but extensive lower lung consolidation on the left with worsening edema. (*C*) Contrast-enhanced CT image 9 days after transplant shows a filling defect in the left inferior pulmonary vein extending into the left atrium (*arrow*). The left lower lobe (*asterisk*) is diffusely consolidated and has low attenuation in contrast to enhancing dependent atelectasis on the right (*arrowhead*). Poor aeration of the left upper lobe was related to extrinsic venous compression, and the upper lobe improved following lower lobectomy.

bronchovascular bundle. The reported incidence after lung resection is less than 1%.[47] Torsion most commonly affects the middle lobe after right upper lobe resection and less commonly the lingula after upper lobe bisegmentectomy (lingular sparing lobectomy).[9] Torsion after lung transplantation is rare.[57] The presence of a large complete interlobar fissure in conjunction with large volume pleural fluid, together with loss of fixation, may facilitate the torsion of the reexpanding parenchyma around the hilum. Complete atelectasis from airway compromise and hemorrhagic infarction due to venous ischemia can ensue.[47,58,59]

Chest radiographic findings of lobar torsion include consolidation or complete atelectasis of the involved lobe, which often has an unusual orientation (**Fig. 14**). CT, especially with sagittal reformations, can confirm torsion by showing

abnormal configuration of the bronchovascular structures. Venous engorgement can cause expansion of and low attenuation consolidation or ground-glass opacity in the affected lobe with reduced or absent venous drainage. Affected pulmonary arteries will be attenuated or have abrupt cutoffs.[9,60]

Cardiac Herniation

Cardiac herniation is an extremely rare complication of intrapericardial pneumonectomy occurring within 24 hours of surgery and having a mortality rate of up to 50%.[61,62] Failed closure of a surgical pericardial defect in conjunction with extubation, cough, changes in patient position, and negative intrathoracic pressure from percutaneous drainage can lead to

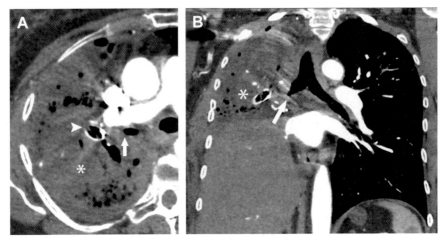

Fig. 14. Woman with middle lobe torsion and venous infarction after upper and lower lobectomy and failed pulmoplasty. Axial (*A*) and coronal reformatted (*B*) contrast-enhanced CT images show an enlarged and consolidated middle lobe (*asterisk*) without enhancement and abrupt cutoff of the remaining bronchus (*arrows*). The pleural drain (*arrowhead*) has an unusual orientation. (*Courtesy of* Seth J. Kligerman, M.D. ,San Diego, CA).

herniation of the heart through the defect. With herniation to the right, compression or torsion of the venae cavae can reduce preload and lead to cardiovascular collapse. With leftward herniation, the ventricles can prolapse, and the coronary arteries can be compressed against the edge of the pericardial defect leading to myocardial infarction.

Radiographic findings include pneumopericardium and displacement of the heart into the pneumonectomy space accompanied by mediastinal shift. With rightward herniation, the cardiac apex will be displaced to the right, and the mediastinal vascular pedicle can widen from engorgement of the superior vena cava (**Fig. 15**). With leftward herniation, the mass of the herniated ventricles will be apparent in the pneumonectomy space and have a fattened boot shape. Findings are more apparent following rightward herniation than leftward herniation. Chest CT is confirmatory, but many patients may be hemodynamically unstable and require emergent reoperation.[9,61,62]

MEDIASTINITIS

Acute mediastinitis occurs in 0.4% to 5.0% of patients undergoing chest surgery, with most cases

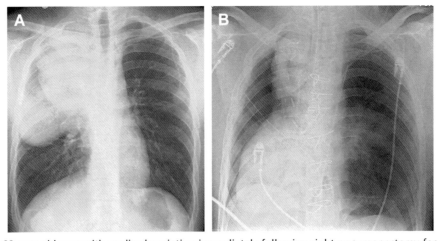

Fig. 15. A 23-year-old man with cardiac herniation immediately following right pneumonectomy for malignant germ cell tumor resection. (*A*) Preoperative PA radiograph shows a large mass in the right hemithorax and normal orientation of the heart. (*B*) AP radiograph obtained immediately after surgery shows dextrorotation of the heart into the right pneumonectomy space. (*Courtesy of* Travis S. Henry, M.D. ,San Francisco, CA).

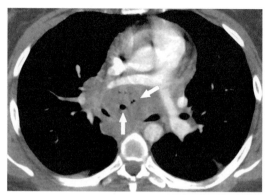

Fig. 16. A 26-year-old woman with mediastinal abscess after mediastinoscopy. Contrast-enhanced CT image shows a large fluid collection with gas pockets (*arrows*) in the subcarinal space with mass effect on the airways and pulmonary arteries.

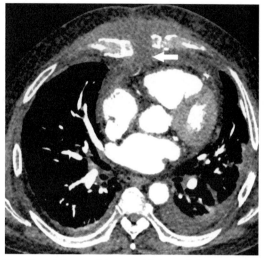

Fig. 17. A 64-year-old man with DSWI following coronary arterial bypass grafting requiring wire removal and debridement. Contrast-enhanced CT image shows diastasis of the sternal osteotomy with fluid tracking from the anterior chest wall through the sternotomy into the prevascular mediastinum (*arrow*). Small pleural and pericardial effusions are present.

occurring after cardiac surgery.[63,64] Imaging findings of acute mediastinitis are usually indistinguishable from the normal postoperative mediastinum during the first 2 to 3 postoperative weeks. However, the presence of mediastinal liquid and gas collections beyond 3 weeks is highly suggestive. Chest radiographic findings suggesting developing mediastinitis include new or worsening pneumomediastinum or loss of normal mediastinal contours and interfaces. CT shows these abnormalities to advantage with better characterization and localization (**Fig. 16**). Collections can organize into abscesses or may be more phlegmonous. Other commonly associated findings include pleural and pericardial effusion and reactive mediastinal lymph node enlargement.[64]

CHEST WALL
Deep Sternal Wound Infection

Deep sternal wound infection (DSWI) occurs in up to 1.8% of patients undergoing cardiac surgery through a median sternotomy approach.[65] Risk factors for DSWI include obesity, diabetes mellitus or hyperglycemia, female sex, and older age. Preoperative antibiotics can greatly reduce the risk of DSWI.[66,67]

Radiographs can show disruption and separation of sternal wires when sternal dehiscence develops. CT is performed for most patients and can show subcutaneous fluid collections, osteolysis, and sternal wire disruption (**Fig. 17**).[60]

Postoperative Lung Hernia

Postoperative lung hernia is a very uncommon complication of chest surgery.[68–70] In the authors'

experience, it is seen occasionally as an incidental finding after thoracotomy for lung transplantation. Lung can herniate through site of rib osteotomy or intercostal muscle and endothoracic fascial defects. Most require no intervention, as complications are quite rare. Entrapment and strangulation of lung tissue is rare and may require reduction and closure.[71,72] Lung hernias are dynamic and may change across serial imaging studies or between inspiration and expiration (**Fig. 18**).

DIAPHRAGM DYSFUNCTION

The exact incidence of phrenic nerve injury leading to diaphragm dysfunction after cardiothoracic surgery is unknown. The reported incidence after cardiac surgery ranges from 1.2% to 60.0%,[73] but in the authors' experience the real incidence is probably on the far lower end of this spectrum. Phrenic nerve injury also can occur after resection of a prevascular mediastinal mass or thymectomy.[74] Mechanisms of injury include hypothermal, mechanical, and possibly ischemic.

The primary finding of phrenic nerve injury is persistent postoperative elevation of the ipsilateral hemidiaphragm. Associated atelectasis may be present. Many patients have no symptoms. Patients with underlying lung disease may develop new or worsening dyspnea, which may be positional. Fluoroscopic evaluation of

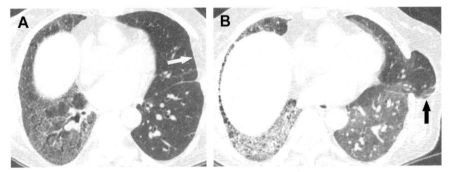

Fig. 18. A 68-year-old man with dynamic left lung hernia after lung transplantation. (*A*) Unenhanced inspiratory CT image shows straightening of the pleura-chest wall interface at the site of the thoracotomy defect (*arrow*). (*B*) On expiration, a large portion of the lingula herniates out of the thoracic cavity (*arrow*).

the diaphragm ("sniff test") can confirm the diagnosis, showing paradoxic upward motion of the affected hemidiaphragm during a short, intense inhalation through the nose. Many phrenic nerve injuries resolve within 6 to 12 months.[73]

RETAINED SURGICAL FOREIGN BODIES

Retained surgical foreign body is rare, and its frequency has been further reduced by proactive strategies including intraoperative checklists and instrument counts. Many institutions also routinely perform postoperative chest radiography to assess for retained foreign bodies. Nevertheless, accidental oversights during prolonged or emergent surgeries and obesity remain risk factors for a retained surgical foreign body (**Fig. 19**).[75] Surgical sponges and gauzes are the most common retained foreign bodies and usually are located in the pleural space. To assist radiographic identification, radiopaque components have been added to most surgical items. Sometimes, these foreign materials may mimic pulmonary neoplasm or parenchymal consolidation, delaying or obstructing the correct diagnosis. Furthermore, new devices are being developed and used and may not be familiar to the radiologist or may be challenging to identify on imaging studies, making the identification of truly undesired items more complicated.

POSTOPERATIVE COMPLICATIONS SPECIFIC TO ESOPHAGEAL SURGERY

Esophagectomy is usually performed with curative intent for esophageal carcinoma. The type of esophagectomy performed depends on tumor extent and location and surgeon preference. Recently, minimally invasive esophagectomy (MIE) and robot-assisted esophagectomy have increased.[76] Ivor Lewis esophagectomy (ILE) is the most commonly performed surgery for

carcinoma of the mid and lower esophagus.[77] ILE consists of an upper abdominal incision to mobilize and tubularize the stomach followed by a thoracic incision to remove the diseased portion of the esophagus and adjacent lymph nodes en bloc and a surgical anastomosis. Transhiatal (transmediastinal) esophagectomy consists of a subxiphoid abdominal incision to tubularize and mobilize the stomach and a left lower cervical incision with a cervical anastomosis, thus avoiding having to enter the chest percutaneously. A McKeown esophagectomy consists of abdominal, right thoracic, and left lower cervical incisions. Selection of technique is beyond the scope of this review. Complications after esophagectomy are common, occurring in up to 60% of patients; however,

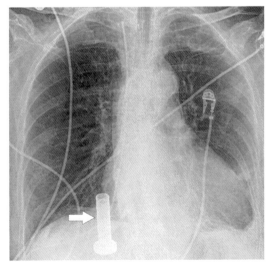

Fig. 19. A 75-year-old woman with retained VATS port in the right pleural space after MIE. AP radiograph right after surgery shows VATS port (*arrow*) in the lower right hemithorax. The port presumably fell into the chest during instrument removal.

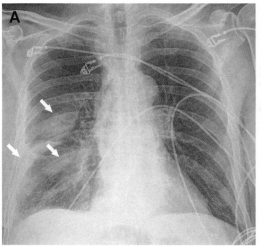

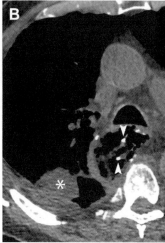

Fig. 20. A 62-year-old man with anastomotic leak after esophagogastrostomy for esophageal carcinoma. (*A*) AP radiograph 7 days after ILE shows a large, loculated right pleural collection (*arrows*). (*B*) Unenhanced CT image show disruption of the surgical staple line with staples (*arrowheads*) and debris within the conduit lumen. A portion of the loculated pleural collection (*asterisk*) is visible.

mortality rates have dropped to approximately 3%.[78]

Anastomotic Leak

Anastomotic leak is a serious complication following esophageal surgery and is reported to have a mortality rate of 3.3%.[79] Early anastomotic leaks, occurring within the first 3 postoperative days are nearly always the result of technical failure, whereas later leaks, occurring within 3 to 7 days after surgery, usually develop because of ischemic injury to the gastric stump or below the anastomosis. Patients with anastomotic leaks can develop fever, leukocytosis, and sepsis, and purulent fluid or frank pus may empty through the surgical drain.[31,78]

Findings on chest radiographs suggesting an anastomotic breakdown or other leak include new gas and liquid collection in the mediastinum, enlarging hydropneumothorax, or worsening lung consolidation from infection (**Fig. 20**). Esophagography with water-soluble contrast can detect, localize, and characterize leaks but can miss small leaks if proper technique is not used. CT scanning has the advantage of detecting abnormal mediastinal collections and can show fistulae. However, small leaks can be occult when the conduit is collapsed, so some investigators recommend administering a small amount of water-soluble oral contrast material immediately before scanning. Leaks can fistulize with the pleural space or central tracheobronchial tree. Tiny leaks may close spontaneously. Small leaks are typically managed conservatively with percutaneous drainage, a

conduit stent, or both. Larger leaks may require surgical repair, often with a muscular flap. Conduit strictures can form as a result of ischemic injury or infection.[31,78]

Ischemic Necrosis

Ischemic necrosis of the gastric conduit is very rare because of the rich blood supply from the

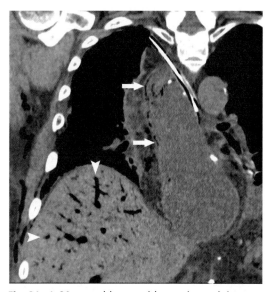

Fig. 21. A 64-year-old man with gastric conduit pneumatosis and portal venous gas from ischemic injury. Coronal reformatted, unenhanced CT image several days after esophagectomy shows gas in the conduit wall (*arrows*) and extensive portal venous gas (*arrowheads*).

right gastric and gastroepiploic arteries brought along into the chest. In addition, part of the omentum is also brought into the chest and wrapped around the anastomosis. However, severe postoperative hypotension or intraoperative injury to the blood supply can lead to ischemic necrosis of the conduit (Fig. 21). Emergent surgical repair is required with resection of the conduit, diverting esophagostomy (spit fistula), and a feeding jejunostomy. Continuity can usually be restored several months later, usually with a retrosternal colonic interposition.[78]

SUMMARY

The radiologist is an important contributor to the postoperative care of patients undergoing cardiothoracic surgery. Early identification of postoperative complications has the potential to reduce morbidity and mortality. Chest imaging can identify postsurgical complications of cardiothoracic surgery before they are clinically apparent and confirm their presence and further characterize them when they are suspected. Knowledge of the spectrum of complications following cardiothoracic surgery and of their respective imaging manifestations is essential for the radiologist to make a meaningful impact on patient care.

REFERENCES

1. Bajwa SS, Kulshrestha A. Diagnosis, prevention and management of postoperative pulmonary edema. Ann Med Health Sci Res 2012;2(2):180–5.
2. Arieff AI. Fatal postoperative pulmonary edema: pathogenesis and literature review. Chest 1999;115(5):1371–7.
3. Lohser J, Slinger P. Lung injury after one-lung ventilation: a review of the pathophysiologic mechanisms affecting the ventilated and the collapsed lung. Anesth Analg 2015;121(2):302–18.
4. O'Gara B, Talmor D. Perioperative lung protective ventilation. BMJ 2018;362:k3030.
5. Mulkey Z, Yarbrough S, Guerra D, et al. Postextubation pulmonary edema: a case series and review. Respir Med 2008;102(11):1659–62.
6. Hirleman E, Larson DF. Cardiopulmonary bypass and edema: physiology and pathophysiology. Perfusion 2008;23(6):311–22.
7. Gluecker T, Capasso P, Schnyder P, et al. Clinical and radiologic features of pulmonary edema. Radiographics 1999;19(6):1507–31 [discussion: 1532–3].
8. Turnage WS, Lunn JJ. Postpneumonectomy pulmonary edema. A retrospective analysis of associated variables. Chest 1993;103(6):1646–50.
9. de Groot PM, Shroff GS, Carter BW, et al. Lung cancer: postoperative imaging and complications. J Thorac Imaging 2017;32(5):276–87.
10. Bernard GR, Artigas A, Brigham KL, et al. The American-European Consensus Conference on ARDS. Definitions, mechanisms, relevant outcomes, and clinical trial coordination. Am J Respir Crit Care Med 1994;149(3 Pt 1):818–24.
11. Fan E, Brodie D, Slutsky AS. Acute respiratory distress syndrome: advances in diagnosis and treatment. JAMA 2018;319(7):698–710.
12. Obadina ET, Torrealba JM, Kanne JP. Acute pulmonary injury: high-resolution CT and histopathological spectrum. Br J Radiol 2013;86(1027):20120614.
13. Carcano C, Okafor N, Martinez F, et al. Radiographic manifestations of transfusion-related acute lung injury. Clin Imaging 2013;37(6):1020–3.
14. Dulu A, Pastores SM, Park B, et al. Prevalence and mortality of acute lung injury and ARDS after lung resection. Chest 2006;130(1):73–8.
15. Desai SR. Acute respiratory distress syndrome: imaging of the injured lung. Clin Radiol 2002;57(1):8–17.
16. Litle VR, Swanson SJ. Postoperative bleeding: coagulopathy, bleeding, hemothorax. Thorac Surg Clin 2006;16(3):203–7, v.
17. Vummidi DR, Chung JH, Stern E. Extrapleural fat sign. J Thorac Imaging 2012;27(5):W101.
18. Hong A, King CS, Brown AW, et al. Hemothorax following lung transplantation: incidence, risk factors, and effect on morbidity and mortality. Multidiscip Respir Med 2016;11:40.
19. Alpert JB, Godoy MC, Degroot PM, et al. Imaging the post-thoracotomy patient: anatomic changes and postoperative complications. Radiol Clin North Am 2014;52(1):85–103.
20. Rotman JA, Plodkowski AJ, Hayes SA, et al. Postoperative complications after thoracic surgery for lung cancer. Clin Imaging 2015;39(5):735–49.
21. Restrepo CS, Lemos DF, Lemos JA, et al. Imaging findings in cardiac tamponade with emphasis on CT. Radiographics 2007;27(6):1595–610.
22. Nicol AJ, Navsaria PH, Beningfield S, et al. A straight left heart border: a new radiological sign of a hemopericardium. World J Surg 2014;38(1):211–4.
23. Ohta Y, Miyoshi F, Kaminou T, et al. The evaluation of cardiac tamponade risk in patients with pericardial effusion detected by non-gated chest CT. Acta Radiol 2016;57(5):538–46.
24. Contou D, Voiriot G, Djibre M, et al. Clinical features of patients with diffuse alveolar hemorrhage due to negative-pressure pulmonary edema. Lung 2017;195(4):477–87.
25. Lichtenberger JP, Digumarthy SR, Abbott GF, et al. Diffuse pulmonary hemorrhage: clues to the diagnosis. Curr Probl Diagn Radiol 2014;43(3):128–39.

26. Alloubi I, Jougon J, Delcambre F, et al. Early complications after pneumonectomy: retrospective study of 168 patients. Interact Cardiovasc Thorac Surg 2010;11(2):162–5.

27. Algar FJ, Alvarez A, Salvatierra A, et al. Predicting pulmonary complications after pneumonectomy for lung cancer. Eur J Cardiothorac Surg 2003;23(2):201–8.

28. Díaz-Ravetllat V, Ferrer M, Gimferrer-Garolera JM, et al. Risk factors of postoperative nosocomial pneumonia after resection of bronchogenic carcinoma. Respir Med 2012;106(10):1463–71.

29. Franquet T, Giménez A, Rosón N, et al. Aspiration diseases: findings, pitfalls, and differential diagnosis. Radiographics 2000;20(3):673–85.

30. Zhou XD, Dong WH, Zhao CH, et al. Risk scores for predicting dysphagia in critically ill patients after cardiac surgery. BMC Anesthesiol 2019;19(1):7.

31. Mboumi IW, Reddy S, Lidor AO. Complications after esophagectomy. Surg Clin North Am 2019;99(3):501–10.

32. Goodman LR. Postoperative chest radiograph: II. Alterations after major intrathoracic surgery. AJR Am J Roentgenol 1980;134(4):803–13.

33. Doerr CH, Allen MS, Nichols FC, et al. Etiology of chylothorax in 203 patients. Mayo Clin Proc 2005;80(7):867–70.

34. Pool KL, Munden RF, Vaporciyan A, et al. Radiographic imaging features of thoracic complications after pneumonectomy in oncologic patients. Eur J Radiol 2012;81(1):165–72.

35. Dougenis D, Walker WS, Cameron EW, et al. Management of chylothorax complicating extensive esophageal resection. Surg Gynecol Obstet 1992;174(6):501–6.

36. Zhao Z, Zhang T, Yin X, et al. Update on the diagnosis and treatment of tracheal and bronchial injury. J Thorac Dis 2017;9(1):E50–6.

37. Paul S, Bueno R. Section VI: complications following esophagectomy: early detection, treatment, and prevention. Semin Thorac Cardiovasc Surg 2003;15(2):210–5.

38. Lim H, Kim JH, Kim D, et al. Tracheal rupture after endotracheal intubation—a report of three cases. Korean J Anesthesiol 2012;62(3):277–80.

39. Ovári A, Just T, Dommerich S, et al. Conservative management of post-intubation tracheal tears—report of three cases. J Thorac Dis 2014;6(6):E85–91.

40. Bagga B, Kumar A, Chahal A, et al. Traumatic airway injuries: role of imaging. Curr Probl Diagn Radiol 2018. [Epub ahead of print].

41. Cardinale L, Priola AM, Priola SM, et al. Radiological contribution to the diagnosis of early postoperative complications after lung resection for primary tumor: a revisional study. J Thorac Dis 2016;8(8):E643–52.

42. Lazarus DR, Casal RF. Persistent air leaks: a review with an emphasis on bronchoscopic management. J Thorac Dis 2017;9(11):4660–70.

43. Bylicki O, Vandemoortele T, Orsini B, et al. Incidence and management of anastomotic complications after bronchial resection: a retrospective study. Ann Thorac Surg 2014;98(6):1961–7.

44. Chae EJ, Seo JB, Kim SY, et al. Radiographic and CT findings of thoracic complications after pneumonectomy. Radiographics 2006;26(5):1449–68.

45. Deschamps C, Bernard A, Nichols FC, et al. Empyema and bronchopleural fistula after pneumonectomy: factors affecting incidence. Ann Thorac Surg 2001;72(1):243–7 [discussion: 248].

46. Hollaus PH, Setinek U, Lax F, et al. Risk factors for bronchopleural fistula after pneumonectomy: stump size does matter. Thorac Cardiovasc Surg 2003;51(3):162–6.

47. Cable DG, Deschamps C, Allen MS, et al. Lobar torsion after pulmonary resection: presentation and outcome. J Thorac Cardiovasc Surg 2001;122(6):1091–3.

48. Seo H, Kim TJ, Jin KN, et al. Multi-detector row computed tomographic evaluation of bronchopleural fistula: correlation with clinical, bronchoscopic, and surgical findings. J Comput Assist Tomogr 2010;34(1):13–8.

49. Mehran RJ, Deslauriers J. Late complications. Postpneumonectomy syndrome. Chest Surg Clin N Am 1999;9(3):655–73, x.

50. Shepard JA, Grillo HC, McLoud TC, et al. Right-pneumonectomy syndrome: radiologic findings and CT correlation. Radiology 1986;161(3):661–4.

51. Soll C, Hahnloser D, Frauenfelder T, et al. The postpneumonectomy syndrome: clinical presentation and treatment. Eur J Cardiothorac Surg 2009;35(2):319–24.

52. Valji AM, Maziak DE, Shamji FM, et al. Postpneumonectomy syndrome: recognition and management. Chest 1998;114(6):1766–9.

53. Shen KR, Wain JC, Wright CD, et al. Postpneumonectomy syndrome: surgical management and long-term results. J Thorac Cardiovasc Surg 2008;135(6):1210–6 [discussion: 1216–9].

54. Chaaya G, Vishnubhotla P. Pulmonary vein thrombosis: a recent systematic review. Cureus 2017;9(1):e993.

55. Ohtaka K, Hida Y, Kaga K, et al. Left upper lobectomy can be a risk factor for thrombosis in the pulmonary vein stump. J Cardiothorac Surg 2014;9:5.

56. Hassani C, Saremi F. Comprehensive cross-sectional imaging of the pulmonary veins. Radiographics 2017;37(7):1928–54.

57. Nguyen JC, Maloney J, Kanne JP. Bilateral whole-lung torsion after bilateral lung transplantation. J Thorac Imaging 2011;26(1):W17–9.

58. Childs L, Ellis S, Francies O. Pulmonary lobar torsion: a rare complication following pulmonary resection, but one not to miss. BJR Case Rep 2017;3(1): 20160010.

59. Masuda Y, Marutsuka T, Suzuki M. A risk factor for kinked middle lobar bronchus following right upper lobectomy. Asian Cardiovasc Thorac Ann 2014; 22(8):955–9.

60. Kang YR, Kim JS, Cha YK, et al. Imaging findings of complications after thoracic surgery. Jpn J Radiol 2019;37(3):209–19.

61. Mehanna MJ, Israel GM, Katigbak M, et al. Cardiac herniation after right pneumonectomy: case report and review of the literature. J Thorac Imaging 2007;22(3):280–2.

62. Ponten JE, Elenbaas TW, ter Woorst JF, et al. Cardiac herniation after operative management of lung cancer: a rare and dangerous complication. Gen Thorac Cardiovasc Surg 2012;60(10):668–72.

63. Exarhos DN, Malagari K, Tsatalou EG, et al. Acute mediastinitis: spectrum of computed tomography findings. Eur Radiol 2005;15(8):1569–74.

64. Katabathina VS, Restrepo CS, Martinez-Jimenez S, et al. Nonvascular, nontraumatic mediastinal emergencies in adults: a comprehensive review of imaging findings. Radiographics 2011;31(4):1141–60.

65. Juhl AA, Hody S, Videbaek TS, et al. Deep sternal wound infection after open-heart surgery: a 13-year single institution analysis. Ann Thorac Cardiovasc Surg 2017;23(2):76–82.

66. Filsoufi F, Castillo JG, Rahmanian PB, et al. Epidemiology of deep sternal wound infection in cardiac surgery. J Cardiothorac Vasc Anesth 2009;23(4): 488–94.

67. Cotogni P, Barbero C, Rinaldi M. Deep sternal wound infection after cardiac surgery: evidences and controversies. World J Crit Care Med 2015; 4(4):265–73.

68. Weissberg D, Refaely Y. Hernia of the lung. Ann Thorac Surg 2002;74(6):1963–6.

69. Athanassiadi K, Bagaev E, Simon A, et al. Lung herniation: a rare complication in minimally invasive cardiothoracic surgery. Eur J Cardiothorac Surg 2008;33(5):774–6.

70. Chaturvedi A, Rajiah P, Croake A, et al. Imaging of thoracic hernias: types and complications. Insights Imaging 2018;9(6):989–1005.

71. Ema T, Funai K, Kawase A, et al. Incarceration hernia of the lung after video-assisted thoracic surgery requiring emergency operation: a case report. J Thorac Dis 2018;10(7):E541–3.

72. Temes RT, Talbot WA, Green DP, et al. Herniation of the lung after video-assisted thoracic surgery. Ann Thorac Surg 2001;72(2):606–7.

73. Aguirre VJ, Sinha P, Zimmet A, et al. Phrenic nerve injury during cardiac surgery: mechanisms, management and prevention. Heart Lung Circ 2013; 22(11):895–902.

74. Jaretzki A. Injury to the phrenic and recurrent nerves needs to be avoided in the performance of thymectomy for myasthenia gravis. Ann Thorac Surg 2002; 74(2):633 [author reply: 4].

75. Hariharan D, Lobo DN. Retained surgical sponges, needles and instruments. Ann R Coll Surg Engl 2013;95(2):87–92.

76. Falkenback D, Lehane CW, Lord RV. Robot-assisted gastrectomy and oesophagectomy for cancer. ANZ J Surg 2014;84(10):712–21.

77. Nichols FC, Allen MS, Deschamps C, et al. Ivor Lewis esophagogastrectomy. Surg Clin North Am 2005;85(3):583–92.

78. Sonavane S, Watts J, Terry N, et al. Expected and unexpected imaging features after oesophageal cancer treatment. Clin Radiol 2014;69(8):e358–66.

79. Lerut T, Coosemans W, Decker G, et al. Anastomotic complications after esophagectomy. Dig Surg 2002; 19(2):92–8.

Imaging of Cardiac Support Devices

Seth Kligerman, MD*, Michael Horowitz, MD, PhD, Kathleen Jacobs, MD, Elizabeth Weihe, MD

KEYWORDS

- Intra-aortic balloon pump (IABP) • Left ventricular assist device
- Extracorporeal membrane oxygenation (ECMO) • Impella • Complications • Physiology • Normal

KEY POINTS

- Numerous technologies are available to provide cardiovascular support in the intensive care unit setting.
- Some of these devices provide temporary support, whereas others serve as a bridge to definitive therapy.
- Knowledge of their function and normal imaging appearance is necessary to recognize device complications that can be life threatening.
- Common complications with these devices include misplacement, migration, device failure, bleeding, vascular injury, stroke, and infection.

INTRODUCTION

Patients hospitalized in the intensive care unit (ICU) often have multiple support lines and devices that need routine imaging evaluation by radiologists. In patients with cardiogenic shock or depressed cardiac function, mechanical circulation support devices are often used in combination with medical therapies to improve patient outcomes and sometimes can stabilize patients for subsequent surgical intervention. This review discusses some of the more commonly encountered mechanical circulation devices seen in ICU patients and reviews both proper placement and commonly encountered device-related complications that can be diagnosed on imaging.

INTRA-AORTIC BALLOON PUMP
Configurations and Physiology

The intra-aortic balloon pump (IABP) is a temporary mechanical circulatory support device used to augment coronary artery perfusion and reduce myocardial oxygen demand. First introduced in the late 1960s to treat cardiogenic shock, the IABP remains the most commonly used mechanical circulatory support device in the United States for acute myocardial infarction (MI), cardiogenic shock, various forms of cardiomyopathy, and in the perioperative cardiac surgery setting.[1] The balloon, typically 20 to 25 cm in length, is mounted on a catheter and connected via external driveline to a control unit. The balloon inflates with helium during diastole, thus displacing blood and increasing arterial pressure in the ascending aorta to yield increased coronary perfusion pressure. Deflation in early systole decreases afterload and slightly reduces myocardial demand.[2,3] The IABP can be placed by either femoral or axillary approach.[4]

IABP use is contraindicated in patients with severe aortic regurgitation, as counterpulsation would significantly worsen regurgitant flow, and severe tachyarrhythmia may reduce IABP effect both by hindering timing of inflation/deflation and decreasing coronary filling time in diastole.[2] Other

Disclosure Statement: The authors have nothing to disclose.
Cardiothoracic Radiology, University of California, San Diego, 9500 Gilman Drive, La Jolla, CA 92093, USA
* Corresponding author.
E-mail address: skligerman@ucsd.edu

contraindications include aortic dissection, severe peripheral vascular disease that prevents safe access, uncontrolled septicemia, and severe bleeding diathesis.[5]

Normal Appearance

On frontal chest radiograph (CXR; **Fig. 1**), the IABP can be most readily identified by an approximately 4-mm linear metallic marker on each end of the balloon, although depending on the field of view, the lower marker may not be seen. For a femoral-approach IABP, the upper marker of the balloon should be located along the inferior aspect of the aortic arch or approximately 2 cm above the carina.[6,7] If seen, the inferior marker typically projects over the T12 or L1 vertebral body. If the CXR is obtained in diastole, the balloon itself may appear as a tubular lucency projecting over the descending aorta (see **Fig. 1**). An axillary-approach IABP may be identified by the associated axillary sheath; positioning of the upper marker should be similar to femoral-approach devices.

On nongated computed tomography (CT), the metallic markers will be evident, and the balloon will typically appear as a linear or gas-filled structure depending on the cardiac cycle. With electrocardiogram (ECG)-gating, the balloon will be more clearly cylindrical, and the process of inflation and deflation may be observed through different phases of the cardiac cycle (**Fig. 2**).

Complications

The most common complication is malposition of the IABP, which may occur in up to 50% of patients.[4] High balloon malposition (**Fig. 3**) may result in cycle-dependent occlusion of the arch vessels with extremity or cerebral diastolic hypoperfusion, whereas low balloon malposition (**Fig. 4**) yields less efficient counterpulsation and may result in occlusion of the renal arteries, celiac, and mesenteric axes with distal organ diastolic hypoperfusion.[1] Dissection is another possible complication of IABP placement and may occur in the aorta or anywhere else along the course of femoral or axillary catheter placement.[8] Other complications include bleeding at the site of placement, distal embolic events, and limb ischemia.[4] Balloon rupture can occur but cannot be diagnosed on radiograph.[9]

IMPELLA
Configurations and Physiology

The Impella (Abiomed Inc., Danvers, MA) device is a newer percutaneous LVAD used to augment cardiac output and reduce myocardial workload in patients with advanced heart failure and/or cardiogenic shock. It has been shown to provide improved hemodynamic support compared with the IABP[10] and is endorsed in certain settings by both European and American guidelines.[11]

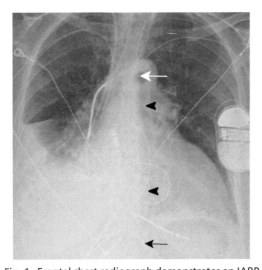

Fig. 1. Frontal chest radiograph demonstrates an IABP in appropriate position with the upper metallic marker (*white arrow*, obliquely imaged) projecting approximately 2 cm above the carina. The lower marker (*black arrow*) projects over the left superior aspect of the L1 vertebral body. The patient was imaged in diastole as evident by the inflated balloon (between *arrowheads*).

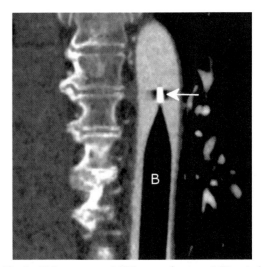

Fig. 2. Oblique coronal CT images from an ECG-gated cardiac CT angiogram (CTA) shows inflation of the balloon (B) during diastole. The superior metallic marker (*white arrow*) is in the mid-descending thoracic aorta, which is too low.

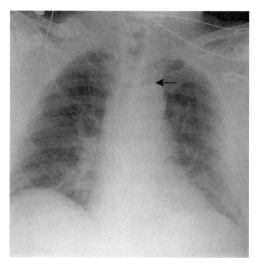

Fig. 3. High malposition of an IABP in a 44-year-old man status post-MI shows the metallic superior marker in the left subclavian artery (*black arrow*).

Meta-analysis of clinical trials has demonstrated mortality benefit in early invention and thus the Impella is often placed before percutaneous coronary intervention (PCI) in acute MI with cardiogenic shock and in high-risk elective PCI procedures.[12,13]

Impella variants exist for both left and right ventricular support, including multiple models for left ventricular (LV) support (**Table 1**).[14] The LV Impella design incorporates a catheter housing an axial

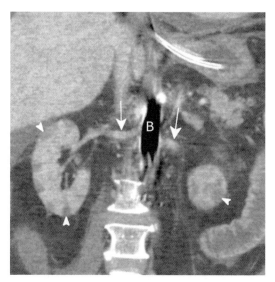

Fig. 4. Oblique coronal CT of the abdomen and pelvis during diastole shows low position of the IABP, with the inflated balloon (B) crossing the renal artery ostia bilaterally (*white arrows*) with multiple renal infarcts (*white arrowheads*).

pump and outlet area at its proximal end and a distal inlet area connected to a thin pigtail providing stabilization for positioning across the aortic valve into the LV.[2,15] The rotational pump delivers nonpulsatile flow and, unlike the IABP, the Impella provides stable hemodynamic support regardless of cardiac rhythm. The Impella is approved by the Food and Drug Administration for 6 hours of use but is often used in off-label applications for days to weeks where it can provide support in the acute setting or serve as a bridge to ventricular assist device (VAD) placement or heart transplantation.[16,17] Contraindications include mechanical aortic valve, severe aortic stenosis, ventricular septal defect, and severe peripheral arterial disease.[2]

Normal Appearance

Impella devices have a distinctive appearance and are easy to recognize on chest radiograph and CT (**Fig. 5**). The metallic pump and inlet/outlet areas are densely radiopaque, and the catheter housing/tip are usually readily apparent. The much more rarely encountered Impella LD lacks the pigtail associated with the other devices and takes a distinct, direct transaortic course. Radiographic evaluation should focus on proper transaortic valve placement with the inlet area and pigtail projecting over the LV contour and the outlet area projecting over the proximal ascending aorta near the aortic root in LV devices. In the right ventricular (RV) Impella device, the inlet area should project over the inferior vena cava and the outlet area over the main pulmonary artery (**Fig. 6**). Evaluation as for any potential complications is also crucial.

Complications

Reported complications associated with the Impella device include device failure (10%–20%), device migration (20%), hemolysis (5%–10%), and bleeding either during or after implantation (5%–10%).[18,19] LV Impella malpositioning may occur either too proximal or distal (**Fig. 7**). Rare complications include aortic valve injury, cardiac tamponade, and acute mitral regurgitation.[20–22] Acute vascular complications including limb ischemia, hematoma, and/or pseudoaneurysm at the site of insertion occur in approximately 15% to 20% of cases.[13]

EXTRACORPOREAL MEMBRANE OXYGENATION
Configurations and Physiology

Extracorporeal membrane oxygenation (ECMO) provides cardiopulmonary support in cases of

Table 1
Types of Impella devices

	Impella 2.5	Impella CP	Impella 5.0	Impella LD	Impella RP
Ventricle	Left	Left	Left	Left	Right
Motor size	12 F	14 F	21 F	21 F	22 F
Insertion	Femoral or axillary artery, percutaneous	Femoral or axillary, percutaneous	Femoral or axillary artery cutdown	Surgical placement into aorta	Femoral vein
Maximum blood flow	2.5 L/min	4.0 L/min	5.0 L/min	5.0 L/min	4.6 L/min

potentially reversible acute respiratory and/or cardiac failure. Venous blood is pumped through an extracorporeal oxygenator that saturates hemoglobin with oxygen and removes carbon dioxide before returning blood to circulation.

There are 2 main configurations of ECMO: venovenous-ECMO (VV-ECMO) and venoarterial-ECMO (VA-ECMO). In VV-ECMO, a single-cannulation or double-cannulation approach may be used. Single-cannulation technique uses a dual-lumen cannula (Avalon Elite; Avalon Laboratories, Rancho Dominguez, CA), which drains venous blood through outer lumen fenestrations in the superior vena cava and inferior vena cava (IVC), and then returns oxygenated blood through a second lumen with a port in the right atrium[23]

(Fig. 8). Double-cannulation technique involves placement of 2 separate cannulas, one via the common femoral vein for drainage and the other via the internal jugular vein or femoral vein for infusion (Fig. 9). In VA-ECMO, a cannula drains venous blood from the vena cava or right atrium and oxygenated blood returns to arterial circulation through the femoral, axillary, or carotid artery in a so-called peripheral ECMO circuit (Fig. 10), or through the aorta in a central ECMO circuit.[24]

Both VV-ECMO and VA-ECMO provide respiratory support by supplementing oxygenation, but a

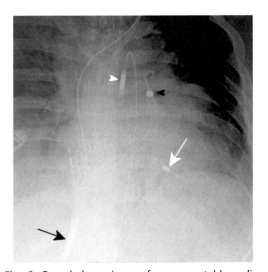

Fig. 6. Coned down image from a portable radiograph shows a right femoral vein approach right ventricular percutaneous assist device and left femoral artery approach left ventricular percutaneous assist device in appropriate position. The right ventricular percutaneous assist device inlet area (*black arrow*) and outlet area (*black arrowhead*) project over the upper IVC and main pulmonary artery, respectively. The left ventricular percutaneous assist device inlet area (*white arrow*) and outlet area (*white arrowhead*) project over the left ventricle and proximal ascending aorta, respectively.

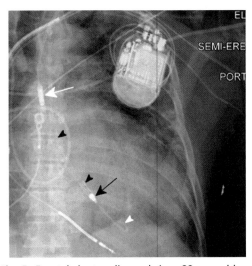

Fig. 5. Frontal chest radiograph in a 38-year-old patient with an axillary-approach percutaneous LVAD in appropriate position with the inlet area (*black arrow*) and pigtail (*white arrowhead*) projecting over the LV and outlet area/pump (*white arrow*) projecting near the aortic root. The catheter housing can be seen between the 2 metallic portions (*black arrowheads*).

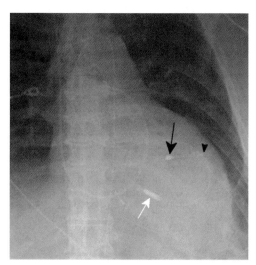

Fig. 7. Frontal chest radiograph demonstrates a distally malpositioned femoral-approach LV percutaneous LVAD with the pigtail tip (*arrowhead*), inlet (*black arrow*) (i) and outlet pump (o/p) (*white arrow*) all projecting over the left ventricle. (*Case courtesy of Dr Travis Henry, UCSF, San Francisco, CA.*)

key distinction is that only VA-ECMO provides hemodynamic support. VA-ECMO bypasses the pulmonary circulation allowing for decreased pulmonary artery pressures and decreased LV

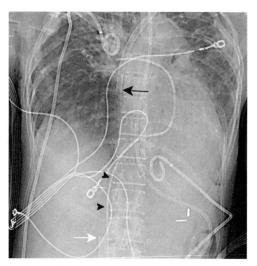

Fig. 9. Double-cannula VV-ECMO in a 50-year-old woman with pleuroparenchymal fibroelastosis and acute respiratory failure. Frontal chest radiograph demonstrates double-cannulation technique with a left transjugular approach venous cannula terminating near the superior cavoatrial junction (*black arrow*) and a left femoral-approach venous cannula terminating in the IVC (*white arrow*). A femoral-approach pulmonary artery catheter follows the same course as the femoral venous cannula (*arrowheads*).

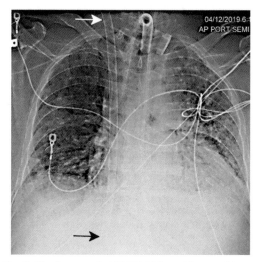

Fig. 8. Single cannula VV-ECMO in a 40-year-old man with ARDS secondary to influenza. Frontal chest radiograph demonstrates right transjugular approach single-cannulation technique with a dual-lumen VV-ECMO cannula (Avalon). The catheter is placed into the right internal jugular vein (*white arrow*) and its tip is in the IVC (*black arrow*). Concurrent transesophageal echocardiogram was performed to confirm jet from the right atrial port oriented toward the tricuspid valve.

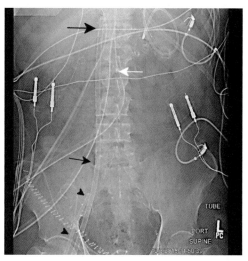

Fig. 10. Peripheral VA-ECMO in a 64-year-old man with ischemic cardiomyopathy status post heart transplantation complicated by cardiogenic and septic shock. Right femoral-approach venous cannula terminates in the abdominal IVC (*black arrows*) and right femoral-approach arterial cannula terminates in the right common iliac vein (*arrowheads*). Note the arterial cannula is positioned lateral to the venous cannula, as expected for correct arterial placement. The inferior metallic marker from an IABP can be seen at the L1-L2 disc interspace (*white arrow*), which is slightly low.

preload, thereby decompressing the LV. Direct arterial blood return also increases systemic pressures, improves end-organ perfusion, and maintains a higher Pao_2 compared with VV-ECMO.[25] Given the different physiology of VV-ECMO versus VA-ECMO, their indications also differ. VA-ECMO is used in the setting of acute cardiogenic shock when low cardiac output and hypotension are refractory to volume resuscitation, vasopressors, inotropic supplementation, or IABP. VA-ECMO also may be used post cardiothoracic surgery in patients unable to be weaned from cardiopulmonary bypass or as a bridge to heart transplantation.[25] However, ECMO is often transitioned to a VAD before heart transplantation as a direct ECMO bridge to transplant is associated with poor 1-year and 5-year posttransplant outcomes.[26]

Either VV-ECMO or VA-ECMO can be used for respiratory support to provide rescue therapy in acute respiratory failure or as a bridge to lung transplantation, although VV-ECMO may be preferred if cardiovascular support is not needed, as it avoids the complications of arterial cannulation. ECMO in the management of acute respiratory distress syndrome (ARDS) provides a significant survival benefit.[27] ECMO allows for "lung rest" and facilitates lung-protective ventilation strategies including decreased tidal volumes and Fio_2 to decrease ventilator-associated injury and oxygen toxicity.[28]

Imaging

Chest and abdominal radiographs are obtained to confirm and monitor cannula placement. Single-cannulation VV-ECMO cannula is placed via an internal jugular approach with distal tip in the IVC above the hepatic veins, outflow port oriented toward the tricuspid valve[29] (see **Fig. 8**). In the double-cannulation VV-ECMO technique, the inflow cannula is placed in the IVC near the inferior cavoatrial junction from a femoral approach and the outflow cannula is positioned in the right atrium near the superior cavoatrial junction from either a femoral or internal jugular approach[30] (see **Fig. 9**).

In central VA-ECMO, the inflow cannula should be positioned in the right atrium and outflow cannula in the ascending aorta. In peripheral VA-ECMO, the inflow cannula tip is again placed in the IVC or right atrium from a femoral approach (internal jugular approach less common), but the arterial cannula is placed via the femoral artery into the common iliac artery (see **Fig. 10**). A distal perfusion catheter connected to the ECMO arterial outflow may be placed at the site of arterial

access. This will appear as a smaller caliber catheter near the arterial ECMO cannula with tip oriented in the opposite direction, retrograde in the femoral or axillary artery.[31]

CT is helpful in the evaluation of patients with ECMO. However, altered hemodynamics in VA-ECMO circulation poses a challenge during contrast-enhanced CT. In full VA-ECMO, there is complete cardiopulmonary bypass with an empty LV and closed aortic valve. Contrast injected peripherally would be drawn into the venous cannula, circulate through the ECMO circuit, then infuse into the arterial cannula. Any contrast opacification of the aorta in this case is a result of retrograde flow from pressure of blood returning from the arterial ECMO cannula, with contrast mixing or layering in the aortic lumen (**Fig. 11**). Mixing artifact and contrast layering can be misinterpreted as an aortic dissection and/or thrombus.[32] A delayed phase of imaging can often provide more homogeneous vascular opacification.

For optimal opacification of the pulmonary arteries, left heart, and aorta, the patient should be on partial VA-ECMO with reduced flow rates.[31–34] As only a fraction of contrast enters the pulmonary circulation and patients on VA-ECMO have reduced cardiac output, contrast will be slow to opacify the pulmonary arteries and aorta. A delayed phase may be obtained in addition to an arterial phase to permit more time for contrast mixing and circulation.[32] Central venous catheter injection or direct injection through the venous or arterial cannula is preferred.[32,34] Temporary cessation of ECMO during injection and CT acquisition also may be considered if the patient is deemed able to tolerate this.

Complications

Due to systemic anticoagulation therapy, platelet dysfunction, and mechanical hemolysis associated with ECMO, the most frequent complication of ECMO is hemorrhage, occurring in 30% to 40% of patients, including bleeding at the cannulation site, pulmonary hemorrhage, intra-abdominal hemorrhage, mediastinal hematoma, hemothorax, and intracranial hemorrhage.[35,36]

Vascular complications occur less frequently, but are the most important cause of patient mortality.[37] Vascular complications related to cannulation/decannulation are more common with VA-ECMO and include vascular perforation, arterial dissection (see **Fig. 11**) or pseudoaneurysm, distal limb ischemia, and arteriovenous fistula[24] (**Fig. 12**). Ischemia is a well-known potential complication of peripheral VA-ECMO, reported in 10% to 70% of VA-ECMO patients.[38] Oxygenated blood

A

B

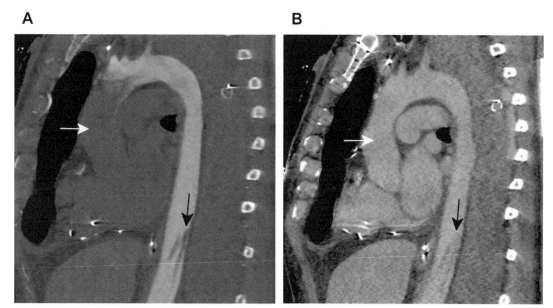

Fig. 11. Dissection and mixing artifact on VA-ECMO. (*A*) Candy-cane image of the aorta during systemic arterial phase shows homogeneous high-contrast opacification of the descending thoracic aorta but no contrast in the ascending aorta (*white arrow*) cardiac chambers. (*B*) A 90-second delay candy-cane image shows more homogeneous opacification of the cardiovascular system (*white arrow*). An iatrogenic aortic dissection is present in the descending thoracic aorta (*black arrows, A, B*) due to VA-ECMO cannulation.

preferentially perfuses organs distal to the arterial cannulation site, but relatively deoxygenated blood from the heart perfuses the myocardium, brain, and upper extremities, placing these organs

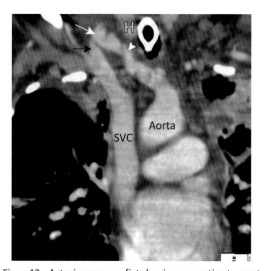

Fig. 12. Arteriovenous fistula in a patient post double-cannula VV-ECMO for ARDS. Coronal contrast-enhanced CT following ECMO decannulation shows a communication between the right internal jugular vein (*black arrow*) and right brachiocephalic artery (*white arrowhead*) compatible with arteriovenous fistula (*white arrow*).

at risk for ischemia. ECMO patients, especially those on VA-ECMO, are also at a significantly increased risk for pulmonary arterial, systemic arterial (**Fig. 13**), and systemic venous thrombus formation including secondary to blood stasis in the setting of low cardiac output, thrombogenic exposure to synthetic surfaces of the ECMO circuit, and chronic endothelial injury.[39] Additional common ECMO complications include infection and acute renal injury.[35]

Although cannula positioning is usually confirmed during fluoroscopic and/or echocardiogram-guided placement, radiologists should monitor for cannula malpositioning, migration, and kinking on ICU CXRs. For instance, a venous cannula placed too low in the IVC can occlude the hepatic veins, resulting in hepatic venous obstruction[40] (**Fig. 14**). Arterial cannula placed too peripherally in the femoral artery increases risk of coronary, cerebral, and distal limb ischemia.[41]

VENTRICULAR ASSIST DEVICES
Configurations and Physiology

Heart transplantation is the gold standard for patients with chronic LV failure. Although the number of transplants performed in the United States continues to increase, limited organ availability often leads to wait times for heart transplants of more than 6 months.[42] In addition, many patients are

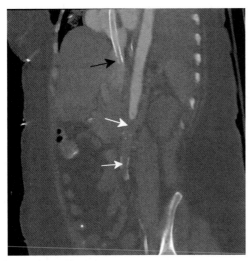

Fig. 13. Aortic thrombosis in a 47-year-old woman with ARDS. Coronal oblique multiplanar reconstruction shows the VV-ECMO cannula in the IVC (*black arrow*). There is abrupt thrombosis of the abdominal aorta (*white arrows*) at the level of the renal arteries without distal opacification.

not eligible for a heart transplant because of various comorbidities.[42,43] In decades past, patients on the transplant wait list or those not eligible to receive a heart transplant were treated with optimized medical therapy alone. In the past 20 years, the widespread development of

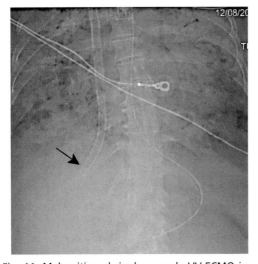

Fig. 14. Malpositioned single cannula VV-ECMO in a 49-year-old woman with ARDS secondary to influenza. Frontal radiograph shows a right transjugular approach venous cannula curving toward the liver at the level of the hepatic veins/hepatic IVC (*black arrow*). Ultrasound confirmed the ECMO catheter was in the middle hepatic vein.

surgically inserted pumps, or VADs, have been shown to reduce mortality compared with optimized medical therapy alone as well as improve quality of life.[44–46] These VADs are implanted for 2 primary reasons: as a bridge to cardiac transplant and as a destination therapy for those not eligible for cardiac transplant.[43,46] A third less common indication is to serve as a bridge to recovery in a select subset of younger patients who develop a nonischemic cardiomyopathy due to acute myocardial injury such as myocarditis or postpartum cardiomyopathy.[47–49] In most instances, VADs are placed into the LV to provide LV support (LVAD) or into both the LV and right atrium to provide biventricular support (BiVAD).

Although there are numerous types of LVADs in commercial use, most share 4 similar mechanical components: (1) inflow cannula that is surgically tunneled into the left ventricular apex; (2) outflow cannula that is anastomosed to the ascending aorta; (3) pump that is, positioned between and connects to both the inflow and outflow cannulas, pulling blood from the LV and pumping it into the ascending aorta; and (4) drive line that connects to the pump, exits through the skin surface, and connects to an external belt controller and battery pack.

Normal Appearance

The normal appearance of an LVAD on radiography depends on the type of device and only certain devices are reviewed. Although the inflow mechanism and pumps differ among the devices, all have an outflow cannula that is anastomosed to the aorta and a drive line that extends inferior over the abdomen. The outflow cannula is nearly invisible on CXR except for the proximal portion near the pump that is surrounded by reinforcing material such as Dacron or Gore-Tex (**Figs. 15–18**).[49]

First generation LVADs will not be discussed as they are rarely seen in clinical practice today. Second generation LVADs include the HeartMate II and Jarvik 200. The HeartMate II (see **Fig. 15**) device has an inflow cannula that is inserted into the LV apex. There are 2 bend reliefs that allow for some flexibility in the system. The inflow bend relief is positioned between the pump and the inflow cannula and is seen as a radiolucent region. The outflow bend relief is positioned between the pump and outflow cannula and is attached to the pump, and on the HeartMate II is connected via a snap ring. One should make sure to inspect the orientations of both bend reliefs to ensure that they are properly connected. For the HeartMate II, a pocket is surgically

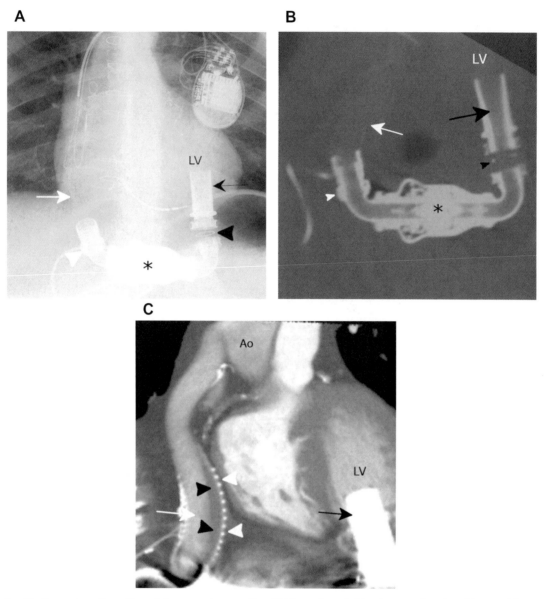

Fig. 15. Normal configuration of the second generation LVAD used as a bridge to transplant in a 44-year-old man with an ischemic cardiomyopathy. Coned down views from posteroanterior radiograph (*A*) and representative coronal oblique multiplanar reconstruction from a CT (*B*) show that the inflow cannula (*black arrows*), which is placed into the LV, is connected to the pump (*asterisk*) via a radiolucent inflow bend relief (*black arrowheads*). The outflow cannula (*white arrows*) is connected to the pump via the outflow bend relief via a snap ring (*white arrowheads*) and is surrounded by Gore-Tex, which allows for it to be partially visualized on CXR. The alignment of the LVAD should be closely evaluated in each patient undergoing radiograph or CT. CT using a soft tissue window (*C*) shows the normal appearance of the inflow (*black arrow*) and outflow (*white arrow*) cannulas, which anastomose with the LV and ascending aorta (Ao), respectively. In-between the cannula and the mesh (*white arrowheads*), it is common to see a thin layer of low-density fluid of soft tissue attenuation material (*black arrowheads*), which is thought to represent blood or other fluid that collects in-between the layers. This should not be mistaken for thrombus.

created in the lower thorax/superior abdomen to house in pump. This can be a site of infection as discussed later in this article.

The Jarvik 2000 (see **Fig. 16**) unlike other LVADs, has the cylindrical pump directly inserted

into the LV and does not have an inflow cannula.[50] On radiograph and CT, the Jarvik appears as a cylindrical device within the LV.

Third generation devices including the Heart-Mate III (see **Fig. 17**) and HeartWare HVAD (see

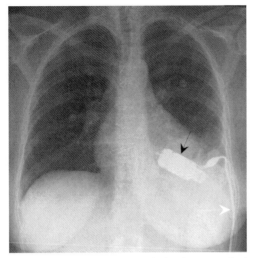

Fig. 16. Normal appearance of the interventricular second generation LVAD in a 47-year-old woman with an ischemic cardiomyopathy. Frontal radiograph shows the small size of the interventricular second generation LVAD. Unlike other devices, the pump of this LVAD is inserted directly into the LV cavity (*black arrow*). The driveline (*white arrow*), which provides power to the device via an external battery, is connected to the pump and courses through the subcutaneous tissues before exiting the skin.

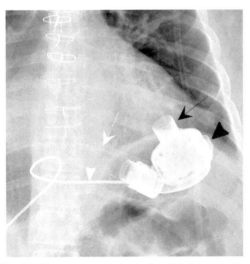

Fig. 17. Normal appearance of a third generation LVAD in a 32-year-old man with a nonischemic dilated cardiomyopathy. Coned down posteroanterior radiograph shows the normal appearance of the LVAD with the inflow cannula seated in the LV (*black arrow*) and the pump (*black arrowhead*) with the adjacent pericardium. The portion of the outflow cannula surrounded by Gore-Tex can be seen (*white arrow*). The driveline is also visualized (*white arrowhead*).

Fig. 18) have the inflow cannula directly connected to the centrifugal pump, which is positioned near the LV apex. In the setting of a BiVAD, the second VAD device is inserted into the right atrium and the outflow cannula anastomoses with the main pulmonary artery (see Fig. 18).

CT allows for more detailed evaluation of device positioning and potential complications, and cardiac gating should be considered if the primary indication for the study is LVAD evaluation. On CT, the inflow cannula should be directed posteriorly toward the mitral valve. The outflow cannula can have bends but should not be kinked.

On CT, it is important to recognize that smooth fluid or soft tissue attenuation is commonly seen along the course of the outflow cannula (see Fig. 15). This low attenuation is thought to represent blood between the protective Gore-Tex material and the wall of the outflow graft. This should not be mistaken for thrombus, although the differentiation is not always easy.

Complications

LVAD complications can occur in both the acute and delayed setting, and LVAD dysfunction is not an uncommon indication for CT. Complications are numerous and include bleeding, malposition or hardware failure, thrombus, stroke, infection, and right heart failure.

Bleeding is a common complication after LVAD placement and can occur either around or distant to the surgical site.[51] Chest CT is used to assess for and possibly localize the site of bleeding in the thorax with common sites including the LV apex and aortic anastomosis.[52] The volume of blood can be quite large leading to cardiac tamponade (Fig. 19).[49]

Gastrointestinal bleeding is also common after LVAD placement. Most of these bleeds occur in the upper gastrointestinal tract and are secondary to use of systemic anticoagulation, activation of the fibrinolytic pathway, acquired von Willebrand factor deficiency, and development of small intestinal angiodysplasias due to increased rotary speed of the pump.[53] Imaging is not routinely used for this complication.

LVAD malposition can be an immediate or delayed complication. The inflow cannula should be positioned pointing posteriorly toward the mitral valve and greater than 7° of angulation off this axis can predispose patients to adverse events.[54] If the LVAD is directed toward or contacts the septum, complications such as low-

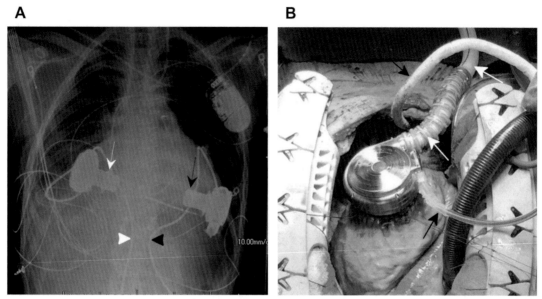

Fig. 18. (*A, B*) Third generation LVADs used for biventricular support (BiVAD) in a 28-year-old man with a non-ischemic cardiomyopathy. (*A*) Frontal radiograph shows 2 assist devices. The left-sided device (*black arrow*) is within the LV and the right-sided device is within the right atrium (*white arrow*). Their respective drivelines are seen (*black* and *white arrowheads*). The third generation LVADs have similar appearances on imaging. (*B*) Surgical image during third generation LVAD placement shows the pump (*black arrowhead*) inserted into the LV apex with the driveline (*black arrows*) and outflow cannula (*white arrows*) emanating from the pump.

flow states, thrombus formation, occlusion, and wall injury can occur (**Fig. 20**).[49,55]

Pronounced bending or kinking in the regions of the bend reliefs of cannula anastomotic sites can lead to complications, such as slow flow or thrombosis. In some instances, the snap ring, which connects the

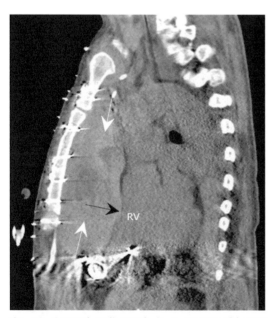

Fig. 19. Coronal radiograph in a 57-year-old man 1 day after LVAD placement shows a large mediastinal hematoma (*white arrows*) leading to compression (*black arrow*) of the RV and tamponade physiology.

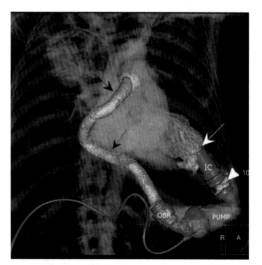

Fig. 20. Malposition of a second generation LVAD inflow catheter in a 60-year-old man with a nonischemic cardiomyopathy. Volume-rendered image from a CTA shows the inflow cannula (IC) is positioned superiorly toward the anterior wall and a portion of the catheter has dislodges from the apex (*white arrow*). The inflow bend relief (*white arrowhead*), pump, outflow bend relief (OBR), and outflow cannula (*black arrows*) are nicely seen on this reformat.

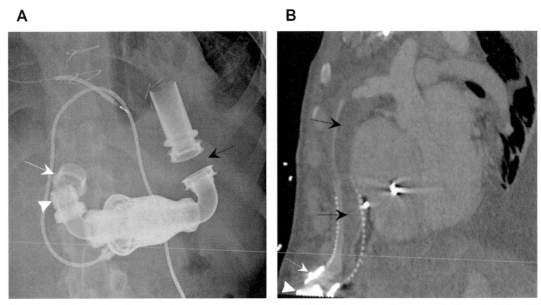

Fig. 21. Partial snap ring disconnection in a second generation LVAD leading to outflow cannula thrombosis in a 39-year-old man with a nonischemic cardiomyopathy. (*A*) Coned down views from posteroanterior radiograph show the normal alignment of the IC and pump (*black arrow*). However, there is marked abnormal angulation of the outflow cannula (*white arrow*) in relation to the outflow portion of the pump (*white arrowhead*) due to partial disconnection of the snap ring. (*B*) Sagittal oblique reformats shows near complete disconnection of the snap ring (*white arrow*) in relation to the outflow portion of the pump (*white arrowhead*), which can be visualized only on the inferior aspect of the study. The outflow cannula has nearly completely thrombosed (*black arrows*), which required repeat surgery.

outflow bend relief to the pump, can become partially or completely disconnected.[52] On radiograph and CT, one can see abnormal malalignment or discontinuity at the level of the snap ring (**Fig. 21**).

In a patient with an LVAD, thrombus can occur in the LVAD system (see **Fig. 21**; **Fig. 22**), dilated LV, or aortic root.[55] Thrombus can lead to pump dysfunction and may embolize to the systemic circulation. Contrast-enhanced chest CT is an excellent tool for the assessment of thrombus in nearly all locations in the thorax except for the extremely radiodense pump itself. A portal venous phase of imaging could be used to further help delineate thrombus from surrounding structures.

Embolic and hemorrhagic strokes are devastating complications of LVAD therapy with an incidence ranging from 12.1% to 28.7%.[56] Both are a common cause of mortality and may prevent the patient from the receiving a transplant.[56,57]

Infection is a common complication of LVAD placement and has been divided into 3 categories by the International Society of Heart and Lung Transplantation: VAD-specific infections, VAD-related infections, and non-VAD infections[58] (**Table 2**). VAD-specific infection includes infections of the pump and/or cannula, infection

of the pocket where the pump is located, or infection of the driveline that courses from the pump through the subcutaneous tissues and exits the skin surface. The rate of LVAD infection

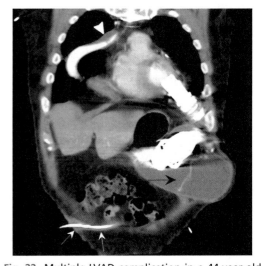

Fig. 22. Multiple LVAD complication in a 44-year-old woman with a second generation LVAD. Coronal oblique image from a CT shows fat-stranding around the driveline (*white arrows*) due to *Escherichia coli* infection as well as a large pocket abscess (*black arrow*). In addition, thrombus formation can be seen in the outflow cannula (*white arrowhead*).

Table 2
Classification of infections in patients with a ventricular assist device (VAD)

VAD-Specific Infections	VAD-Related Infections	Non-VAD Infections
Pump infection	Infective endocarditis	Lower respiratory tract infection
Cannula infection	Sternal wound infection	Cholecystitis
Pocket infection	Mediastinitis	*Clostridium difficile* infection
Drive line infection–superficial	Bloodstream infections (thought to be due to VAD)	Urinary tract infection
Drive line infection–deep		Bloodstream infections (thought to be not due to VAD)

varies with a prevalence that ranges from 14% to 80%.[49,52] Percutaneous driveline infections are the most common infection and can be isolated or denote deeper infection along the driveline, pocket, or hardware.[58]

Contrast-enhanced CT is the primary tool for assessment of infection with imaging manifestations that range from fat-stranding around the driveline to rim-enhancing abscess formation around component of the LVAD (see **Fig. 22**; **Fig. 23**). The presence or development of gas of fluid around LVAD components weeks after surgery should raise concern for infection.

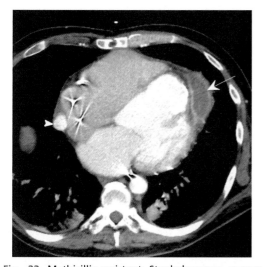

Fig. 23. Methicillin-resistant Staphylococcus aureus (MRSA) abscess formation in a 51-year-old man 1 month following LVAD implantation. Repeat CT shows a pericardial abscess (*white arrow*). The outflow cannula of the LVAD can be partially visualized (*white arrowhead*). MRSA was cultured from the driveline.

SUMMARY

Cardiovascular support devices, including the IABP, Impella, ECMO, and VAD are commonly encountered in the ICU setting. Knowledge of their configuration and function allows for one not only to recognize their normal appearance on imaging but also allow for accurate and rapid diagnosis when complications occur.

REFERENCES

1. de Waha S, Desch S, Eitel I, et al. Intra-aortic balloon counterpulsation—basic principles and clinical evidence. Vascul Pharmacol 2014;60(2): 52–6.
2. Ergle K, Parto P, Krim SR. Percutaneous ventricular assist devices: a novel approach in the management of patients with acute cardiogenic shock. Ochsner J 2016;16(3):243–9.
3. Dahlslett T, Karlsen S, Grenne B, et al. Intra-aortic balloon pump optimizes myocardial function during cardiogenic shock. JACC Cardiovasc Imaging 2018;11(3):512–4.
4. Estep JD, Cordero-Reyes AM, Bhimaraj A, et al. Percutaneous placement of an intra-aortic balloon pump in the left axillary/subclavian position provides safe, ambulatory long-term support as bridge to heart transplantation. JACC Heart Fail 2013;1(5): 382–8.
5. Trost JC, Hillis LD. Intra-aortic balloon counterpulsation. Am J Cardiol 2006;97(9):1391–8.
6. Kim JT, Lee JR, Kim JK, et al. The carina as a useful radiographic landmark for positioning the intraaortic balloon pump. Anesth Analg 2007;105(3):735–8.
7. Godoy MC, Leitman BS, de Groot PM, et al. Chest radiography in the ICU: part 2, evaluation of cardiovascular lines and other devices. AJR Am J Roentgenol 2012;198(3):572–81.
8. Trabattoni P, Zoli S, Dainese L, et al. Aortic dissection complicating intraaortic balloon pumping:

percutaneous management of delayed spinal cord ischemia. Ann Thorac Surg 2009;88(6):e60–2.

9. Bhamidipaty M, Mees B, Wagner T. Management of intra-aortic balloon pump rupture and entrapment. Aorta (Stamford) 2016;4(2):61–3.

10. Meyns B, Dens J, Sergeant P, et al. Initial experiences with the Impella device in patients with cardiogenic shock - Impella support for cardiogenic shock. Thorac Cardiovasc Surg 2003;51(6):312–7.

11. Ouweneel DM, Eriksen E, Sjauw KD, et al. Percutaneous mechanical circulatory support versus intra-aortic balloon pump in cardiogenic shock after acute myocardial infarction. J Am Coll Cardiol 2017;69(3):278–87.

12. Flaherty MP, Khan AR, O'Neill WW. Early Initiation of Impella in acute myocardial infarction complicated by cardiogenic shock improves survival: a meta-analysis. JACC Cardiovasc Interv 2017;10(17): 1805–6.

13. Abaunza M, Kabbani LS, Nypaver T, et al. Incidence and prognosis of vascular complications after percutaneous placement of left ventricular assist device. J Vasc Surg 2015;62(2):417–23.

14. Burzotta F, Trani C, Doshi SN, et al. Impella ventricular support in clinical practice: collaborative viewpoint from a European expert user group. Int J Cardiol 2015;201:684–91.

15. Miller PE, Solomon MA, McAreavey D. Advanced percutaneous mechanical circulatory support devices for cardiogenic shock. Crit Care Med 2017; 45(11):1922–9.

16. Griffith BP, Anderson MB, Samuels LE, et al. The RECOVER I: a multicenter prospective study of Impella 5.0/LD for postcardiotomy circulatory support. J Thorac Cardiovasc Surg 2013;145(2):548–54.

17. Higgins J, Lamarche Y, Kaan A, et al. Microaxial devices for ventricular failure: a multicentre, population-based experience. Can J Cardiol 2011;27(6):725–30.

18. Gaudard P, Mourad M, Eliet J, et al. Management and outcome of patients supported with Impella 5.0 for refractory cardiogenic shock. Crit Care 2015;19:363.

19. Lemaire A, Anderson MB, Lee LY, et al. The Impella device for acute mechanical circulatory support in patients in cardiogenic shock. Ann Thorac Surg 2014;97(1):133–8.

20. Hong E, Naseem T. Color doppler artifact masking iatrogenic aortic valve injury related to an Impella device. J Cardiothorac Vasc Anesth 2019;33(6): 1584–7.

21. Elhussein TA, Hutchison SJ. Acute mitral regurgitation: unforeseen new complication of the Impella LP 5.0 ventricular assist device and review of literature. Heart Lung Circ 2014;23(3):e100–4.

22. Lauten A, Engstrom AE, Jung C, et al. Percutaneous left-ventricular support with the Impella-2.5-assist device in acute cardiogenic shock: results of the Impella-EUROSHOCK-registry. Circ Heart Fail 2013; 6(1):23–30.

23. Hirose H, Yamane K, Marhefka G, et al. Right ventricular rupture and tamponade caused by malposition of the Avalon cannula for veno-venous extracorporeal membrane oxygenation. J Cardiothorac Surg 2012;7:36.

24. Makdisi G, Wang IW. Extra corporeal membrane oxygenation (ECMO) review of a lifesaving technology. J Thorac Dis 2015;7(7):E166–76.

25. Lim HS, Howell N, Ranasinghe A. Extracorporeal life support: physiological concepts and clinical outcomes. J Card Fail 2017;23(2):181–96.

26. Stehlik J, Edwards LB, Kucheryavaya AY, et al. The Registry of the International Society for Heart and Lung Transplantation: 29th official adult heart transplant report–2012. J Heart Lung Transplant 2012; 31(10):1052–64.

27. Peek GJ, Mugford M, Tiruvoipati R, et al. Efficacy and economic assessment of conventional ventilatory support versus extracorporeal membrane oxygenation for severe adult respiratory failure (CESAR): a multicentre randomised controlled trial. Lancet 2009;374(9698):1351–63.

28. Brodie D, Bacchetta M. Extracorporeal membrane oxygenation for ARDS in adults. N Engl J Med 2011;365(20):1905–14.

29. Bermudez CA, Rocha RV, Sappington PL, et al. Initial experience with single cannulation for venovenous extracorporeal oxygenation in adults. Ann Thorac Surg 2010;90(3):991–5.

30. Shaheen A, Tanaka D, Cavarocchi NC, et al. Veno-venous extracorporeal membrane oxygenation (V V ECMO): indications, preprocedural considerations, and technique. J Card Surg 2016;31(4): 248–52.

31. Lee S, Chaturvedi A. Imaging adults on extracorporeal membrane oxygenation (ECMO). Insights Imaging 2014;5(6):731–42.

32. Liu KL, Wang YF, Chang YC, et al. Multislice CT scans in patients on extracorporeal membrane oxygenation: emphasis on hemodynamic changes and imaging pitfalls. Korean J Radiol 2014;15(3): 322–9.

33. Acharya J, Rajamohan AG, Skalski MR, et al. CT angiography of the head in extracorporeal membrane oxygenation. AJNR Am J Neuroradiol 2017; 38(4):773–6.

34. Lidegran MK, Ringertz HG, Frenckner BP, et al. Chest and abdominal CT during extracorporeal membrane oxygenation: clinical benefits in diagnosis and treatment. Acad Radiol 2005;12(3): 276–85.

35. Cheng R, Hachamovitch R, Kittleson M, et al. Complications of extracorporeal membrane oxygenation for treatment of cardiogenic shock and cardiac

arrest: a meta-analysis of 1,866 adult patients. Ann Thorac Surg 2014;97(2):610–6.

36. Zangrillo A, Landoni G, Biondi-Zoccai G, et al. A meta-analysis of complications and mortality of extracorporeal membrane oxygenation. Crit Care Resusc 2013;15(3):172–8.

37. Tanaka D, Hirose H, Cavarocchi N, et al. The impact of vascular complications on survival of patients on venoarterial extracorporeal membrane oxygenation. Ann Thorac Surg 2016;101(5):1729–34.

38. Pillai AK, Bhatti Z, Bosserman AJ, et al. Management of vascular complications of extra-corporeal membrane oxygenation. Cardiovasc Diagn Ther 2018;8(3):372–7.

39. Menaker J, Tabatabai A, Rector R, et al. Incidence of cannula-associated deep vein thrombosis after veno-venous extracorporeal membrane oxygenation. ASAIO J 2017;63(5):588–91.

40. Victor K, Barrett N, Glover G, et al. Acute Budd-Chiari syndrome during veno-venous extracorporeal membrane oxygenation diagnosed using transthoracic echocardiography. Br J Anaesth 2012;108(6): 1043–4.

41. Hosmane SR, Barrow T, Ashworth A, et al. Extracorporeal membrane oxygenation: a radiologists' guide to who, what and where. Clin Radiol 2015;70(5): e58–66.

42. Goldstein BA, Thomas L, Zaroff JG, et al. Assessment of heart transplant waitlist time and pre- and post-transplant failure: a mixed methods approach. Epidemiology 2016;27(4):469–76.

43. Sajgalik P, Grupper A, Edwards BS, et al. Current status of left ventricular assist device therapy. Mayo Clin Proc 2016;91(7):927–40.

44. Rose EA, Gelijns AC, Moskowitz AJ, et al. Long-term use of a left ventricular assist device for end-stage heart failure. N Engl J Med 2001;345(20):1435–43.

45. Health Quality O. Left ventricular assist devices for destination therapy: a health technology assessment. Ont Health Technol Assess Ser 2016;16(3):1–60.

46. Rogers JG, Aaronson KD, Boyle AJ, et al. Continuous flow left ventricular assist device improves functional capacity and quality of life of advanced heart failure patients. J Am Coll Cardiol 2010; 55(17):1826–34.

47. Birks EJ, George RS, Hedger M, et al. Reversal of severe heart failure with a continuous-flow left ventricular assist device and pharmacological therapy: a prospective study. Circulation 2011;123(4): 381–90.

48. Birks EJ, Tansley PD, Hardy J, et al. Left ventricular assist device and drug therapy for the reversal of heart failure. N Engl J Med 2006;355(18):1873–84.

49. Carr CM, Jacob J, Park SJ, et al. CT of left ventricular assist devices. Radiographics 2010;30(2):429–44.

50. Siegenthaler MP, Martin J, van de Loo A, et al. Implantation of the permanent Jarvik-2000 left ventricular assist device: a single-center experience. J Am Coll Cardiol 2002;39(11):1764–72.

51. Slaughter MS, Rogers JG, Milano CA, et al. Advanced heart failure treated with continuous-flow left ventricular assist device. N Engl J Med 2009; 361(23):2241–51.

52. Mohamed I, Lau CT, Bolen MA, et al. Building a bridge to save a failing ventricle: radiologic evaluation of short- and long-term cardiac assist devices. Radiographics 2015;35(2):327–56.

53. Gurvits GE, Fradkov E. Bleeding with the artificial heart: gastrointestinal hemorrhage in CF-LVAD patients. World J Gastroenterol 2017;23(22):3945–53.

54. Chivukula VK, Beckman JA, Prisco AR, et al. Left ventricular assist device inflow cannula angle and thrombosis risk. Circ Heart Fail 2018;11(4): e004325.

55. Shroff GS, Ocazionez D, Akkanti B, et al. CT imaging of complications associated with continuous-flow left ventricular assist devices (LVADs). Semin Ultrasound CT MR 2017;38(6):616–28.

56. Willey JZ, Gavalas MV, Trinh PN, et al. Outcomes after stroke complicating left ventricular assist device. J Heart Lung Transplant 2016;35(8):1003–9.

57. Parikh NS, Cool J, Karas MG, et al. Stroke risk and mortality in patients with ventricular assist devices. Stroke 2016;47(11):2702–6.

58. Hannan MM, Husain S, Mattner F, et al. Working formulation for the standardization of definitions of infections in patients using ventricular assist devices. J Heart Lung Transplant 2011;30(4):375–84.

Neuroimaging of Patients in the Intensive Care Unit
Pearls and Pitfalls

Judith A. Gadde, DO, MBA*, Brent D. Weinberg, MD, PhD,
Mark E. Mullins, MD, PhD

KEYWORDS

- ICU (Intensive Care Unit) • Imaging • Neurosurgical • Pearls • Pitfalls

KEY POINTS

- Attention to quality, safety, utilization, and appropriateness is paramount when evaluating imaging of patients in the intensive care unit (ICU).
- Carefully scrutinizing all the provided images in critically ill patients, such as scouts and localizers, is crucial to answering the clinical question.
- When evaluating imaging, one must be aware of potential postprocedural complications in the ICU patient.

BACKGROUND AND IMPORTANCE

Patients in the intensive care unit (ICU) often are some of the sickest in the hospital. There are many reasons why diagnostic imaging or image-guided invasive procedures are requested, with a wide range of pathology possible.

BRIEF INTRODUCTION OF IMAGING MODALITIES

The first step in imaging an ill patient is to determine which modality to choose, if any. Attention to quality, safety, utilization, and appropriateness is paramount.[1,2] The most pertinent imaging modalities are introduced briefly. Catheter angiography, transcranial sonography, and nuclear medicine brain death scans are not discussed due to space constraints. Diagnostic imaging is also focused on and not invasive procedures, for similar reasons.

Computed Tomography

Computed tomography (CT) is a widely utilized method due to its availability, speed of use, and presence in some ICUs. Noncontrast head CT scans are performed to evaluate patients for urgent intracranial pathologies, such as hemorrhage, herniation, infection/inflammation, infarction, and hydrocephalus. Severe trauma, stroke, and altered mental status are common scenarios where CT may be used.

Computed Tomography Angiography

CT angiography (CTA) uses intravenous contrast with imaging during the arterial phase for detailed evaluation of potential arterial pathology, including aneurysms, vasospasm, infarction, and vascular malformations. CTA of the neck often is performed to evaluate for vascular injuries, including traumatic arterial injury, dissection, transections, and arterial stenosis.

Disclosure Statement: The authors have no disclosures.
Department of Radiology and Imaging Services, Emory University School of Medicine, 1364 Clifton Road Northeast, Suite BG20, Atlanta, GA 30319, USA
* Corresponding author.
E-mail address: jagadde@emory.edu

Radiol Clin N Am 58 (2020) 167–185
https://doi.org/10.1016/j.rcl.2019.08.003
0033-8389/20/© 2019 Elsevier Inc. All rights reserved.

radiologic.theclinics.com

Computed Tomography Venography

CT venography (CTV), like CTA, uses intravenous contrast but instead images the venous phase to evaluate pathologies, such as venous sinus thrombosis, cortical vein thrombosis, and thrombophlebitis. CTV of the neck can be performed to evaluate extent of clot, stenosis, and occlusion. CTV also can be beneficial in the posttraumatic setting to evaluate for injury from blunt or penetrating trauma.

Computed Tomography Perfusion

CT perfusion (CTP) also requires administration of iodinated contrast with dynamic imaging during contrast passage to evaluate for acute ischemia, acute infarction, or vasospasm. Quantitative parameters, including cerebral blood flow, cerebral blood volume, mean transit time, time to peak, and Tmax, are calculated from contrast curves to evaluate for specific pathology.[3]

Iodinated Contrast

Iodinated contrast should only be used when it is required for decisions that affect clinical management. Allergies and impaired renal function can affect their use in ICU patients. The American College of Radiology *Manual on Contrast Media* and *Appropriateness Criteria* provide excellent evidence-based resources on when and how contrast is used, which is especially important in ICU patients.[4,5]

Portable Computed Tomography

Portable CT scanners can increase scan availability and reduce the need to transport critically ill patients,[6] which can be challenging because of the need for portable ventilation, intravenous sedation, and extensive supportive tubes, lines, and drains.[7] Portable CT can be useful in patients too unstable to travel, including those on extracorporeal membrane oxygenation or ventricular assist device. Challenges to interpreting portable CTs include decreased spatial and contrast resolution and increased motion artifact.

Radiographs/Scouts

Use of radiographs is limited to evaluation of lines and tubes, such as a ventricular catheter.[8,9] Radiographs have advantages, including rapid examination times, ready availability, and low radiation exposure.[9] Scout radiographs, performed as part of CT examinations, also are important for evaluating support apparatus, craniocervical alignment, craniotomies, and surgical hardware.

Magnetic Resonance

Indications for performing magnetic resonance (MR) include further investigating a CT finding, evaluating a patient with persistent neurologic symptoms despite normal CT/prior imaging, and post-treatment follow-up. MR imaging has myriad challenges in ICU patients. MR scanners often are spatially distant from the ICU, requiring stability for transport. Safety-related patient considerations are paramount, and patients require MR safety clearance in regard to devices, implants, foreign bodies, prior surgeries, and so forth. Monitoring equipment must be switched to MR-compatible equipment. Implanted cardiac devices, including pacemakers and defibrillators, pose a special imaging situation, but patients with these devices can sometimes be scanned after consultation with an electrophysiologist and appropriate changes to device settings if local protocols allow for this.[10] On MR images, localizer/scout sequences should be reviewed for any unexpected findings.

Magnetic Resonance Angiography

MR angiography (MRA) is performed to evaluate the arterial vasculature and usually includes the brain and/or neck. Time-of-flight (TOF) technique allows MRA to be performed without the administration of intravenous gadolinium contrast agents. Contrast-enhanced or time-resolved (4-dimensional) MRA may be useful, however, to evaluate specific entities, such as vascular malformations, dissection, and pseudoaneurysm.[11,12]

Magnetic Resonance Venography

MR venography (MRV) can be performed to evaluate the venous vasculature of the brain and/or neck. Like MRA, MRV can be performed without contrast via the TOF technique or after the administration of gadolinium. TOF MRV is prone to artifacts; therefore, MRV with contrast is preferred to evaluate for dural venous sinus thrombosis.[13]

Gadolinium

As with iodinated contrast, gadolinium agents should be used only when necessary to answer the desired clinical question. Patients' renal function is a consideration but less of an issue today than years ago.[14] Patients also must be evaluated for potential allergic reactions to gadolinium. Pregnant patients typically are not given gadolinium agents because this has been shown to cross the placenta into the fetus with uncertain effects.[4,15]

SPECTRUM OF INTRACRANIAL NEUROLOGIC PATHOLOGY
Intracranial Trauma

Traumatic injury is a common indication for brain imaging in the ICU setting, with noncontrast head CT usually the first line of imaging. It is crucial to understand the different intracranial compartments in order to understand the types of pathology that can occur (**Fig. 1**). It is not always possible to place extra-axial hemorrhage into a specific compartment. A subdural hematoma typically is more crescent-shaped and can cross sutures. Subdural hematomas are usually due to tearing of crossing bridging veins. In comparison, epidural hematomas are commonly biconvex or lens-shaped, do not cross sutures, and may cross the midline. Epidural hematomas are associated with calvarial fractures, classically described with middle meningeal artery or midline venous injury.[16]

Trauma is the most common cause of subarachnoid hemorrhage (SAH).[17] When traumatic in etiology, it is typically located in the peripheral cerebral sulci rather than in the sylvian fissures and basal cisterns. Traumatic SAH also may be located adjacent to fractures or cerebral contusions, rather than adjacent to the circle of Willis.

Diffuse axonal injury (DAI) is another entity that may be seen in patients with high-energy trauma and results in altered mental status. These abnormalities usually occur at the grey-white matter junction, corpus callosum, and brainstem, presumably due to differences in mechanical properties at tissue interfaces. CT may show small hemorrhages, although CT is normal in 50% or more cases of DAI.[18] MR imaging, in particular susceptibility-weighted imaging and T2-weighted images, is traditionally more sensitive than CT for DAI.[19] The degree of injury often is underestimated by imaging.[20]

Intracranial Vascular Pathology

ICU patients can have a range of intracranial vascular pathologies, including aneurysm, vascular malformation, ischemia, and vasospasm. When a noncontrast head CT reveals acute intracranial hemorrhage, CTA of the head usually is the most appropriate next examination to evaluate for an underlying vascular lesion, such as ruptured intracranial aneurysm. This hemorrhage is sometimes (although not always) centered around the site of rupture. Other vascular malformations, such as arteriovenous malformations or dural arteriovenous fistulas, can result

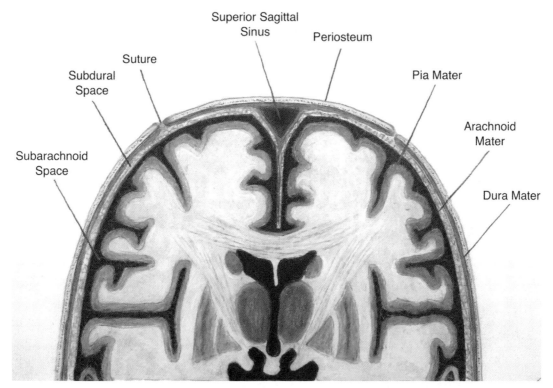

Fig. 1. The various intracranial compartments are illustrated, including epidural, subdural, subarachnoid, and intra-axial.

in single-compartment or multiple-compartment hemorrhage.

Ischemic stroke is another common indication for imaging. This indication may arise in the inpatient setting due to altered mental status or new acute neurologic deficit. Evaluation usually begins with a noncontrast head CT to identify those acute ischemic stroke patients who are candidates for thrombolysis. This noncontrast head CT is used mainly to evaluate for acute intracranial hemorrhage, but this scan also is an opportunity to evaluate for additional potential causes of a patient's symptoms (eg, metastatic disease and brain tumor) as well as the size, density, and extent of ischemic infarction. If acute intracranial hemorrhage is identified, CTA may be considered to evaluate for an underlying vascular malformation or a site of active bleeding. Depending on institutional preference, stroke patients go on to be evaluated by a combination of CTA and CTP or MR imaging.

Dural venous thrombosis is another pathology that can be seen in ICU patients. The dural venous sinus may appear hyperdense on a noncontrast head CT or there may be concern

for a hemorrhagic venous infarction, classically manifested as parenchymal hemorrhages in an unusual location for hemorrhagic transformation of ischemic infarction. Presence and extent of venous thrombosis can be characterized further with CTV or MRV.[13]

Vasospasm is reactive narrowing of the intracranial arteries, commonly after SAH with peak at 5 days to 14 days after initial hemorrhage.[21] If severe enough, the vasospasm can result in alternations in cerebral perfusion, leading to ischemia/infarction (**Fig. 2**). Patients usually are evaluated at the bedside with transcranial doppler, but CT/CTA/CTP can be used for further evaluation, often varying with local practice patterns.[22,23] CTA typically shows interval (that is, recently acquired) intracranial arterial narrowing.

Brain Herniation Patterns and Complications/ Low Tonsils

It is crucial to be aware of the various types of brain herniation patterns and their often associated complications (**Fig. 3**).[24,25] Subfalcine herniation

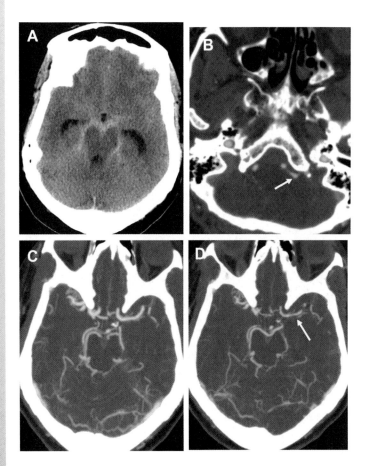

Fig. 2. A 57-year-old woman with worst headache of her life. CT head without contrast (A) shows SAH and obstructive hydrocephalus. Initial CTA head (B) demonstrates a left posterior inferior cerebellar artery fusiform aneurysm (arrow). CTA head performed 3 days after coiling of left PICA aneurysm (C) demonstrates normal caliber of the intracranial arteries. CTA head performed 7 days after initial presentation (D) shows moderate narrowing of the intracranial arteries, for example, the left middle cerebral artery (arrow).

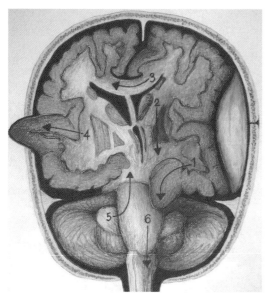

Fig. 3. A left-sided epidural hematoma demonstrates the various types of herniation patterns, including (1) uncal herniation, (2) downward transtentorial herniation, (3) subfalcine herniation, (4) extracranial herniation, (5) ascending transtentorial herniation, and (6) tonsillar herniation.

is characterized by the frontal lobe, commonly the cingulate gyrus, sliding underneath the falx cerebri. Potential complications include compression of the anterior cerebral artery, resulting in acute ischemia or hydrocephalus due to compression at the foramen of Monro.

Transtentorial herniation can be unilateral or bilateral, involves brain crossing the tentorium at the level of the incisura/notch, and has several subtypes. Uncal herniation is when the medial portion of the anterior temporal lobe, the uncus, is shifted into the suprasellar cistern. Effacement of the ambient cisterns often can occur, with complications including posterior cerebral artery or brainstem compression. Duret hemorrhages usually are small hemorrhages within the medulla or pons as a result of descending transtentorial herniation. A cerebellar hemisphere crossing the tentorium at the level of the incisura/notch characterizes ascending/upward transtentorial herniation.

Extracranial/transcranial brain herniation can be seen in the setting of trauma with an open calvarial fracture but more commonly (at least in the authors' experience) is an expected finding after decompressive hemicraniectomy in the setting of increased intracranial pressure (eg, after middle cerebral artery stroke).

Cerebellar tonsillar herniation is manifested as crowding at the level of the foramen magnum due to descent of the cerebellar tonsils. Low-lying cerebellar tonsils extending through the foramen magnum are not synonymous with acute brain herniation, because there are other potential causes of this finding including Chiari I malformation, idiopathic intracranial hypertension, and cerebrospinal fluid (CSF) hypotension[26] (**Fig. 4**).

Hydrocephalus

Hydrocephalus is active distension of the ventricular system due to inadequate CSF flow from its origin to the point of absorption. Hydrocephalus can be communicating or

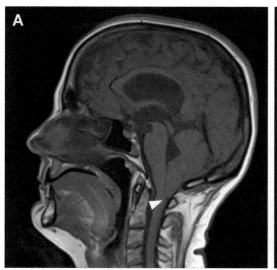

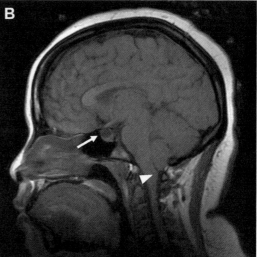

Fig. 4. (*A*) A 55-year-old woman with headache. Midline T1 image shows cerebellar tonsils 1.5 cm below the foramen magnum (*arrowhead*). (*B*) A 31-year-old woman with headache. In addition to low-lying cerebellar tonsils (*arrowhead*), note the partially empty and expanded sella (*arrow*).

noncommunicating/obstructive and acute or nonacute. Communicating hydrocephalus demonstrates enlargement of all ventricles, whereas noncommunicating hydrocephalus involves only ventricles proximal to a point of obstruction within the ventricular system. Acute or uncompensated hydrocephalus is characterized by periventricular edema on CT and MR. Noncontrast head CT is the usual initial imaging modality in patients with known or suspected hydrocephalus. A short brain MR imaging is an alternative used at some institutions, especially pediatric hospitals to evaluate the ventricular size in patients with hydrocephalus. These studies typically consist of a fast T2-weighted sequence (such as a T2 HASTE) in 1 or more planes as well as a diffusion-weighted sequence, depending on the institution. For patients with a shunt, the visualized portions of shunt hardware on CT and MR imaging should be scrutinized carefully for discontinuities or unexpected abnormalities (Fig. 5).

Intracranial Infections/Inflammatory

Intracranial infections, including meningitis, encephalitis, and focal abscess, can be challenging to diagnose and are a significant concern in the ICU patient. These all can cause changes in mental status, which can lead to hospitalization in the ICU or develop in patients already hospitalized for other reasons.

Meningitis can occur spontaneously or be iatrogenic, such as after an intracranial surgery or spinal procedure. When there is suspicion for meningitis, initial imaging typically is performed with CT of the head without contrast, which, despite low sensitivity for intracranial infection, is useful for excluding masses and hemorrhage and assessing for mass effect. In some cases of infection, edema may be visualized on CT. MR imaging of the brain with contrast is the mainstay of imaging for intracranial infection.[27]

Imaging findings of meningitis include leptomeningeal enhancement, brain swelling, hydrocephalus, and altered CSF intensity on T1 and fluid-attenuated inversion recovery (FLAIR).[28] In severe cases, CSF can be T1 hyperintense and fail to suppress on FLAIR, commonly in the prepontine cistern and cerebral sulci. Meningitis can progress to frank involvement of CSF within the ventricles or ventriculitis. Other ominous signs include FLAIR hyperintensity, restricted diffusion (implying frank pus), and periventricular edema or enhancement (Fig. 6).[29] Abnormal appearance of the CSF also can be artifactual, particularly when patients are on supplemental oxygen. Performing FLAIR postcontrast can increase sensitivity for leptomeningeal disease.[30] Basal meningitis, when abnormal imaging enhancement is centered on the basal cisterns, prepontine cisterns, and sylvian fissures (Fig. 7), suggests unusual causes, such as tuberculosis, fungi, or sarcoidosis.[31]

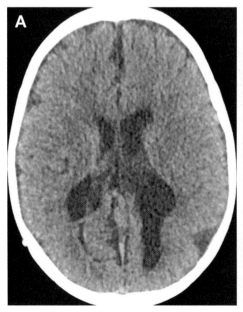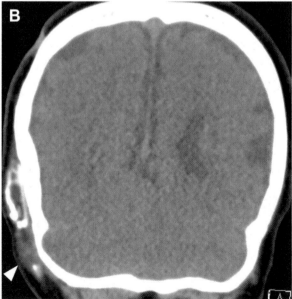

Fig. 5. A 5-year-old boy presents with severe headache and nausea. Axial CT head without contrast (A) shows dysmorphic and enlarged lateral ventricles. Coronal CT reformats in soft tissue windows (B) demonstrate discontinuity with a focal collection just inferior to the shunt reservoir (arrowhead).

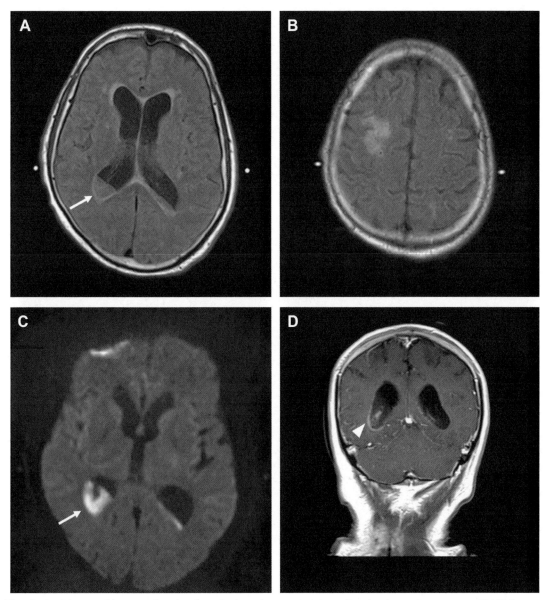

Fig. 6. An 81-year-old man who developed altered mental status after lumbar spine surgery. FLAIR images through the ventricles (*A*) and cerebral hemispheres (*B*) demonstrate layering debris in the ventricles (*A* [*arrow*]) and parenchymal abnormalities in the cerebral hemispheres. DWI (*C*) shows restricted diffusion in the debris (*arrow*), consistent with pus. T1 postcontrast imaging (*D*) shows subtle enhancement of the ventricular margin (*arrowhead*), consistent with ventriculitis.

Encephalitis is the presence of intracranial infection with parenchymal involvement, which can include the cerebral hemispheres (cerebritis) or cerebellum manifested by abnormal T2/FLAIR hyperintensity and swelling. Cerebritis of the medial temporal lobes, either unilateral or bilateral, has a special differential diagnosis, which includes herpes encephalitis (**Fig. 8**).[32] Limbic encephalitis is an immune-mediated encephalitis sometimes associated with a systemic malignancy and has an overlapping appearance with herpes encephalitis, although it often does not enhance.[33] Patients with suspected limbic encephalitis should be evaluated for systemic malignancies.

Abscess is intracranial infection that has been walled off into a single location or compartment. Pyogenic parenchymal abscess is characterized by 1 or more fluid collections with centrally reduced diffusion surrounded by a wall with

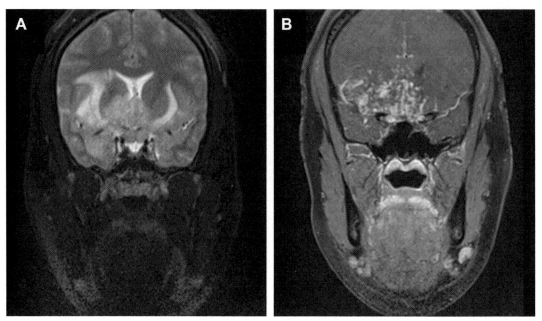

Fig. 7. A 32-year-old woman with headache and right visual changes. Coronal T2 fat-saturated (*A*) and T1 post-contrast fat-saturated (*B*) images show marked edema and swelling in the inferior frontal lobes and avid enhancement along the sulci and basal cisterns. This patient had a hilar lymph node biopsy consistent with sarcoidosis.

T2 hypointensity and postcontrast enhancement (Fig. 9). Abscesses may have a thinner wall along the ventricular margin and can rupture into the ventricles, causing ventriculitis, as described previously.[34] Multiple abscesses suggest a central source of infection, such as endocarditis or bacteremia. Nonbacterial causes of infection, such as toxoplasmosis, may have a similar appearance but often lack abnormal diffusion. Abscesses outside of the brain parenchyma, most commonly in the epidural space (empyema) or subdural space, often are related to local spread of infection from frontal sinusitis or mastoiditis.[34] Their imaging appearance is similar, with a central area of reduced diffusion and surrounding rim of thick enhancement. A concerning complication of epidural empyema is dural venous sinus thrombosis.

Postsurgical Complications

Patients undergoing intracranial procedures are at risk of early (eg, 48 hours or less) and late (days to weeks) complications. Changes in mental status after a neurosurgical procedure are usually investigated with noncontrast CT, whereas MR imaging may be considered to follow CT if needed. Early complications,

including hemorrhage or infarct, can occur from direct injury during the procedure.[35] Patients undergoing resection of highly vascular masses, such as glioblastoma or breast, renal, thyroid, and melanoma metastases, are at particular risk for hemorrhage. Infarction can occur from damage to the parenchymal arterial supply or draining veins, manifested by hypodensity and loss of gray-white differentiation on CT and areas of reduced diffusion on MR imaging, which can occur adjacent to or remote from the resection.[36] Although a thin rim of devitalized tissues is expected surrounding the resection bed, larger or focal areas of restricted diffusion adjacent to or distant from the resection bed are concerning (Fig. 10). Venous occlusion and infarction also sometimes occur. Another less common, although significant, postoperative complication is tension pneumocephalus, when air from the surrounding environment or sinuses is drawn intracranially before becoming trapped by a ball valve mechanism (Fig. 11).[37] This type of intracranial air may result in brain herniation. Intracranial infection can also occur as a delayed postsurgical complication.

Thrombolytic treatment for stroke, including both intravenous tissue plasminogen activator and intra-arterial interventions, can have

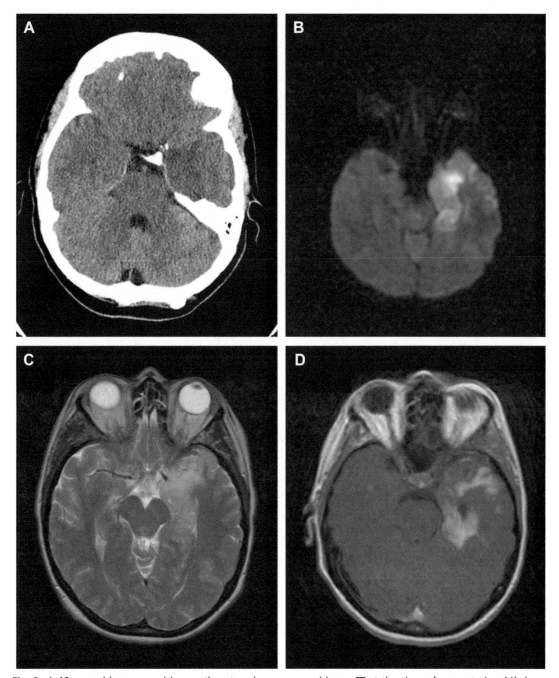

Fig. 8. A 46-year-old woman with sore throat and memory problems. CT at the time of presentation (*A*) shows abnormal hypodensity in the left medial temporal lobe. Follow-up MR imaging shows abnormal elevated diffusion (*B*), T2 hyperintensity (*C*), and avid T1-postcontrast enhancement (*D*) consistent with herpes encephalitis.

complications best evaluated with noncontrast CT. Intracranial hemorrhage is the most significant major complication after stroke treatment.[38] Contrast staining is a phenomenon in which previously administered intravenous contrast leaks from abnormal vessels in the region, obscuring areas of infarction and mimic hemorrhage. Contrast staining is less dense than hemorrhage, confined to anatomic areas of infarct, and significantly decreases in density within 24 hours.[39] Stroke patients should be considered for further evaluation with brain MR imaging, including diffusion and FLAIR, to evaluate for infarction.

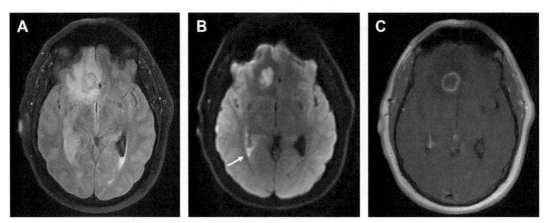

Fig. 9. A 50-year-old man with multiple odontogenic infections presenting with diplopia, ataxia, and headache. FLAIR (*A*) demonstrates an isointense mass in the inferior right frontal lobe with surrounding edema. DWI (*B*) has central hyperintensity compatible with pus. Pus is also seen in the right ventricle (*arrow*). Postcontrast T1 (*C*) shows peripheral enhancement compatible with abscess.

Postprocedure ischemia, ranging from punctate infarcts to diffuse hypoxic injury, also is a significant concern in the ICU patient. Although CT may be a useful initial screen, MR imaging with diffusion frequently is needed to assess for small infarcts and subtle manifestations of diffuse hypoxia. Small infarcts may not be seen on CT, whereas more diffuse injury may be seen as brain swelling, loss of gray-white differentiation, and parenchymal hypodensities. MR imaging findings include abnormal diffusion in areas sensitive to oxygen deprivation, including the basal ganglia and cortex.[40] It can be challenging to see diffuse hypoxic injury, because the findings can often be subtle and bilaterally symmetric.

Spine procedures can also lead to intracranial complications. When intradural procedures are performed, shifts in CSF can lead to hemorrhages at locations that are spatially remote from the surgical site. The characteristic manifestation of this process is (spatially) remote

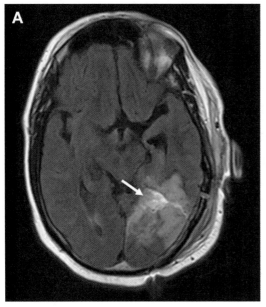
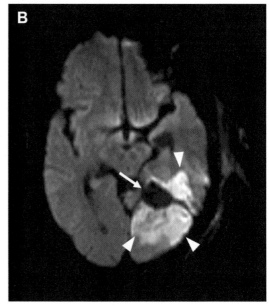

Fig. 10. A 35-year-old male status post–resection of a glioblastoma. Postoperative FLAIR (*A*) and DWI (*B*) images show a small resection cavity in the left occipital lobe (*arrows*) with a significantly larger area of surrounding diffusion restriction (*arrowheads*).

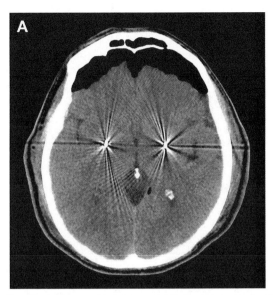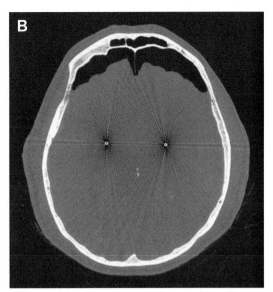

Fig. 11. A 61 year old status post–bilateral deep brain stimulator placement for Parkinson disease. During surgery, the patient developed a prominent amount of pneumocephalus with peaking of the bilateral frontal lobes, the Mt. Fuji sign, as shown on brain (*A*) and bone window (*B*) CT.

cerebellar hemorrhage (**Fig. 12**), in which a cerebellar hemorrhage occurs after a spinal surgery.[41] Similar findings can be seen after surgeries in the intracranial compartment.[42] A search for associated dural sinus thrombosis, and thus hemorrhagic venous infarction, is prudent. Spinal complications of procedures are discussed later.

Delayed postoperative complications, from approximately 2 days to weeks after the

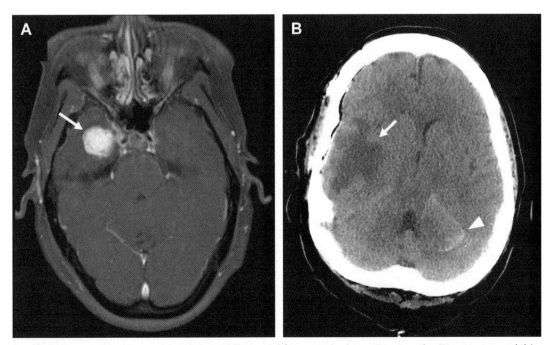

Fig. 12. A 56-year-old woman with a right middle cranial fossa meningioma. Preoperative T1 postcontrast (*A*) imaging demonstrates an extra-axial mass in the right middle cranial fossa (*arrow*). Postoperative CT (*B*) demonstrates edema in the surgical bed (*arrow*) as well as subarachnoid and parenchymal hemorrhage in the left posterior fossa (*arrowhead*) remote form the operative site.

procedure, include a separate range of conditions. Postoperative hemorrhage remains a consideration, although the probability decreases with time. The peak time for postoperative infection is weeks to months after surgery.[43] Findings are similar to those described for other infections of the neural axis (eg, meningitis, encephalitis, and abscess), with the site of infection centered around the surgical site. Diffusion-weighted imaging (DWI) and postcontrast MR imaging imaging is imperative, because focal sites of infection frequently are hyperintense on DWI. Postoperative blood products also are hyperintense on DWI, mimicking infection and confounding imaging interpretation; a combination of blood and infection also is possible. Postoperative infection should be suspected in the following situations: increasing fluid collection, area of DWI hyperintensity exceeding suspected blood products on T1 and gradient-weighted imaging, increasing mass effect, and worsening edema within the parenchyma or soft tissues.

Another late complication of intracranial surgery is the sunken (skin) flap syndrome, which can occur after craniectomy (**Fig. 13**). There is associated paradoxic mass effect, with the midline shifting away from the side of the craniectomy.[44]

Tumors

Aside from complications of surgery, discussed previously, patients with brain tumors, including both primary tumors and metastases, are subject to complications, such as intracranial hemorrhage. Tumors, which are commonly highly vascular, are subject to spontaneous hemorrhage (**Fig. 14**). Another significant complication in tumor patients is worsening mass effect. Other related complications include herniation, hydrocephalus, and ventricular entrapment. Noncontrast CT typically is sufficient to evaluate for tumor complications, although MR imaging of contrast may be needed to further evaluate the extent of tumor.

Immunocompromised Patients

Immunocompromised patients are susceptible to a range of neurologic abnormalities including unusual infections (eg, toxoplasmosis, tuberculosis, and fungal disease) and lymphoma. Imaging manifestations also may differ between immunocompetent and immunocompromised individuals. For example, CNS lymphoma in an HIV patient can have a much more varied appearance and may lack the solid nodular enhancement typical in immunocompetent patients (**Fig. 15**).[45] Progressive multifocal encephalopathy is a rare but serious virus-mediated demyelinating

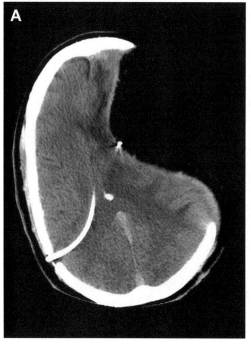
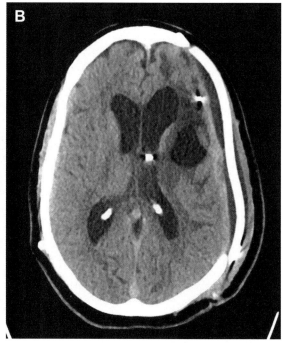

Fig. 13. A 30-year-old man with history of craniectomy for gunshot wound presenting with altered mental status. Initial CT demonstrates sunken skin flap with paradoxic left to right midline shift and cerebral edema (*A*), which improves after cranioplasty (*B*).

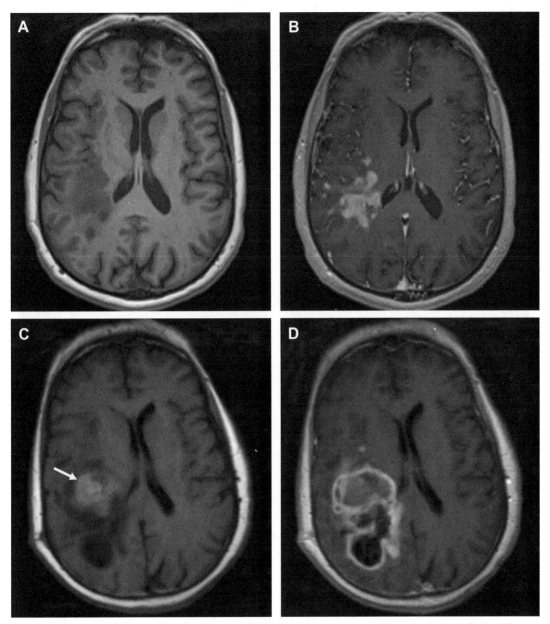

Fig. 14. A 67-year-old man with glioblastoma and worsening symptoms 3 weeks into radiation therapy. Precontrast (*A*) and postcontrast (*B*) T1 images prior to radiation therapy show a right parietal enhancing mass. Precontrast (*C*) and postcontrast (*D*) T1 images 3 weeks into radiation therapy show a central area of T1 hyperintensity compatible with hemorrhage into the tumor (*arrow*) with resulting worsening mass effect.

syndrome in immunocompromised patients with imaging manifestations, including progressively worsening bilateral white matter abnormalities, which are characteristically T1 hypointense and T2 hyperintens, and lack postcontrast enhancement.[46]

Immunocompromised patients also are particularly susceptible to sinus disease, the most

aggressive of which is invasive fungal sinusitis (IFS). IFS is characterized by infection, which begins in the nasal cavity and rapidly spreads along vascular structures and can extend intracranially to involve the cavernous sinus and brain. Emergent MR imaging without and with contrast material is usually the test of choice, with findings including nonenhancing nasal mucosa,

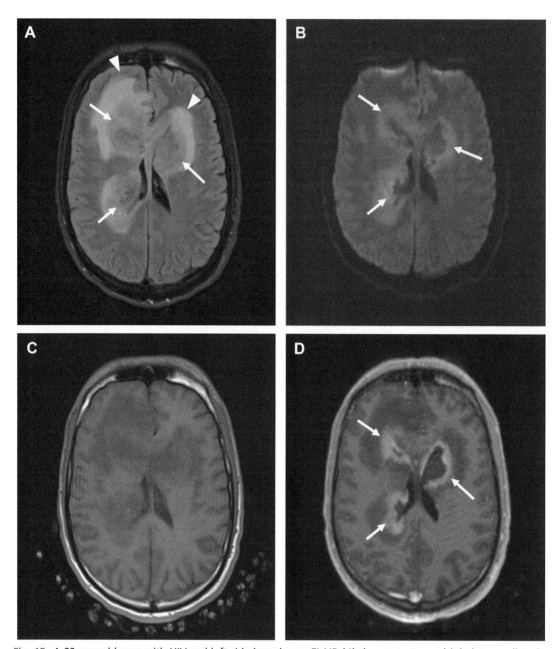

Fig. 15. A 32-year-old man with HIV and left-sided weakness. FLAIR (*A*) demonstrates multiple intermediate intensity masses along the margins of the ventricles (*arrows*) with surrounding edema (*arrowheads*). They have a rim of high intensity on DWI (*B* [*arrows*]). Precontrast T1 (*C*) and postcontrast T1 (*D*) demonstrate peripherally enhancing masses along the ventricle margin (*arrows*).

enhancement/invasion outside of the sinus involving such structures as the retroantral and/or orbital fat, and potential intracranial enhancement along the leptomeninges and cavernous sinus. A routine evaluation for manifestations of IFS on CT scans performed in immunocompromised patients is prudent, especially in the setting of fever and neutropenia.

Toxic/Metabolic

Toxic or metabolic conditions are frequently bilateral, involve the basal ganglia, and are symmetric.[47] Patients with hepatic encephalopathy may have bilaterally symmetric T1 hyperintensities in the basal ganglia, sometimes called hepatocerebral degeneration.[48] Wernicke encephalopathy, a condition of thiamine deficiency, is characterized by bilaterally symmetric T2 hyperintense abnormalities in the basal ganglia, thalamus, and tissue surrounding the cerebral aqueduct the fourth ventricle[49]; involvement of the mammillary bodies is highly suggestive.

Osmotic demyelination is an inflammatory condition, which occurs in the setting of abnormalities of serum osmolality, in particular low sodium that has been rapidly corrected. Central pontine myelinolysis is a subset of osmotic demyelination associated with bilaterally symmetric T2 hyperintense demyelinating lesions in the pons (**Fig. 16**).[47] Similar abnormalities can be seen outside the pons (extrapontine myelinolysis), particularly in the basal ganglia and subcortical white matter.

Glucose abnormalities, including profound hypoglycemia and hyperglycemia, are common in ICU patients. Very low blood sugars can be accompanied by seizures, with the more common MR imaging findings being subtle T2 hyperintensities in the basal ganglia and cortex.[50] Cortical abnormalities may overlap with the imaging appearance of seizure. On the other hand, marked hyperglycemia, in particular nonketotic acidosis, has its own imaging findings of T1 hyperintensities in the basal ganglia (**Fig. 17**).[50] Imaging findings of both hypoglycemia and hyperglycemia can be reversible. The unifying theme behind toxic/metabolic abnormalities is that they should be considered any time bilaterally symmetric brain abnormalities are seen.

Brief Overview of Spine Imaging in Intensive Care Unit Patients

Routine imaging of the spine in ICU patients is not common. Suspicion for infection, specifically bacterial discitis osteomyelitis, is an indication for imaging the spine. CT of the spine is limited in this context because of overlap between imaging findings of degenerative changes and infection. MR imaging is traditionally preferable to CT in this setting. Infection in the spine most often arises in the disk and spreads to the adjacent bone, with imaging findings including abnormal fluid signal within the disk and surrounding soft tissues, abnormal enhancement, and paraspinal or epidural abscess (**Fig. 18**). Tuberculous osteomyelitis also can occur and should be considered in patients with relevant risk factors and spinal osteomyelitis with relative sparing of the underlying disk.[51]

Postsurgical complications in the spine include hematoma and infection. Postoperative hematoma into the surgical bed can cause compression of the remaining spinal canal. CT is the first-line test in a patient with postoperative symptoms, although hematoma can be challenging to visualize, particularly in the setting of surgical hardware. MR imaging usually is superior to CT for evaluating postoperative hematoma, although it also can be degraded by metallic artifacts. Intravenous contrast is usually not necessary in the immediate postoperative period.

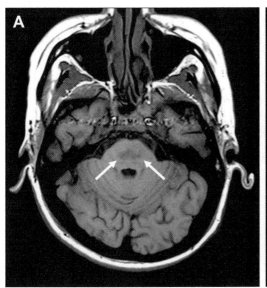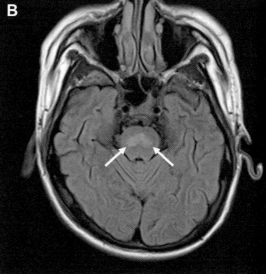

Fig. 16. A 51 year old with fever and lower extremity pain. Precontrast T1 (*A*) and FLAIR (*B*) images show bilaterally symmetric abnormalities in the pons (*arrows*), compatible with osmotic demyelination.

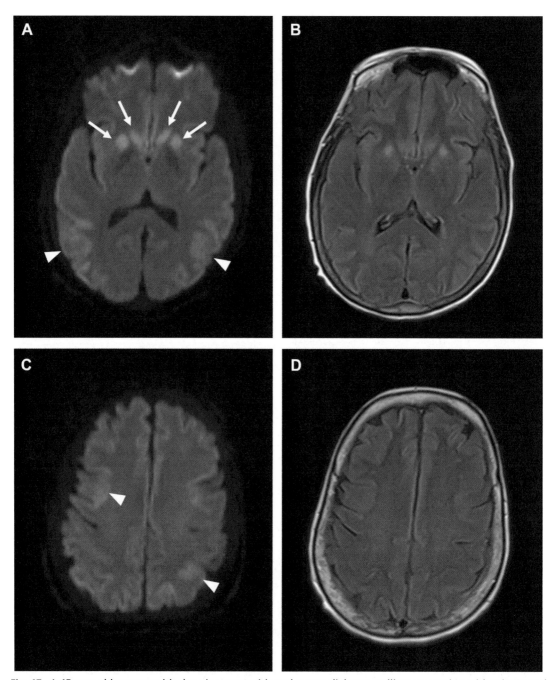

Fig. 17. A 45-year-old woman with chronic pancreatitis and severe diabetes mellitus presenting with seizure and profoundly low glucose. MR imaging demonstrated bilaterally symmetric diffusion (*A*) and FLAIR (*B*) abnormalities in the basal ganglia (*A* [*arrows*]) with more subtle areas of abnormality in the cortex (*arrowheads*). Additional areas of cortical diffusion (*C* [*arrowheads*]) and FLAIR (*D*) abnormalities were present more superiorly in the cerebral hemispheres.

In the days to weeks after surgical intervention, postoperative fluid collections both in the surgical bed and epidural space can cause complications.[52] Postoperative seroma, evolving hematoma, and abscess share imaging features, because they commonly are T2 hyperintense fluid collections within the surgical bed. Intravenous contrast can be useful, because abscess more typically has more robust surrounding enhancement, and enhancement of the descending nerve

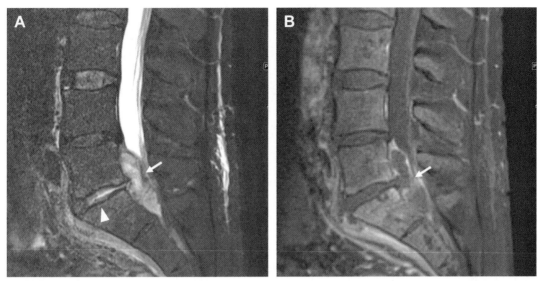

Fig. 18. A 52-year-old man with back pain and bacteremia. Sagittal T2 fat-saturated (*A*) demonstrate abnormal hyperintensity within the L5-S1 disk space (*arrowhead*) with an adjacent epidural abscess (*arrow*). T1 postcontrast fat-saturated images (*B*) demonstrate peripheral enhancement of the epidural abscess (*arrow*).

roots or spinal cord is suspicious for infectious arachnoiditis (in this time frame). DWI is an excellent troubleshooting technique, because abscess features reduced diffusion (see caveat about hemorrhage and DWI discussed previously). In the spine, any collection that is more hyperintense than the spinal cord on DWI is concerning.

Spinal cord infarction is a rare but serious complication of surgeries, including primarily aortic repair and long segment fusions involving the thoracic spine (**Fig. 19**). Spinal cord infarction is characterized by acute onset of symptoms shortly after the intervention, with MR imaging findings of long segment T2 hyperintensity that can include the complete, central, and ventral portions of the cord cross-section. Dorsal location of spinal cord infarction is uncommon. Abnormal DWI hyperintensity is critical in making this diagnosis, and it is important to image a long enough segment of the spine so that normal cord can be compared with the infarcted portion.

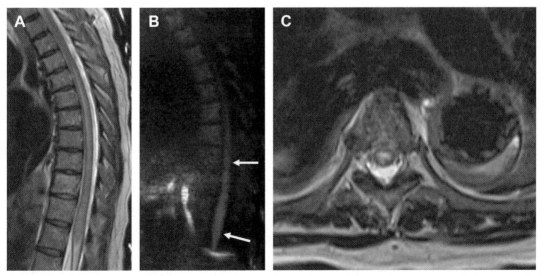

Fig. 19. A 64-year-old woman with lower extremity weakness after aortic dissection repair. Sagittal (*A*) and axial T2 (*C*) images show a long segment central hyperintensity, which has abnormal hyperintensity on DWI (*B* [*arrows*]), consistent with cord infarct.

SUMMARY

In summary, neuroimaging of patients from the ICU may seem daunting but can be surmountable with awareness of the potential pathology and complications commonly seen in these patients.

ACKNOWLEDGMENTS

Thank you to Travis Healey, MD, from Indiana University School of Medicine, Department of Vascular and Interventional Radiology, for the illustrations for Figs. 1 and 3.

REFERENCES

1. Vijayasarathi A, Hawkins CM, Hughes DR, et al. How much do common imaging studies cost? A nationwide survey of radiology trainess. Am J Roentgenol 2015;205:929–35.
2. Hollingsworth TD, Duszak R Jr, Vijayasarathi A, et al. Trainee knowledge of imaging appropriateness and safety: results of a series of surveys from a large academic medical center. Curr Probl Diagn Radiol 2019;48(1):17–21.
3. de Lucas EM, Sánchez E, Gutierrez A, et al. CT protocol for acute stroke: tips and tricks for general radiologists. Radiographics 2008;28(6):1673–87.
4. Radiology ACo. ACR manual on contrast media. In: 2018. Available at: https://www.acr.org/Clinical-Resources/Contrast-Manual.
5. Radiology ACo. ACR appropriateness criteria. In: 2019. Available at: https://www.acr.org/Clinical-Resources/ACR-Appropriateness-Criteria.
6. Mangla S, Chaloopka JC, Huddle DC. Early clinical experience with a dedicated portable computer tomography scanner in a biplane neuroangiography suite: assessment of feasibility and utility in neurointerventional practice. Interv Neuroradiol 2000;6(3): 211–20.
7. Parmentier-Decrucq E, Poissy J, Favory R, et al. Adverse events during intrahospital transport of critically ill patients: incidence and risk factors. Ann Intensive Care 2013;3(1):10.
8. Wallace AN, McConathy J, Menias CO, et al. Imaging evaluation of CSF shunts. Am J Roentgenol 2014;202(1):38–53.
9. Lee MJ, Streicher DA, Howard BM, et al. Ventricular shunt radiographs: still relevant in the cross-sectional era? Pictorial review of the radiographic appearance of ventricular shunt and approach to interpreting shunt series radiographs. Neurographics 2016;6(4):202–12.
10. Camacho JC, Moreno CC, Shah AD, et al. Safety and quality of 1.5-T MRI in patients with conventional and mri-conditional cardiac implantable electronic devices after implementation of a standardized protocol. AJR Am J Roentgenol 2016;207(3):599–604.
11. Saindane AM, Boddu SR, Tong FC, et al. Contrast-enhanced time-resolved MRA for pre-angiographic evaluation of suspected spinal dural arterial venous fistulas. J Neurointerv Surg 2015;7(2): 135–40.
12. Boddu SR, Tong FC, Dehkhaghani S, et al. Contrast-enhanced time-resolved MRA for follow-up of intracranial aneurysms treated with the pipeline embolization device. Am J Roentgenol 2014;35(11): 2112–8.
13. Sadigh G, Mullins ME, Saindane AM. Diagnostic performance of MRI sequences for evaluation of dural venous sinus thrombosis. Am J Roentgenol 2016; 206(6):1298–306.
14. Kaewlai R, Abujudeh H. Nephrogenic systemic fibrosis. Am J Roentgenol 2012;199(1):W17–23.
15. Webb JA, Thomsen HS, Morcos SK. The use of iodinated and gadolinium contrast media during pregnancy and lactation. Eur Radiol 2005;15(6): 1234–40.
16. Aurangzeb A, Ahmed E, Afridi EA, et al. Frequency of extradural hematoma in patients with linear skull fracture. J Ayub Med Coll Abbottabad 2015;27(2): 314–7.
17. Long B, Koyfman A, Runyon MS. Subarachnoid hemorrhage: updates in diagnosis and management. Emerg Med Clin North Am 2017;35(4):803–24.
18. Currie S, Saleem N, Straiton JA, et al. Imaging assessment of traumatic brain injury. Postgrad Med J 2016;92(1083):41–50.
19. Mittl RL, Grossman RI, Hiehle JF, et al. Prevalence of MR evidence of diffuse axonal injury in patients with mild head injury and normal head CT findings. AJNR Am J Neuroradiol 1994;15(8): 1583–9.
20. Ma J, Zhang K, Wang Z, et al. Progress of research on diffuse axonal injury after traumatic brain injury. Neural Plast 2016;2016:9746313.
21. Bederson JB, Connolly ES Jr, Batjer HH, et al. Guidelines for the management of aneurysmal subarachnoid hemorrhage: a statement for healthcare professionals from a special writing group of the Stroke Council, American Heart Association. Stroke 2009;40(3):994–1025.
22. Djelilovic-Vranic J, Basic-Kes V, Tiric-Campara M, et al. Follow-up of Vasospasm by Transcranial Doppler Sonography (TCD) in Subarachnoid Hemorrhage (SAH). Acta Inform Med 2017;25(1):14–8.
23. Stecco A, Fabbiano F, Amatuzzo P, et al. Computer tomography perfusion and computed tomography angiography in vasoaspm after subarachnoid hemorrhage. J Neurosurg Sci 2018;62(4):397–405.
24. Johnson PL, Eckard DA, Chason DP, et al. Imaging of acquired cerebral herniations. Neuroimaging Clin N Am 2002;12(2):217–28.

25. Young GB. Impaired consciousness and herniation syndromes. Neurol Clin 2011;29(4):765–72.

26. Schievink WI. Misdiagnosis of spontaneous intracranial hypotension. Arch Neurol 2003;60(12):1713–8.

27. Foerster BR, Thurnher MM, Malani PN, et al. Intracranial infections: clinical and imaging characteristics. Acta Radiol 2007;48(8):875–93.

28. Hazany S, Go JL, Law M. Magnetic resonance imaging of infectious meningitis and ventriculitis in adults. Top Magn Reson Imaging 2014;23(5):315–25.

29. Fujikawa A, Tsuchiya K, Honya K, et al. Comparison of MRI sequences to detect ventriculitis. AJR Am J Roentgenol 2006;187(4):1048–53.

30. Mathews VP, Caldemeyer KS, Lowe MJ, et al. Brain: gadolinium-enhanced fast fluid-attenuated inversion-recovery MR imaging. Radiology 1999;211(1):257–63.

31. Meltzer CC, Fukui MB, Kanal E, et al. MR imaging of the meninges. Part I. Normal anatomic features and nonneoplastic disease. Radiology 1996;201(2):297–308.

32. Rabinstein AA. Herpes virus encephalitis in adults: current knowledge and old myths. Neurol Clin 2017;35(4):695–705.

33. Kelley BP, Patel SC, Marin HL, et al. Autoimmune encephalitis: pathophysiology and imaging review of an overlooked diagnosis. AJNR Am J Neuroradiol 2017;38(6):1070–8.

34. Mohan S, Jain KK, Arabi M, et al. Imaging of meningitis and ventriculitis. Neuroimaging Clin N Am 2012;22(4):557–83.

35. Wong JM, Panchmatia JR, Ziewacz JE, et al. Patterns in neurosurgical adverse events: intracranial neoplasm surgery. Neurosurg Focus 2012;33(5):E16.

36. Gempt J, Gerhardt J, Toth V, et al. Postoperative ischemic changes following brain metastasis resection as measured by diffusion-weighted magnetic resonance imaging. J Neurosurg 2013;119(6):1395–400.

37. Clement AR, Palaniappan D, Panigrahi RK. Tension pneumocephalus. Anesthesiology 2017;127(4):710.

38. Charidimou A, Turc G, Oppenheim C, et al. Microbleeds, cerebral hemorrhage, and functional outcome after stroke thrombolysis. Stroke 2017;48(8):2084–90.

39. Amans MR, Cooke DL, Vella M, et al. Contrast staining on CT after DSA in ischemic stroke patients progresses to infarction and rarely hemorrhages. Interv Neuroradiol 2014;20(1):106–15.

40. Muttikkal TJ, Wintermark M. MRI patterns of global hypoxic-ischemic injury in adults. J Neuroradiol 2013;40(3):164–71.

41. Sturiale CL, Rossetto M, Ermani M, et al. Remote cerebellar hemorrhage after supratentorial procedures (part 1): a systematic review. Neurosurg Rev 2016;39(4):565–73.

42. Sturiale CL, Rossetto M, Ermani M, et al. Remote cerebellar hemorrhage after spinal procedures (part 2): a systematic review. Neurosurg Rev 2016;39(3):369–76.

43. Dashti SR, Baharvahdat H, Spetzler RF, et al. Operative intracranial infection following craniotomy. Neurosurg Focus 2008;24(6):E10.

44. Akins PT, Guppy KH. Sinking skin flaps, paradoxical herniation, and external brain tamponade: a review of decompressive craniectomy management. Neurocrit Care 2008;9(2):269–76.

45. Brandsma D, Bromberg JEC. Primary CNS lymphoma in HIV infection. Handb Clin Neurol 2018;152:177–86.

46. Horger M, Beschorner R, Beck R, et al. Common and uncommon imaging findings in progressive multifocal leukoencephalopathy (PML) with differential diagnostic considerations. Clin Neurol Neurosurg 2012;114(8):1123–30.

47. Chokshi FH, Aygun N, Mullins ME. Imaging of acquired metabolic and toxic disorders of the basal ganglia. Semin Ultrasound CT MR 2014;35(2):75–84.

48. Ferrara J, Jankovic J. Acquired hepatocerebral degeneration. J Neurol 2009;256(3):320–32.

49. Manzo G, De Gennaro A, Cozzolino A, et al. MR imaging findings in alcoholic and nonalcoholic acute Wernicke's encephalopathy: a review. Biomed Res Int 2014;2014:503596.

50. Bathla G, Hegde AN. MRI and CT appearances in metabolic encephalopathies due to systemic diseases in adults. Clin Radiol 2013;68(6):545–54.

51. Gouliamos AD, Kehagias DT, Lahanis S, et al. MR imaging of tuberculous vertebral osteomyelitis: pictorial review. Eur Radiol 2001;11(4):575–9.

52. Jain NK, Dao K, Ortiz AO. Radiologic evaluation and management of postoperative spine paraspinal fluid collections. Neuroimaging Clin N Am 2014;24(2):375–89.

Imaging of Altered Mental Status

Alina Uzelac, DO

KEYWORDS

- Hypoxic-anoxic injury • Hydrocephalus • Hypertensive encephalopathy • Fat emboli
- Duret hemorrhage • Osmotic demyelination • Pituitary apoplexy

KEY POINTS

- The clinical history of altered mental status implies a broad differential, and can be a challenge to the managing physicians. It refers to either disturbed consciousness or decreased arousal.
- There are numerous etiologies underlying altered mental status, either related to systemic illnesses or central nervous system processes (organic or psychiatric).
- Neuroimaging is an important tool for solving the clinical dilemma and gleaning through the vast array of etiologies of consciousness perturbations.
- Given the serious consequences of a delay in diagnosis, obtaining brain imaging early is crucial.
- Noncontrast computerized tomography of the brain provides a rapid screening, whereas MR imaging is reserved for more complex presentations unsolved by CT.

INTRODUCTION

Altered mental status (AMS) is one of the most common indications for brain imaging of both emergency room and hospitalized patients. AMS is a broad term, and can imply either changes in consciousness (supratentorial function) or in arousal (executed by the brainstem). Underlying etiologies includes both systemic illnesses and central nervous system processes, the latter encompassing both organic and psychiatric causes. The long and varied differential diagnosis can make AMS a potentially vexing clinical problem.[1]

AMS (or encephalopathy) can be generally divided into the following 2 broad categories:

- *Systemic etiologies,* such as infections, metabolic derangements, side effects of medications, vasculitis, autoimmune encephalitis, and, at our institution, polysubstance abuse.
- *Organic brain causes,* such as new or worsening intracranial hemorrhage, traumatic brain injury, central nervous system infections, mass effect/herniation related to a tumor or to new/increasing size of an infarction, reversible posterior encephalopathy syndrome, nonconvulsive seizures, and acute hydrocephalus.[2]

AMS is often an acute or subacute event, and the timely identification of potentially treatable intracranial pathology is paramount to its management. Several nonimaging diagnostic tests have been proposed to predict imaging findings, but their utility is generally limited due to the urgency of the clinical situation. In mild traumatic brain injury, serum biomarkers, such as glial fibrillary acidic protein and ubiquitin C-terminal hydrolase-1, have been established as predictors of intracranial hemorrhage. In atraumatic scenarios, various tentative criteria have been advocated as foretelling of a positive brain scan, such as elevated diastolic blood pressure, focal weakness, low Glasgow Coma Scale score, antiplatelet/

Disclosure Statement: None.
Neuroradiology, Department of Radiology, Zuckerberg San Francisco General Hospital, University of California, 1001 Potrero Avenue, Room 1X56, San Francisco, CA 94110, USA
E-mail addresses: alina.uzelac@ucsf.edu; Alina.uzelac@icloud.com

Radiol Clin N Am 58 (2020) 187–197
https://doi.org/10.1016/j.rcl.2019.08.002

anticoagulant use, plantar reflexes, presence of headache, dilated pupils, and low C-reactive protein.[3,4]

Neuroimaging, particularly noncontrast head computed tomography (CT), provides the most rapid and effective screening tool for AMS. Although sometimes criticized for its "overuse," the gravity of delay leaves managing physicians little leeway to forfeit brain imaging.

Given the breadth of the subject, this article focuses on some common clinical problems and a select group of interesting presentations underlying AMS. Related clinical diagnoses and indications for neuroimaging are further discussed in the Judith Ann Gadde and colleagues' article, "Neuroimaging of Patients in the ICU: Pearls and Pitfalls," in this issue.

HYPOXIC-ANOXIC BRAIN INJURY, ALSO KNOWN AS HYPOXIC-ISCHEMIC BRAIN INJURY

Encephalopathy due to hypoxic-anoxic brain injury, also known as hypoxic-ischemic brain injury (HIBI), is the result of decreased perfusion and oxygenation of the brain and is due to hypotension/hypoperfusion from cardioembolic phenomenon or drastically decreased cardiac output.

The leading etiology of HIBI is cardiac arrest (also known as pulseless electrical activity, PEA arrest). Interestingly, these patients with cardiac arrest are most likely to die because of the hypoxic-anoxic brain injury (HIBI is the primary cause of death in 68% of inpatient cardiac arrests).[5]

The spectrum of imaging findings of HIBI is broad, with appearance from subtle to striking. In the hyperacute injury, the head CT findings can be nearly imperceptible (**Fig. 1**A), and clinical history is important. Conversely, the HIBI is sometimes not suspected clinically and is apparent on imaging.

Mild Hypoxic-Anoxic Injury

Symptoms and imaging findings can be reversible in milder cases, particularly if the gray matter (basal ganglia and cortex) is spared. The patients who develop only early supratentorial deep white matter involvement (**Fig. 1**B) have a better prognosis and the imaging findings mirror the clinical course.[6] A delayed post-hypoxic leukoencephalopathy has also been described, and patients could re-present with symptoms 2 to 3 weeks after an initial recovery.

Infratentorial involvement in HIBI (**Fig. 1**C) is much less common. The cerebellar white matter symmetric involvement has been usually associated with toxic-metabolic insults and is seen with spongiform leukoencephalopathy related to illicit drug use such as heroin, and particularly with inhalation of heated heroin vapors (also known as "chasing the dragon").[7] The imaging diagnosis challenge lies in discerning between HIBI and toxic-metabolic injury.

Severe Hypoxic-Ischemic Injury

In severe hypoxic-ischemic injury, the brain injury is due to decreased blood flow and impaired removal of harmful cellular metabolites, such as lactate and glutamate, which accumulate and have deleterious effects.[8]

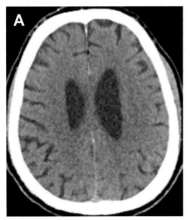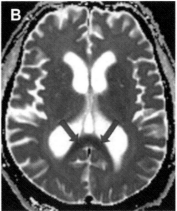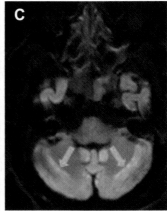

Fig. 1. Subtle hypoxic-anoxic injury. An 82-year-old man status post cardiac arrest. (*A*) Noncontrast brain CT (NCCT) obtained on the day of admission shows diffuse slight blurring of the gray-white differentiation. (*B*) Apparent diffusion coefficient (ADC) map associated with a DWI sequence from MR imaging obtained 9 days later for prognostication shows low ADC in the splenium of corpus callosum (*arrows* in *B*) and reduced diffusion in the cerebellar hemispheres (*arrows* in *C*) on the DWI.

The severe HIBI can result in florid edema (**Figs. 2** and **3**), causing hyperdense appearance of the subarachnoid space,[9] and can eventually result in downward brain herniation (see **Fig. 3**C). Of course, the prognosis is guarded.

At our institution, many of the HIBI cases are imaged with MR imaging in the delayed subacute stages, when the lack of clinical improvement becomes evident. These patients are not regaining consciousness as expected after treatment of other conditions for which they were admitted. Delayed MR imaging diagnosis can be a challenge, as the acute findings of cytotoxic edema (reduced diffusion and T2 hyperintensity of the basal ganglia and cortex) subside and only subtle residua can be perceived. Arterial spin labeling perfusion and MR spectroscopy may be helpful in some cases.

Hypoglycemia

Hypoglycemia is well-known to cause central nervous system sign and symptoms, from focal neurologic deficits to coma and death, and its imaging manifestations can mirror the clinical severity. Characteristic involvement of the hippocampus, cerebral cortex, and basal ganglia with sparing of the posterior fossa has been described on MR imaging.[10] Isolated deep supratentorial white matter involvement also can occur (**Fig. 4**A, B).

With profound hypoglycemia, cerebral fullness can develop due to vasogenic edema related to decreased osmolality of the parenchyma. The blood-brain barrier has been demonstrated to remain intact.[11] The CT appearance may be confused with hypoxic-anoxic injury or edema related to traumatic brain injury. The distinction can be made by the observation that even though the cerebrospinal fluid (CSF) spaces can be completely effaced, the gray-white differentiation remains preserved in hypo-osmolality-induced cerebral edema (**Fig. 4**C, D).

Teaching point
Sulcal and ventricular effacement can be related to markedly decreased cerebral parenchymal osmolality, such as seen with profound hypoglycemia, hyponatremia, or with volume overload (ie, polydipsia). The imaging findings are usually reversible, the gray-white differentiation is preserved, and the appearance should not be confused with hypoxic-anoxic or traumatic brain injury.

Hydrocephalus

There are several etiologies for the development of acute hydrocephalus, such as meningitis, subarachnoid hemorrhage from aneurysmal rupture, enlarging lesions producing mass effect at the foraminae (of Monro, of Luschka or Magendie,

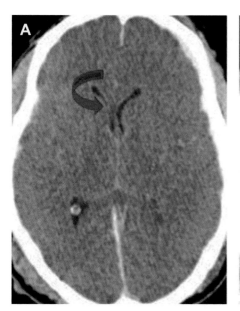
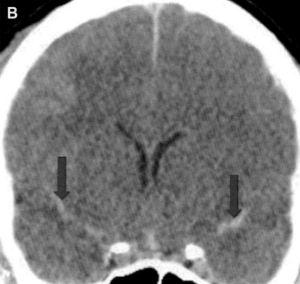

Fig. 2. Severe hypoxic-anoxic injury. A 30-year-old man found at the bottom of 15 stairs. (*A*) NCCT shows diffuse sulcal and lateral ventricles effacement (*curved arrow*) and loss of gray-white differentiation. (*B*) Coronal reformation shows hyperdense subarachnoid space: "pseudosubarachnoid hemorrhage" (*arrows*), which is mostly due to compression of distended vessels against a low attenuation edematous cerebrum. The urine toxicology screen was positive for benzodiazepines and alcohol.

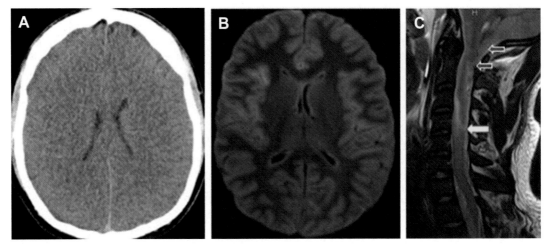

Fig. 3. Severe hypoxic-anoxic injury. A 29-year-old man found down. (A) CT shows compressed sulci and ventricle and loss of gray-white differentiation. (B) MR imaging DWI sequence shows reduced diffusion throughout the cortex. (C) Sagittal T2-weighted image of cervical spine shows downward cerebellar tonsillar herniation (*red arrows*) that leads to buckling of the cervical cord (*yellow arrow*).

magnum), fourth ventricle, or Sylvian aqueduct (**Fig. 5**). The compressive effect of the enlarged ventricles on the adjacent parenchyma causes interstitial edema and axonal hypoxia and results in subsequent retrograde neuronal damage, which is thought to be responsible for the alteration in level of consciousness. A dysregulation due to altered innervation or disruption of local cell interactions has also been implicated.[12]

HYPERTENSIVE ENCEPHALOPATHY

Patients with severe hypertension can present with headache, confusion, seizures, and, if left untreated, could progress to coma. An edematous pons, such as seen in severe hypertension, can alter the normal CSF flow in the posterior fossa and result in hydrocephalus (**Fig. 6**), which can further worsen the hypertensive encephalopathy. Hypertension is complex in its causation of disturbed consciousness. The increased cerebral perfusion likely leads to the perturbation of the blood-brain barrier with resultant edema. An older theory postulates that high blood pressure leads to cerebral autoregulatory vasoconstriction, ischemia, and subsequent edema.[13] The acute obstructive hydrocephalus due to posterior fossa edema and the diffuse abnormal vascular perfusion of cerebrum due to hypertension can synchronously and additively cause AMS.

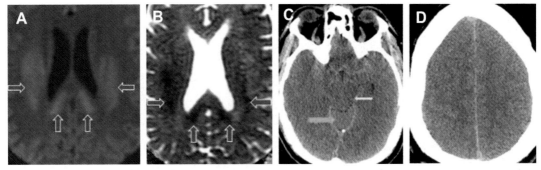

Fig. 4. Profound hypoglycemia. (A, B) DWI obtained in a 30-year-old woman with an episode of severe hypoglycemia. Note the deep white matter and splenium of corpus callosum reduced diffusion (*arrows* in A) and corresponding low ADC (*arrows* in B). (C, D) Head CT of 47-year-old man with AMS who was found to have severe hypoglycemia. (C) Note upward transtentorial herniation of superior cerebellar vermis (*blue arrow*) and effacement of the basilar cisterns (*red asterisk* marks the suprasellar cistern and the *yellow arrow* the perimesencephalic cistern). (D) The cerebral sulci and basilar cisterns are completely effaced, but the gray-white differentiation is intact.

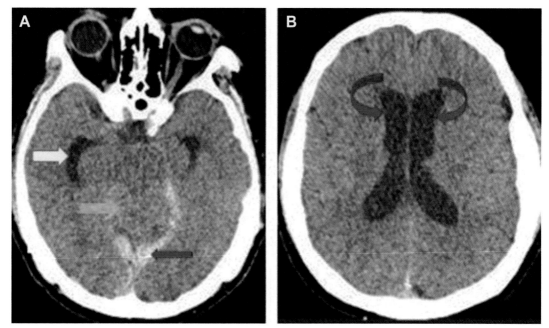

Fig. 5. Acute obstructive hydrocephalus from posterior fossa subdural hematoma. A 63-year-old man on warfarin for atrial fibrillation with markedly elevated international normalized ratio had waxing and waning mental status. (*A*) NCCT shows enlarged temporal horns of the lateral ventricles (*yellow arrow*) and upward transtentorial cerebellar superior vermian herniation (*blue arrow*) due to posterior fossa subdural hematoma (*red arrow*). (*B*) The lateral ventricles are large compared with the cerebral sulci due to acute obstruction from the posterior fossa mass effect on the fourth ventricle and Sylvian aqueduct.

Diffuse Traumatic Hemorrhagic Axonal Injury and Fat Emboli

Diffuse axonal injury (DAI) leads to impairments in cognitive, motor, and sensory functions because of the disruption of neuronal connections. Distinguishing between DAI and fat emboli can have prognostic and sometimes treatment implications, therefore the imaging diagnosis plays an important role. The patients with DAI can have serious long-term neurologic impairment, and MR imaging is confirmatory of the diagnosis.[14]

The axonal injury lesions are neither symmetric in distribution, nor uniform in size, and occur in

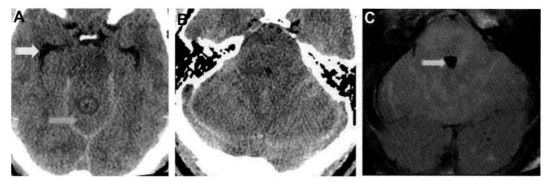

Fig. 6. Obstructive hydrocephalus due to hypertensive encephalopathy. A 45-year-old man with hypertension, headache, and AMS. (*A*) Note the dilated temporal horns of lateral ventricles (*yellow arrow*), upward transtentorial herniation (*blue arrow*), and compressed Sylvian aqueduct (*circled in red*) on NCCT. (*B*) Red arrow points to the effaced fourth ventricle. (*C*) On the T2 fluid-attenuated inversion recovery (FLAIR) sequence from MR imaging obtained 2 days later after treatment of his hypertension, the fourth ventricle has improved in size (*green arrow*), and there is residual T2 pontine hyperintensity reflecting edema. This patient subsequently presented to the emergency room several times for hypertensive emergency with similar imaging findings.

characteristic locations (such as the superior cerebellar peduncles, parasagittal subcortical white matter of frontal and parietal lobes, and corpus callosum), which have been described decades ago.[15] Axonal injury hemorrhages are clumpy and of various sizes, some with a linear configuration due to venular hemorrhages paralleling and surrounding the injured axons (Fig. 7A).

Cerebral fat embolism should not be confused with DAI. Even though showering of fat emboli is not common, it is a known complication of traumatic long bone fractures or orthopedic surgery, and is also occasionally seen with bone marrow infarction in patients with sickle cell disease (Fig. 7). The fat emboli are punctate and diffusely spread in the cerebrum and cerebellum (see Fig. 7B). The appearance of the so-called "starfield" (Fig. 8A, B) is not so conspicuous on the diffusion-weighted image (DWI), but is dramatic on the susceptibility weighted sequence (SWI). The patients with cerebral fat emboli are generally expected to have a better chance at neurologic recovery than the patients with DAI.[16]

Ischemia/Cytotoxic Edema Due to Arterial Vasospasm

Any form of ischemic injury can cause altered arousal, particularly if the thalamus, hypothalamus, basal forebrain, and brainstem are involved.

Cerebral edema and vasospasm leading to ischemia have been implicated in delayed encephalopathy that affects patients with aneurysmal subarachnoid hemorrhage (SAH) (Fig. 9). Vasospasm is mostly associated with aneurysmal SAH, but can also occur with infectious meningitis, and seldom with traumatic SAH. The occurrence of vasospasm has been more recently attributed to systemic inflammation from other concomitant conditions. Several inflammatory markers in the CSF have been linked to vasospasm, and the risk of SAH-delayed complications also markedly increases in patients with elevated levels of inflammatory mediators in the serum.[17]

However, it is still unclear which patients are prone to traumatic SAH-related vasospasm leading to ischemia (Fig. 10), but younger patients (who have more reactive arteries) seem to be more affected. And, because of the infrequent occurrence of vasospasm in patients with traumatic SAH, the clinical suspicion, obtaining the imaging confirmatory tests, and the treatment can all be delayed. At our institution, if clinical concern is high, after an initial transcranial Doppler ultrasound, a digital subtraction angiogram (DSA) for definitive diagnosis and possible treatment (with intra-arterial calcium channel blocker, verapamil) is obtained. An interim CT angiogram brain with CT perfusion imaging may sometimes also be obtained before proceeding to the DSA.

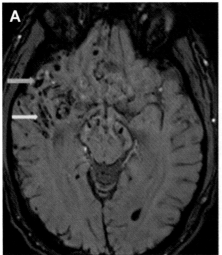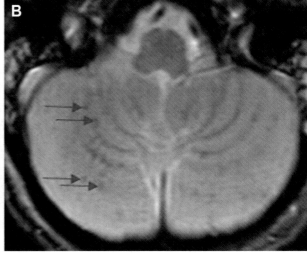

Fig. 7. Traumatic hemorrhagic axonal injury versus fat emboli. (*A*) A 25-year-old man status post motorcycle collision. SWI from a 3 T MR imaging obtained for persistent AMS shows clumpy (*blue arrow*) and linear (*yellow arrow*) low signal in the temporal stem consistent with DAI. (*B*) MR imaging of an 18-year-old woman status post pedestrian versus automobile accident not returning to normal level of consciousness. On 1.5-T T2*-weighted gradient-recalled echo sequence (GRE), the bilateral cerebellar subtle punctate foci of susceptibility (*red arrows*) are equal in size and in a location *not* typical for DAI. Patient had long bone fractures. The MR imaging appearance and eventual recovery were consistent with fat emboli.

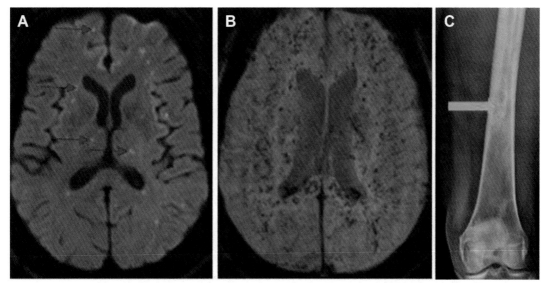

Fig. 8. Cerebral fat emboli. MR imaging of a persistently altered 58-year-old man with a reported history of sickle cell trait. (*A*) Punctate foci of reduced diffusion on the DWI sequence are scattered in deep white matter and thalami (*red arrows*). (*B*) Innumerable foci of susceptibility throughout the brain stand out on the iron sensitive sequence (SWI). (*C*) Femur radiograph shows the sclerosis of the midshaft from bone infarcts related to sickle cell disease (*blue arrow*).

Other Posterior Fossa Causes

Basilar artery thrombosis
Basilar artery occlusions are challenging given the variable presentation and waxing and waning of symptoms. Symptoms range from ataxia to dizziness, but can progress to lethargy, locked-in state, and coma. The relatively common delay in diagnosis implies postponed treatment and high morbidity and mortality. The hyperdensity of the basilar artery (**Fig. 11**A) on noncontrast head CT may be overlooked or misinterpreted as artifact. CT angiogram can confirm lack of luminal contrast opacification. The definitive diagnosis and the intra-arterial treatment/embo-lectomy are done by conventional angiogram (**Fig. 11**B).[18]

Pontine also Known as duret hemorrhage
Pontine hemorrhages can occur with primary or secondary injury to the brainstem. A sudden change in intracranial pressure can lead to abrupt downward herniation, and tearing of the small arterial perforators with secondary pontine hemorrhage (**Fig. 12**), known as Duret hemorrhage. The downward herniation can occur from mass effect from high intracranial pressure (ie, supratentorial lesions or extra-axial hemorrhages) or from low CSF pressure with sudden sagging of the brainstem. The affected patients can become obtunded, and their prognosis used to be deemed guarded. In our experience, some patients can improve with minimal residual deficits, and several cases of good recovery have been reported in the literature. The consensus has emerged that the severity of injury leading to the downward herniation may have been the cause of high morbidity and mortality in patients with poor outcomes, and not the pontine hemorrhage itself.[19,20]

Osmotic Demyelination Syndrome and Wernicke Encephalopathy

Osmotic demyelination (pontine)
Central pontine osmotic demyelination also known as myelinolysis is a known cause of impaired consciousness with indeterminate chances (quoted at approximately 50%) of complete recovery, regardless of the severity of the initial neurologic impairment.[21,22] Cirrhotic/chronic alcoholic individuals have been found to have a worse prognosis. During osmotic disturbances (hyponatremia and hypernatremia, hyperglycemia, hypokalemia) and their inadvertently rapid correction (most commonly encountered in the hospitalized hyponatremic patients), the myelin of white matter tracts undergoes injury. During the acute phase, reduced diffusion in the central pons is present (**Fig. 13**A, B), whereas, in chronic cases, volume loss of the central pons and cystic encephalomalacia can be seen (**Fig. 13**C).

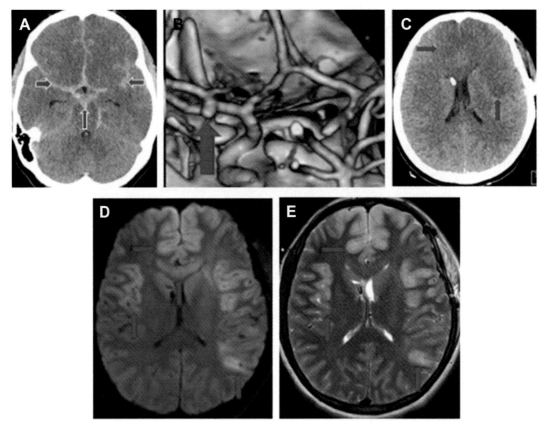

Fig. 9. Infarction as result of vasospasm due to aneurysmal SAH. This 20-year-old woman initially presented to the emergency room with seizure. (*A*) Note the SAH in the basilar cisterns (*red arrows*) on the initial head CT. (*B*) An aneurysm of the middle cerebral artery bifurcation was confirmed on CT angiography and is shown on the 3-dimensional reformation. (*C*) Bilateral anterior circulation territory infarction was diagnosed on CT obtained at 7 days post aneurysm clipping because of sudden change in mental status and elevated intracranial pressure. (*D*) DWI sequence obtained the following day shows cytotoxic edema in the frontal lobes, genu of corpus callosum, and head of caudate due to the anterior circulation vasospasm. (*E*) The anterior circulation cortical edema is also apparent on the T2 fast spin echo sequence (T2 FSE).

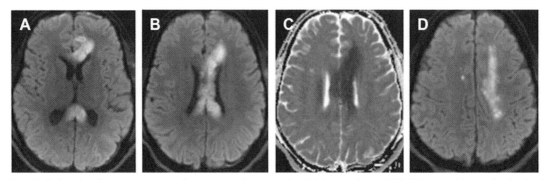

Fig. 10. Infarction from vasospasm after traumatic subarachnoid hemorrhage. This 25-year-old man had spinal cord transection and traumatic intracranial hemorrhage from a motorcycle accident. Borderzone reduced diffusion involves the corpus callosum and deep white matter on DWI (*A*, *B*, and *D*) with corresponding low ADC (*C*) on MR imaging obtained a week later for delayed change in mental status. DSA (not included) confirmed vasospasm.

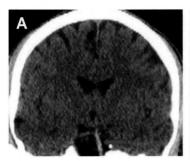

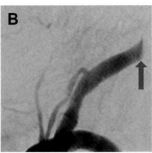

Fig. 11. Basilar artery thrombosis. A 47-year-old man presented with dysmetria, and was found to have cerebellar strokes on MR imaging (not shown here). Patient was treated with intravenous tissue plasminogen activator for vertebral artery dissection. (A) The basilar artery is hyperdense (red arrow) on an NCCT obtained a few hours later when the patient developed agitation and left hemiparesis. (B) DSA shows an occluded vertebral artery with characteristic flameshape configuration of the intraluminal contrast. The patient underwent embolectomy with recanalization of the basilar artery.

Wernicke encephalopathy

Encephalopathy caused by thiamine (vitamin B_1) deficiency is not rare, but is likely often an overlooked diagnosis. It occurs most frequently in elderly and patients with decreased absorption (malnutrition, bariatric surgery), increased metabolism (malignancy), or high carbohydrate intake (intravenous dextrose administration).[23] At our hospital, the number of patients with alcohol abuse is high, so our physicians are on alert regarding the possibility of Wernicke encephalopathy. Consequently, we rarely image and make this diagnosis on MR imaging. The periaqueductal gray high T2 signal on MR imaging is characteristic (Fig. 14A, B), although supratentorial structures (medial thalami) can also be involved. Other associated imaging findings may also point to alcohol abuse, such as T1 hyperintensity of globi pallidi related to hepatic encephalopathy (Fig. 14C), superior vermian atrophy, enlarged parotids/sialadenosis, and peculiar deposition and configuration of neck fat (Madelung neck).

Other Less Common Etiologies (but Worthy of Mention) of Altered Mental Status

Pituitary adenoma hemorrhage leading to apoplexy

The clinical presentation of waxing and waning level of consciousness due pituitary adenoma hemorrhage or necrosis is known to endocrinologists as a manifestation of acute hormonal insufficiencies. These patients need emergent corticosteroid replacement and hemodynamic stabilization.[24] Hemorrhage into pituitary adenomas is not uncommon, and more frequently occurs in middle-aged men. The neurologic findings can also sometimes be related to infarction due to vasospasm caused by the blood products spreading into the subarachnoid space. The hemorrhage into the pituitary adenoma is frequently inconspicuous on CT (Fig. 15A, C), as this imaging modality is only approximately 20% sensitive in diagnosing the hemorrhage.[25] So, in patients whose symptoms could be related to pituitary dysfunction and hemorrhage, an MR imaging sella should be obtained for evaluation of the macroadenoma for possible hemorrhage. On MR imaging, fluid-fluid levels are considered

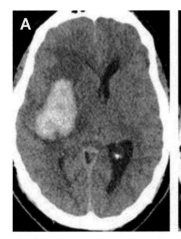

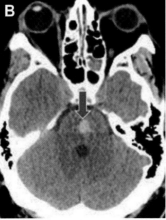

Fig. 12. Pontine Duret hemorrhage. (A) NCCT of a 64-year-old man who was admitted for hypertensive basal ganglia hemorrhage. (B) NCCT obtained 7 days later because of acute change in mental status and blown pupil. The central pontine hemorrhage (red arrow) was a result of downward herniation (due to sudden enlargement of the supratentorial hematoma) leading to injury to the pontine arterial perforators. The blown pupil was due to the uncal herniation compressing the parasympathetic peripheral fibers of the right third nerve.

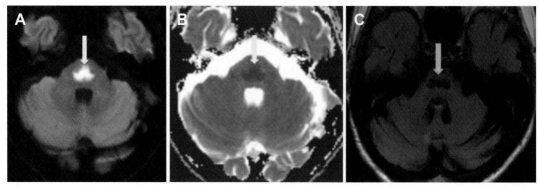

Fig. 13. Osmotic demyelination: acute and sequela. (*A* and *B*) MR imaging of 51-year-old man admitted for cognitive amnestic syndrome and waxing and waning mental status. Reduced diffusion (*arrow* in *A*) with corresponding low ADC (*arrow* in *B*) in the central pons in a characteristic "trident" configuration of osmotic pontine demyelination. (*C*) Sequela of central pontine myelinolysis on T2 FLAIR in a 52-year-old woman with chronic alcohol abuse. The pontine encephalomalacia (*blue arrow*) is dramatic. Note also the accompanying atrophied cerebellar folia.

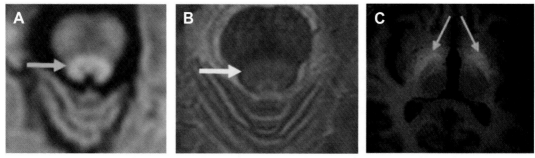

Fig. 14. Wernicke and hepatic encephalopathy. MR imaging of a 45-year-old man with history of alcohol abuse and persistent AMS. The periaqueductal gray/dorsal midbrain is high signal on both DWI (*arrow* in *A*) and T2 FSE (*arrow* in *B*). (*C*) The globi pallidi are high signal intensity on the T1-weighted sequence consistent with hepatic encephalopathy.

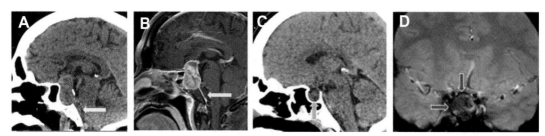

Fig. 15. Hemorrhagic adenoma. (*A, B*) A 58-year-old woman with waxing and waning level of consciousness, somnolence, and headache for which she underwent repeat CT stroke protocols (NCCT, CT angiogram, and CT perfusion) during her hospital stay. (*A*) Sagittal reformation from stroke protocol CT shows the sella turcica is enlarged and a sellar slightly heterogeneous mass with suprasellar extension is present. (*B*) The hyperintensity of the mass on subsequent gadolinium (Gd)-enhanced T1-weighted sequence is due mostly to Gd extravasation into the acute hematoma and can be misinterpreted as tumor enhancement. Small/subtle volume of extra-axial blood is posterior to the clivus on both CT and MR imaging (*yellow arrows*). (*C*) Example of an "unremarkable" macroadenoma (*blue arrow*) on CT in a 28-year-old man woken up from sleep by a sudden headache. (*D*) Hemorrhage is confirmed by the susceptibility artifact in the sella (*red arrows*) on the high-resolution coronal GRE obtained a few hours later. On MR imaging the adenoma is larger compared with earlier CT.

pathognomonic for acute hemorrhage. However, our neurosurgeons describe the intraoperative gross appearance of most hemorrhagic tumors as "swiss cheese," and, in our experience, the fluid-fluid level finding is rare, whereas a heterogeneous appearance of the tumor on MR imaging is common (**Fig. 15B**). Hence, the correct imaging interpretation of hemorrhagic adenoma can be elusive, unless the films are diligently scrutinized.

SUMMARY

Neuroimaging is an invaluable diagnostic tool for sorting through the vast array of etiologies that underlie AMS. Head CT without contrast is the primary modality for evaluation of AMS and should be complemented by MR imaging in cases of negative CT but high clinical concern. Studies to maximize brain imaging efficiency and improve the yield of positive scans through the utilization of clinical and laboratory pre-scan diagnostics are ongoing. However, imaging remains the gold standard due to its rapidity with which certain diagnoses can be made or excluded.

REFERENCES

1. Luttrull MD, Boulter DJ, Kirsch CFE, et al. ACR appropriateness criteria acute mental status change, delirium, and new onset psychosis. J Am Coll Radiol 2019;16(5S):S26–37.
2. Douglas VC, Josephson SA. Altered mental status. Neurologic consultation in the hospital. Continuum (Minneap Minn) 2011;17(5):967–83.
3. Leong LB, Wei Jian KH, Vasu A, et al. Identifying risk factors for an abnormal computed tomographic scan of the head among patients with altered mental status in the Emergency Department. Eur J Emerg Med 2010;17(4):219–23.
4. Shin S, Lee HJ, Shin J, et al. Predictors of abnormal brain computed tomography findings in patients with acute altered mental status in the emergency department. Clin Exp Emerg Med 2018;5(1):1–6.
5. Laver S, Farrow C, Turner D, et al. Mode of death after admission to an ICU following cardiac arrest. Intensive Care Med 2004;30(11):2126–8.
6. Chalela JA, Wolf RL, Maldjian JA, et al. MRI identification of early white matter injury in anoxic–ischemic encephalopathy. Neurology 2001;56(4):481–5.
7. Cheng MY, Chin SC, Chang YC. Different routes of heroin intake cause various heroin-induced leukoencephalopathies. J Neurol 2019;266(2):316–29.
8. Howard RS, Holmes PA, Siddiqui A, et al. Hypoxic–ischaemic brain injury: imaging and neurophysiology abnormalities related to outcome. Q J Med 2012;105(6):551–61.
9. Yuzawa H, Higano S, Mugikura S, et al. Pseudo-subarachnoid hemorrhage found in patients with postresuscitation encephalopathy: characteristics of CT findings and clinical importance. AJNR Am J Neuroradiol 2008;29(8):1544–9.
10. Kang EG, Jeon SJ, Choi SS, et al. Diffusion MR imaging of hypoglycemic encephalopathy. AJNR Am J Neuroradiol 2010;31(3):559–64.
11. Gisselsson L, Smith ML, Siesjö BK. Influence of hypoglycemic coma on brain water and osmolality. Exp Brain Res 1998;120(4):461–9.
12. Del Bigio MR, Di Curzio DL. Nonsurgical therapy for hydrocephalus: a comprehensive and critical review. Fluids Barriers CNS 2016;13:3.
13. Lamy C, Oppenheim C, Méder JF, et al. Neuroimaging in posterior reversible encephalopathy syndrome. J Neuroimaging 2004;14(2):89–96.
14. Moen KG, Brezova V, Skandsen T, et al. Traumatic axonal injury: the prognostic value of lesion load in corpus callosum, brain stem, and thalamus in different magnetic resonance imaging sequences. J Neurotrauma 2014;17:1486–96.
15. Adams JH, Graham DI, Murray LS, et al. Diffuse axonal injury due to nonmissile head injury in humans: an analysis of 45 cases. Ann Neurol 1982;12(6):557–63.
16. Morales-Vidal SG. Neurologic complications of fat embolism syndrome. Curr Neurol Neurosci Rep 2019;19(3):14.
17. Miller BA, Turan N, Chau M, et al. Inflammation, vasospasm, and brain injury after subarachnoid hemorrhage. Biomed Res Int 2014;2014:384342.
18. Ausman JI, Liebeskind DS, Gonzalez N, et al. A review of the diagnosis and management of vertebral basilar (posterior) circulation disease. Surg Neurol Int 2018;9:106.
19. Ishizaka S, Shimizu T, Ryu N. Dramatic recovery after severe descending transtentorial herniation-induced Duret haemorrhage: a case report and review of literature. Brain Inj 2014;28(3):374–7.
20. Bonow RH, Bales JW, Morton RP, et al. Reversible coma and Duret hemorrhage after intracranial hypotension from remote lumbar spine surgery: case report. J Neurosurg Spine 2016;24(3):389–93.
21. Singh TD, Fugate JE, Rabinstein AA. Central pontine and extrapontine myelinolysis: a systematic review. Eur J Neurol 2014;21(12):1443–50.
22. Alleman AM. Osmotic demyelination syndrome: central pontine myelinolysis and extrapontine myelinolysis. Semin Ultrasound CT MR 2014;35(2):153–9.
23. Day GS, del Campo CM. Wernicke encephalopathy: a medical emergency. Can Med Assoc J 2014; 186(8):E295.
24. Bi WL, Dunn IF, Laws ER. Pituitary apoplexy. Endocrine 2015;48(1):69–75.
25. Glezer A, Bronstein MD. Pituitary apoplexy: pathophysiology, diagnosis and management. Arch Endocrinol Metab 2015;59(3):259–64.

Moving?

Make sure your subscription moves with you!

To notify us of your new address, find your **Clinics Account Number** (located on your mailing label above your name), and contact customer service at:

Email: journalscustomerservice-usa@elsevier.com

800-654-2452 (subscribers in the U.S. & Canada)
314-447-8871 (subscribers outside of the U.S. & Canada)

Fax number: 314-447-8029

**Elsevier Health Sciences Division
Subscription Customer Service
3251 Riverport Lane
Maryland Heights, MO 63043**

ELSEVIER